A Clinical
Manual of
Obstetrics

Appleton Clinical Manuals

Ayres, et al.: Medical Resident's Manual, 4th edition
Ellis and Beckmann: A Clinical Manual of Gynecology
Ellis and Beckmann: A Clinical Manual of Obstetrics
Gomella, et al.: The Clinician's Pocket Reference,
4th edition

Forthcoming titles

A Clinical Manual of Cardiology
A Clinical Manual of Nephrology
A Clinical Manual of Nuclear Medicine
Surgical Resident's Manual, 2nd edition

A Clinical Manual of Obstetrics

Jeffrey W. Ellis, M.D.

Assistant Professor of Obstetrics and Gynecology
Department of Obstetrics and Gynecology
Director, Section of Obstetrics and Gynecology
Northwestern Foundation for Research and Education
Northwestern University School of Medicine
Chicago, Illinois

Charles R.B. Beckmann, M.D.

Assistant Professor of Obstetrics and Gynecology
Director, Undergraduate Medical Education
Department of Obstetrics and Gynecology
University of Illinois College of Medicine-Chicago
Chicago, Illinois

 APPLETON-CENTURY-CROFTS/Norwalk, Connecticut

Copyright © 1983 by Appleton-Century-Crofts, a Publishing Division of Prentice-Hall, Inc., except Chapter 13 Copyright © 1981 by Diane R. Gomez.

83 84 85 86 87 / 10 9 8 7 6 5 4 3 2 1

Prentice-Hall International, Inc., London
Prentice-Hall of Australia, Pty. Ltd., Sydney
Prentice-Hall Canada Inc.
Prentice-Hall of India Private Limited, New Delhi
Prentice-Hall of Japan, Inc., Tokyo
Prentice-Hall of Southeast Asia (Pte.) Ltd., Singapore
Whitehall Books Ltd., Wellington, New Zealand
Editora Prentice-Hall do Brasil Ltda., Rio de Janeiro

Library of Congress Cataloging in Publication Data
Main entry under title:
A Clinical manual of obstetrics.
    Companion vol. to: A Clinical manual of gynecology.
    Bibliography: p.
    Includes index.
    1. Obstetrics—Handbooks, manuals, etc.   I. Ellis,
Jeffrey W.   II. Beckmann, Charles R. B.   [DNLM:
1. Obstetrics.   WQ 100   C641]
RG531.C5   1983   618.2   82-20612
ISBN   0-8385-1140-6

Design: Jean M. Sabato

PRINTED IN THE UNITED STATES OF AMERICA

Contributors

Barbara M. Barzansky, Ph.D., M.H.P.E.
Assistant Professor of Health Professions Education
Center for Education Development
University of Illinois - Chicago
Chicago, Illinois

Charles R.B. Beckmann, M.D.
Assistant Professor of Obstetrics and Gynecology
Director, Undergraduate Medical Education
Department of Obstetrics and Gynecology
University of Illinois College of Medicine - Chicago
Chicago, Illinois

Maureen Bocian, M.D.
Assistant Professor of Pediatrics
Department of Pediatrics
University of California School of Medicine at Irvine
Irvine, California

Sandra A. Carson, M.D.
Fellow, Reproductive Endocrinology
Department of Obstetrics and Gynecology
Michael Reese Hospital
University of Chicago
Chicago, Illinois

Jeffrey W. Ellis, M.D.
Assistant Professor of Obstetrics and Gynecology
Department of Obstetrics and Gynecology
Director, Section of Obstetrics and Gynecology
Northwestern Foundation for Research and Education
Northwestern University School of Medicine
Chicago, Illinois

Diane R. Gomez, M.D.
Attending Physician
Section of Pediatrics
Department of Health
City of Chicago
Chicago, Illinois

William Gottschalk, M.D.
Professor of Obstetrics and Gynecology
Department of Obstetrics and Gynecology
Professor of Anesthesiology
Department of Anesthesiology
Rush Medical College
Rush Presbyterian-St. Luke's Medical Center
Chicago, Illinois

Jeffrey C. King, M.D.
Assistant Professor of Obstetrics and Gynecology
Division of Maternal-Fetal Medicine
Department of Obstetrics and Gynecology
Georgetown University
Washington, D.C.

Henry W. Lahmeyer, M.D.
Assistant Professor of Psychiatry
Chief-Consult-Liaison Service
Department of Psychiatry
University of Illinois College of Medicine-Chicago
Chief-Sleep Disorders Clinic
University of Illinois Hospital
Chicago, Illinois

Trusten P. Lee, D.D.S.
Adjunct Attending Staff
Rush-Presbyterian St. Luke's Medical Center
Chicago, Illinois

Frank W. Ling, M.D.
Associate Professor of Obstetrics and Gynecology
Division of Gynecology
Department of Obstetrics and Gynecology
The University of Tennessee Center for the Health Sciences
Memphis, Tennessee

Edward F. Lis, M.D.
Professor of Pediatrics
University of Illinois College of Medicine-Chicago
Director, Division of Services for Crippled Children
Director of Center for Handicapped Children
University of Illinois Hospital
Chicago, Illinois

Katherine Y. Look, M.D.
Chief Resident, Instructor
Department of Obstetrics and Gynecology
University of Illinois College of Medicine-Chicago
Chicago, Illinois

Michael Parsons, M.D.
Fellow, Maternal-Fetal Medicine
Instructor of Obstetrics and Gynecology
Division of Maternal-Fetal Medicine
Department of Obstetrics and Gynecology
University of Illinois College of Medicine-Chicago
Chicago, Illinois

Ronald W. Richards, M.A., Ph.D.
Professor of Health Professions Education
Director, Center for Education Development
University of Illinois College of Medicine-Chicago
Chicago, Illinois

Rudy E. Sabbagha, M.D.
Professor of Obstetrics and Gynecology
Director-Section of Ultrasonography
Department of Obstetrics and Gynecology
Northwestern University School of Medicine
Chicago, Illinois

Milo B. Sampson, B.S.E., M.S., M.D.
Assistant Professor of Obstetrics and Gynecology
Director, Ob-Gyn Ultrasound
Division of Maternal-Fetal Medicine
Department of Obstetrics and Gynecology
University of Illinois College of Medicine-Chicago
Chicago, Illinois

William N. Spellacy, M.D.
Professor and Head
Department of Obstetrics and Gynecology
University of Illinois College of Medicine-Chicago
Chicago, Illinois

Jessica L. Thomason, M.D.
Assistant Professor of Obstetrics and Gynecology
Division of Maternal-Fetal Medicine
Department of Obstetrics and Gynecology
University of Illinois College of Medicine-Chicago
Chicago, Illinois

Anna Tomasi, M.D.
Assistant Professor of Obstetrics and Gynecology
Division of Maternal-Fetal Medicine
Department of Obstetrics and Gynecology
University of Illinois College of Medicine-Chicago
Chicago, Illinois

Ralph K. Tumura, M.D.
Assistant Professor of Obstetrics and Gynecology
Section of Ultrasonography/Section of Maternal-Fetal Medicine
Department of Obstetrics and Gynecology
Northwestern University School of Medicine
Chicago, Illinois

Gayle Wager, M.D.
Attending in Maternal-Fetal Medicine
Abbott-Northwestern Hospital
Minneapolis, Minnesota

Linda A. Wheeler, R.N., C.N.M., Ed.D.
Associate Professor and Director of
Nurse-Midwifery Service
Department of Obstetrics and Gynecology
School of Medicine
University of Tennessee Center for the Health Sciences
Memphis, Tennessee

Bruce A. Work, Jr., M.D.
Professor of Obstetrics and Gynecology
Director, Division of Maternal-Fetal Medicine
Department of Obstetrics and Gynecology
University of Illinois College of Medicine-Chicago
Chicago, Illinois

Contents

Preface

The companion books, *A Clinical Manual of Obstetrics* and *A Clinical Manual of Gynecology*, are designed to bridge the gap between the small pocket guidebooks and "core textbooks" and the large reference textbooks, using an outline format for maximum usability and a pocket size to facilitate availability. They will be of use of the many health professionals involved in the care of women, including medical and nursing students, resident physicians in many disciplines (medicine, surgery, emergency medicine, family practice, pediatrics, etc., as well as obstetrics and gynecology), and practicing physicians and nurses. In each chapter we have struck a balance between too much and too little detail—of pathophysiology, differential diagnosis, evaluation, and management—while at the same time including many of the "practical pearls" so useful in daily health care activities but so often left to be "learned by doing." We trust the resulting books are helpful.

We wish to thank our many authors, the excellence of whose contributions provides the basis for these manuals. We also wish to thank our chairmen, John Sciarra at Northwestern University and William Spellacy at the University of Illinois, for their patience and support. Finally, thanks to Marla Ellis for her forebearance during the long hours of editing; Jeannette West for her tireless typing efforts; and Richard Lampert, John Morgan, Elizabeth Stueck, and Richard Warner of Appleton-Century-Crofts for their support and guidance.

Jeffrey W. Ellis
Charles R.B. Beckmann
Chicago, Illinois
December, 1982

Foreword

This new manual on obstetrics for residents and other health professionals involved in women's health care is unique and innovative. It provides a review of the obstetrical problems that will be faced on a busy service in a format that can be carried and used at all times. The authors selected to write for the manual provide a broad background of experience and expertise with these many problems and their information content is current and comprehensive. The manual will help to improve learning for residents and other health professionals, teaching and patient care—all of which are the ultimate goals for health care and training programs. This manual will become the "Spock" book for the obstetrical resident.

W.N. Spellacy, M.D.
Professor and Head
Department of Obstetrics and Gynecology
University of Illinois College of Medicine-Chicago
Chicago, Illinois

A Clinical
Manual of
Obstetrics

1

The House Officer as Teacher, Learner, and Health Team Manager*

Barbara M. Barzansky, Ph.D., M.H.P.E.
Charles R.B. Beckmann, M.D.
Ronald Richards, Ph.D.
William Spellacy, M.D.
Katherine Look, M.D.

PRACTICE PRINCIPLES

A house officer's daily activities often reflect three closely interwoven functions: (1) a responsibility for coordinating patient care services in outpatient and inpatient settings; (2) a continuing need to acquire skills, knowledge, and clinical experience; and (3) a responsibility for supervising the learning of students and more junior house staff. While teaching is an important function of the resident physician, very few are given

*This chapter appears in both *A Clinical Manual of Obstetrics* and *A Clinical Manual of Gynecology*.

formal training in this area. This chapter will outline some of the instructional techniques that can be used in clinical settings.

A. House staff generally are involved in informal, task-oriented teaching. Most time with students is spent in operating rooms, labor and delivery rooms, clinics, ward work, and rounds.[1]
B. A number of factors have been identified as contributing to effective teaching in clinical settings.[2,3] These will not be discussed in order of priority. All appear to be important in creating an environment where learning can occur.
C. Throughout this discussion, the term "student" will be used to refer to any learners for whom the house officer has responsibility. These may include medical students in an Ob-Gyn clerkship, more advanced medical students in specialty rotations, or junior house staff in Ob-Gyn or other specialties. Usually, junior house officers will teach and supervise medical students, while senior house staff have responsibilities for both medical students and junior house staff.

GENERAL INSTRUCTIONAL SKILLS

It is important that medical students be accepted as rightful members of the health care team,[4] and therefore, the resident should encourage student participation. This will be facilitated by recognizing that students are at the beginning of their education and require chances to ask questions. Students deserve correct explanations. This requires that the resident both know the material and be able to convey the information clearly. Teaching forces the resident to be critical of the knowledge base that he or she has acquired.

A. *Explain the basis of your actions and decisions.*
    1. It is important when explaining complex content to emphasize the main points.
    2. Summarize the explanation and check to see if students have understood what was conveyed.
    3. Give students a chance to make decisions and critique their thought processes and approaches.

B. *Allow time for discussion and questions.*
   1. Listen carefully to student questions. Rephrase the question if you are unsure what was really being asked.
   2. Answer questions clearly. Make sure the student is familiar with the terminology that has been used.
   3. If time and circumstances permit, allow other students a chance to answer a student's question. Intervene if the group is unable to respond or if incorrect information is being presented.
C. *Teach to the level of the student.*
   1. The needs of third- and fourth-year medical students are quite different. Third-year students should be introduced to their expected role on the clinical management team with increasing responsibility as their knowledge and skills develop.
   2. Fourth-year students can be given responsibilities more commensurate with what will be expected of them as interns.

TEACHING PROBLEM-SOLVING

Often the objective of a formal or informal teaching session is to sharpen the learner's ability to solve clinical problems (e.g., differential diagnoses, management plans). To facilitate this, stress approaches rather than solutions. Guide the session so that generalizations are drawn from specific cases. This makes the most efficient use of instructional time and available patient material.

A. *Whenever possible, "ask" rather than "tell."* Appropriate questioning actively involves the student, and this improves learning and retention.
   1. There are two general types of questions. Each has its proper use as a teaching tool.[5]
      a) *Closed questions* ask the student to recall specific facts (e.g., normal values, definitions). They are best used to check whether students have learned basic information. Problem-solving cannot be done without this base of specific facts.

b) *Open questions* require students to integrate information in order to address a problem (e.g., identify relevant variables, develop a hypothesis, suggest possible actions, or defend a position). This type of question is used to determine if the student can approach a clinical problem in the correct way.

2. *Include both closed and open questions* in a teaching session. Usually it is best to start with a few closed questions to make sure the students have learned the relevant facts. Then use open questions to determine whether they can apply the facts to the clinical situation.

3. Use of hypothetical, *"what if,"* questions allows the teacher to generalize from a specific finding or situation to a broader category (e.g., What would you do if her blood pressure had been elevated rather than normal? What if the placenta were located over the os rather than in the fundus?). This gives students a chance to think about clinical cases they may not have the opportunity to actually observe.

4. *Questioning should be done in a nonthreatening, nonjudgmental manner.* Avoid high-pressure quiz sessions and undue penalty for not knowing. Make students realize that questioning is a teaching as well as an evaluation strategy. They should be encouraged to admit when they are unsure of an answer and taught that this attitude is a mark of a maturing professional.

PROVIDING CLINICAL SUPERVISION

The success of a student's learning experience on a clinical rotation may in a large part depend on the house officer's skills as a clinical supervisor.[6]

A. Often students and junior house staff learn new procedures under the supervision of a more senior house officer. There is a general method for teaching manual clinical skills that maximizes both students' learning and comfort with doing the technique.[5]

1. Ideally, for common procedures write out the basic steps

in the order and manner they are done. Check with attending physicians to determine if there is general agreement about how to do the procedure. Make this guide available to students. If there is no time to write out the procedure, describe it verbally to the student and allow time for questions.

2. *Demonstrate* the procedure in its entirety. *Describe* the steps as they are being performed. *Highlight* any deviations from the commonly accepted manner of performing the technique that are necessary because of specific patient characteristics.

3. Allow the student to *practice* the technique as soon after the demonstration as possible. If it is feasible, try to arrange practice with models or simulators before students begin to work with patients.

4. *Observe* the student performing the procedure and provide feedback. Determine when the student has achieved competence and then permit some independence.

5. Periodically observe the student to ensure that performance is still satisfactory.

B. Providing *feedback* to students is an important function of a house officer. There are ways to provide the information that make the feedback most useful and effective.

1. Refer to specific behaviors or actions that were either incorrect or well done. Do not just comment on performance in a general way. For example, tell the student "you ignored the patient's question about birth control," rather than saying "you did not deal with the patient well."

2. Identify both strengths and weaknesses in the student's performance.

3. Give the feedback as close to the actual time of performance as possible. However, use discretion in giving feedback in the presence of patients or peers, especially if it is critical.

4. Check to make sure that the student understood what was communicated. Ask the student to repeat and/or rephrase the comments.

C. After giving students a chance to work up patients, review their history and physical write-up with them. Ask for explanations about their management plan and correct any misconceptions.[6]

D. It is important to decide how much control or supervision to exercise over a particular student. Make an assessment of the level of expertise displayed in particular areas and use this as a guide.

HOUSE OFFICER AS ORGANIZER

House officers are responsible for organizing a service or clinic so that it functions as a site where both patient care and student learning can take place. Certain *management techniques* can help to make this difficult balance easier to maintain.

A. *Set realistic goals for learners.*[2]
1. Often there are general, written objectives for student educational activities. Be aware of these objectives and attempt to design experiences for students that will address them. Try to ensure that each student is exposed to information about the procedures, disease states, and types of patients that are considered important.
2. Give feedback to a student about how well each objective is being met.
3. If formal objectives do not exist for an educational experience, develop an explicit set of informal expectations. Share these with faculty for their input. Make sure students are aware that these expectations exist and that they understand them.
B. *Include students in discussions* with consultants. Teach students how to use these resource persons appropriately.
C. *Familiarize students with the functions of other health professionals* (e.g., nurses, social workers, nutritionists, physical and vocational therapists, health educators). Include them, where appropriate, in discussions with students about patient problems.
D. *Teach efficiency by example.* Make efficient use of both time and personnel. Avoid duplication of activities unless it

serves an educational function. For example, a student and house officer separately examining a patient and comparing results is an educational experience, while two students making separate trips to the same place to deliver samples or to obtain supplies is not.

E. The efficient running of a ward or clinic allows more time to teach informally. Use short blocks of free time to discuss general concepts related to a patient who has just been seen or to review core material (e.g., dating a pregnancy, diagnosis and treatment of infertility).

F. When *"scut" work* must be done, make sure the duty does not always fall on the same individual. Encourage students to be helpful but not to the detriment of other aspects of their education. Stress that routine chores can both increase students' skills and help them learn to organize their time, as well as being part of their new "professional" responsibilities as health care team members.

G. The senior house officer should familiarize junior house staff and students with the setting in which they will be working. This responsibility consists of two general elements.

   1. As soon as possible, inform newcomers about the physical environment of the service or clinic (e.g., location of labs, equipment, supplies) and the general procedures to be followed in order to get things done (e.g., how to order tests, get results, and obtain consults). Introduce new staff to others who will be working with them.

   2. Acquaint students with the preferences of individual attending physicians. Many faculty have definite ways they want their services to operate, and students are often not sophisticated enough to discover these on their own.

DEVELOPMENT OF A PROFESSIONAL ORIENTATION

Clinical training from medical school through residency has been described as a continuum with the objective of sequentially increasing the learner's knowledge, skills, and responsibilities.[4] Paralleling this maturation is the development of a professional identity, which requires the adoption of certain attitudes and behaviors consistent with the practice of medicine. Attending physicians serve as role models for both house staff and students. House officers are also important as models, since students are in contact with and observe them in many different situations. Therefore, teaching by example is an important strategy to employ while working with other house staff and students.

A. The clinical environment can be a stressful one for students. Create an atmosphere where feelings and emotions can be expressed and shared.
B. Teach students to recognize and display sensitivity to patient needs and concerns while they are providing care.[2] Model the ways to establish rapport with patients and give students advice and feedback about their interaction skills.
C. Encourage students to accept other health professionals as colleagues and to deal with them in a respectful and friendly manner.[2,3]
D. Model those behaviors that students, house staff, and supervisors consider to be characteristic of a good clinician.[3]
   1. Display self-confidence and be ready to assume responsibility, without being arrogant.
   2. Be self-critical and willing to admit lack of knowledge.
E. Maintain rapport with peers and supervisors. Be flexible and responsive. Assist colleagues in getting things done when necessary and encourage students to act similarly.
F. Help students develop a sense of perspective. Convey the feeling that though the task of learning medicine is difficult, it is also rewarding.

ATTITUDE TOWARD TEACHING

Students consider teacher enthusiasm and interest as an important factor in their learning.[2,3] The house officer should be concerned with facilitating learning in all interactions with students, not just those formally designated as teaching sessions.

A. *Remain accessible to students.* Be receptive to questions and give explanations when time permits. If it is not possible to respond to a student immediately, make sure to return to the subject later.
B. *Foster in students an attitude of independence and responsibility for their own learning.* When appropriate, rather than immediately providing answers, have students research their questions and report their findings.
C. *Have students share information.* If one student has seen a specific pathology or normal variant, have him or her report on it to the other students in the group.
D. *Use teaching as an instrument for self-diagnosis.* The process of explaining things to others is often a useful way of determining your own information base.

CONTENT EXPERTISE/KNOWLEDGE

The senior house officer is still in the process of acquiring the knowledge and skills necessary for independent practice. This learning can come from a variety of sources: faculty, peers, the published literature, and direct clinical experience.

A. Share appropriate references with junior house staff and students.
B. Encourage beginning students to concentrate their reading on their own patients' problems. This strategy makes the information more relevant and more likely to be retained.

REFERENCES
1. Stenchever MA, Irby D, O'Toole B: A national survey of undergraduate teaching in obstetrics and gynecology. J Med Educ 54:467–470, 1959
2. Stritter FT, Hain JD, Grimes DA: Clinical teaching reexamined. J Med Educ 50:876–882, 1975
3. Irby D: Clinical teacher effectiveness in medicine. J Med Educ 53:808–815, 1978

4. Tonesk X: The house officer as a teacher: what schools expect and measure. J Med Educ 54:613–616, 1979
5. Foley RP, Smilansky J: Teaching Techniques: A Handbook for Health Professionals. New York, McGraw-Hill, 1980
6. Byrne N, Cohen R: Observational study of clinical clerkship activities. J Med Educ 48:919–927, 1973

2

History and Physical Examination*

Jeffrey W. Ellis, M.D.
Charles R.B. Beckmann, M.D.
Linda A. Wheeler, R.N., C.N.M., Ed.D.
Frank W. Ling, M.D.

MEDICAL HISTORY

Practice Principles

The patient's medical history should be obtained in an orderly sequence. When dealing with the obstetric or gynecologic patient, *pertinent gynecologic information is emphasized,* although care should be taken to obtain information regarding the patient's entire medical history in order to detect and treat other intercurrent medical problems.

Chief Complaint

The patient's chief complaint (CC) may be recorded either as a quote of the patient's response or as a description of the patient's response using medical terminology, although care must be

*This chapter appears in both *A Clinical Manual of Obstetrics* and *A Clinical Manual of Gynecology*.

Format of the Gynecologic History
Identifying Data
  Age
  Menarche
  Last Menstrual Period (LMP)
  Previous Menstrual Period (PMP)
  Obstetric Profile   Gravida ＿＿ Para ＿＿ ＿＿ ＿＿ ＿＿

    Number of Pregnancies————

    Number of Term Pregnancies————

    Number of Premature Pregnancies————

    Number of Aborted Pregnancies ————

    Number of Living Children ————

Birth Control History (past and present methods,
sterilization)
Gynecologic Surgery

---

taken to avoid obscuring the patient's true meaning by the use of
technical terminology.

History of Present Illness (HPI)
The following information should be obtained according to the
patient's presenting symptoms.

A. *Bleeding Symptoms*
   1. Changes in the menstrual period interval; duration of
      bleeding; relative amount of bleeding (determine by
      assessing the number of tampons or perineal pads used);
      passage of clots

2. Intermenstrual bleeding: amount, duration, relative time within the menstrual cycle
3. Contact bleeding: after douching, sexual intercourse
4. Postmenopausal bleeding: amount, duration, time interval from last menstrual period, history of hormonal (estrogen) therapy
5. Changes in menstrual pattern in relation to exogenous steroids; estrogen, progesterone, birth control pills

B. *Pain Symptoms*
1. Date of onset
2. Relation to the menstrual period
3. Location
4. Radiation
5. Character: sharp, dull, constant, intermittent
6. Degree: whether the pain incapacitates the patient
7. Factors that decrease or increase pain: position, urination, defecation
8. Use of analgesics, muscle relaxants, etc. (type, frequency, amount, duration of use)
9. Associated gastrointestinal and urinary symptoms

C. *Mass Symptoms*
1. Date of onset
2. Relation to the menstrual period
3. Location
4. Associated symptoms: pain, bleeding, gastrointestinal or urinary disturbance
5. Growth: stable, slow, rapid (measured by such things as "changes" in clothing size, "bloated" sensation, etc.)

D. *Vaginal Discharge*
1. Date of onset
2. Relation to the menstrual period
3. Color, odor, consistency, quantity
4. Associated rectal or urethral discharge
5. Associated symptoms: pain, pruritus
6. Relation to use of medications: antibiotics, exogenous steroids
7. History of previous treatment

E. *Ulceration or Persistent Lesion*
 1. Date of onset
 2. Location
 3. Growth: stable, slow, rapid
 4. Associated symptoms: pain, pruritus, bleeding, discharge
 5. Other body sites with a similar lesion
 6. History of previous treatment
F. *Pelvic Relaxation*
 1. Pressure
 2. Prolapse ("falling out")
 3. Urinary symptoms: urgency, frequency, inability to void, incontinence
 4. Lower gastrointestinal symptoms: constipation, tenesmus, incontinence
G. *Infertility*
 1. Duration
 2. Frequency of intercourse
 3. Prior investigation
 4. Medical or surgical disorders of partner (previous children?)
H. *Pelvic ("Tubal") Infection (Pelvic Inflammatory Disease, PID)*
 1. History consistent with PID: fever (with or without chills), abdominopelvic pain, foul discharge; use of parenteral antibiotics with relief within 48 hours.
 2. History of positive GC culture or documented exposure.

Gynecologic History
The following detailed information is obtained regarding the patient's gynecologic history.
A. Age at menarche
B. Normal interval between menstrual periods
C. Normal durations of menstrual flow
D. Normal amount of menstrual flow (number of perineal pads or tampons)

E. Associated menstrual symptoms: pain, edema, headache
F. Past gynecologic problems treated medically
G. Past gynecologic surgery
H. Contraceptive use: method, side effects, complications

Sexual History
A. Regularity of intercourse
B. Associated symptoms: pain, bleeding
C. Sexual dysfunction

Medical History
A. Chronic diseases: treatment, results
B. Infectious diseases: venereal diseases, exposure to infectious diseases
C. Current medications
D. Past medications
E. Allergies *(include symptoms of allergic reactions)*
F. Use of drugs, alcohol, tobacco
G. Exposure to toxic agents and radiation

Surgical History
A. Dates of procedures
B. Diagnosis
C. Type of surgical procedures
D. Results

Family History
A. Malignancy, chronic illness
B. Hereditary disease
C. Multiple gestation
D. Pertinent obstetric and gynecologic histories of family members

Social History
A. Occupation and financial status
B. Marital status
C. Education

Review of Systems (ROS)
In general, the standard format of the review of systems should be followed. Pertinent "negatives" should be noted in the following systems:

A. Gastrointestinal
   1. Indigestion
   2. Nausea, vomiting, diarrhea
   3. Constipation
   4. Incontinence, tenesmus, rectal bleeding
   5. Abdominal pain
B. Urinary
   1. Urgency, frequency, dysuria, nocturia, incontinence
   2. Hematuria
   3. Inability to void

Format of the Obstetric History (page 12)

THE PELVIC EXAMINATION

Practice Principles

1. A relaxed and comfortable patient is essential for the performance of the pelvic examination.
2. The patient in the lithotomy position with drapes across her knees is blind to the pelvic examination. Eye contact between the patient and the examiner decreases some of the anxiety about the pelvic examination.
3. It is necessary to alleviate the patient's anxiety and enlist her cooperation.
4. Principles to be followed during the pelvic exam include:

• Assure the patient that all procedures will be demonstrated and explained prior to being performed.
• Inform the patient before an area is examined.
• Use slow and deliberate motions to allow the patient to maintain relaxation.

- Inform the patient of any deep palpation or uncomfortable procedures.
- Warm speculum before insertion if possible.

Format of the Pelvic Examination. The following outline should be used when reporting the pelvic examination into the medical record:

- External genitalia
- Vagina
- Cervix
- Corpus
- Adnexa
- Rectovaginal

Physical Findings
The following physical findings should be noted and recorded.

A. *External Genitalia*
   1. Hair distribution
   2. Labia majora/minora: lesions, ulcerations, masses, induration, areas of different color
   3. Clitoris: size, lesions, ulcerations
   4. Urethra: discharge, lesions, ulcerations
   5. Skene's glands/Bartholin's glands: masses, discharge, tenderness
   6. Perineum: lesions, ulcerations, masses, induration
   7. Anus: lesions, ulcerations, fissures, hemorrhoids
B. *Vagina*
   1. Inflammation or atrophy
   2. Lesions, ulceration, excoriation
   3. Masses, induration or nodularity
   4. Discharge (KOH and saline preparation results; vaginal pH)
   5. Septa, status of hymen/introitus
   6. Relaxation of support: rectocele, cystocele, urethrocele, enterocele, uterine prolapse

C. *Cervix*
   1. Size and position; position of transformation zone
   2. Color
   3. Ulcerations, lesions, lacerations (old, new; size, location)
   4. Consistency (firm, hard, soft, nodular)
   5. Pain on motion
   6. Contact bleeding (after pap smear or contact with the speculum)
   7. Discharge
   8. Parous or nulliparous
D. *Corpus*
   1. Position
   2. Size (describe in weeks size as though pregnant)
   3. Contour (smooth, irregular)
   4. Consistency
   5. Mobility
   6. Pain on motion
E. *Adnexa*
   1. Size
   2. Consistency (solid, soft, "thickened")
   3. Contour (smooth, irregular)
   4. Mobility (if not, fixed to what structure)
   5. Position
   6. Pain on motion
F. *Rectovaginal*
   1. Cul de sac: mass, flutulence
   2. Rectovaginal septum: mass, flutulence, nodularity, induration
   3. Parametria: induration, nodularity
   4. Rectum: mass, bleeding
   5. Uterosacral ligaments: nodularity

PROCEDURE GUIDE: PELVIC EXAMINATION

Procedure	Comments
1. Place a glove on one hand.	See comments at end of this section regarding one- and two-glove technique.
2. Make patient as comfortable as possible. If the examiner is male, a female assistant should be present. If the examiner is female, many people also advocate the presence of an assistant who is female.	A female assistant protects the examiner from charges of improper sexual advances and provides the patient with a same-sex support person.
3. Drape the woman so that her knees are covered. The head of the table should be elevated enough that you will have eye contact with the patient.	Covering a woman's knees helps her feel you have some concern for her modesty. Some women feel a drape is unnecessary. However, it is usually best to proceed with the assumption that the patient prefers a drape.
4. Arrange the drape so that it is flat on the patient's abdomen yet covers the patients knees.	A sheet placed flat on the abdomen allows for eye contact between patient and examiner.
5. Sit down. Adjust the light.	
6. Tell the patient you are going to touch the back of her leg. Touch the back of your hand to the inside of the patient's thigh.	This action is relatively noninvasive, assures her you are concerned for her comfort, and involves no discomfort. Watch the muscles around her vagina and rectum. If they contract, make extra efforts to go slowly and be gentle.

7. Observe the perineum and external genitalia. "Chattering" or complete silence at this point will often make the patient anxious.

8. Tell the woman you are going to touch her external genitalia, "privates," "outside," etc. Separate the labia majora from the labia minora. Inspect the urethra.

Normal labia minora may be asymmetrical, and either larger or smaller than the labia majora.

9. Tell the woman you are going to put one finger inside. Insert your index finger to the last phalanx (approximately 1 inch). With palm up, "milk" the urethra.

You are looking for purulent discharge. Most often it is gonorrhea.

10. Using the thumb and index finger, palpate the area at 7 and 8 o'clock, as well as at 4 and 5 o'clock for a Bartholin cyst.

You will feel nothing in the absence of a cyst.

11. Show the patient the speculum if she has not seen one before and tell her you are going to insert it. If you wish, moisten it with warm water to make insertion easier. However, the speculum should be moistened/lubricated for prepubertal girls and postmenopausal women.

Lubricants such as KY Jelly should not be used as they will affect the reading of the Pap smear. If the speculum has not been warmed, warn the patient that it will be cold. Warming the speculum, however, greatly increases patient acceptance of the examination and ease of examination.

12. The speculum can be inserted in many ways. Here are three that are commonly used. Hold the speculum in your ungloved hand:

   a) Insert the index and middle fingers of your examining hand into the vagina and press down posteriorly. Insert the speculum on top of your fingers and rotate it so that the handle is down. Remove your fingers from the vagina.

   b) Place the index and middle fingers of your examining hand just inside the vaginal orifice on either side. Roll them back onto the external genitalia and press posteriorly and laterally to enlarge the vaginal orifice. Insert the speculum.

   c) Place the index and middle fingers of your examining hand on either side of the vagina on the outside. Exert pressure downwards and laterally to

Whatever technique is used, ask the patient to relax (have the patient relax the muscle she uses to cut off her urine stream). It is not unusual for a woman to unconsciously tighten her pelvis muscles at this time. Observe for a cystocele or rectocele as you get ready to insert the speculum.

enlarge the vaginal opening.

Insert the speculum. Whichever method is used remember pressure "posteriorly" presses soft tissue against soft tissue, whereas "anteriorly" soft tissue is "caught" between a hard metal speculum and the bony pelvis.

13. Transfer the handle of the speculum to your other hand. Remember that the vagina angles toward the hollow of the sacrum. Open the speculum. The cervix will appear smooth in comparison with the rugaeted vagina. Its position varies.

The most common reason for not "finding" the cervix is failure to insert the speculum far enough before opening the instrument.

Once the cervix is found, insert the speculum far enough so that the cervix rests within the blades. Set the screw with your ungloved hand.

In most instances it will not be necessary to adjust the lower screw located on the handle of the speculum. Adjusting this screw allows for greater visualization, needed for procedures such as IUD insertion.

14. Observe the vagina and cervix. Saline and KOH preparations should be done on any discharge and pH obtained with litmus paper.

15. Perform a Pap smear and obtain a specimen for the

gonorrhea culture (see procedure guide).

16. Tell the patient you are going to turn and remove the speculum. Unscrew the screw but do not remove the speculum. Rotate the speculum 90° so that you can see the anterior and posterior walls of the vagina. Remove the speculum.

17. Place a small amount of lubricant on the index and middle fingers of your gloved hand. Tell the woman that you are going to examine her internally.

If you obtain the lubricant from a multiple-use tube, be sure you do not touch your fingers to the tube's opening. If you touch the opening, the tube must be thrown away as it may be contaminated with secretions on your gloved hand.

18. Tell the woman you are going to touch the back of her leg again. Then gently and slowly insert your middle and index fingers into the vagina. Turn your palm up and feel for the cervix.

The cervix may be found posteriorly, anteriorly, or any where in between. Its position is most often related to the postion of the uterus: a posterior cervix with an anteverted uterus and an anterior cervix with a retroverted uterus. The cervix will feel like the tip of your nose. Note its shape and consistency. Feel for growths.

19. Now feel the body of the uterus. Place your fingers palm up on top of the cervix. Place your abdom-

It is important to start at the umbilicus with your abdominal hand until you become skilled to avoid missing a

inal hand at the umbilicus. Slowly work your abdominal hand down toward the symphysis trying to trap the anteverted uterus between your two hands (Fig. 2–1).

uterus enlarged by fibroids or pregnancy.

20. If you cannot feel the uterus with this maneuver, place your fingers *under* the cervix and advance them along the posterior part of the cervix as far as they will go. Move your abdominal hand as in step 21, following.

This time you are trying to trap a retroverted uterus between your fingers.

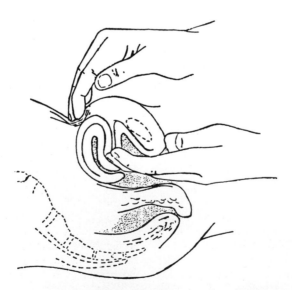

Figure 2–1. Bimanual palpation of the uterus.

21. If you still cannot find the uterus, it is probably in a midposition, i.e., not tilted in either direction. Keep your fingers, palm up, under the cervix and work them toward the patient's head. Place the flat part of the fingers of your abdominal hand above the symphysis. Press toward the examining table trying once again to trap the uterus between your fingers (Fig.2–2).

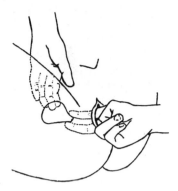

Figure 2–2. Palpation of the uterus in midposition.

22. Once located there are six things about the uterus to be noted; size, shape, position, consistency, mobility, and tenderness.

23. The ovaries and fallopian tubes are located posterior to the broad ligament, which is attached to the uterus. Place your vaginal fingers to the side of the cervix deep in the cul-de-sac (lateral fornix). Move your abdominal hand to the same side just inside the flare of the pelvis. Press down and move your abdominal hand toward the symphysis. Reach up with your vaginal fingers. Bring them together the rest of the

Feeling ovaries is a skill that takes much practice to develop. As a beginner, it is neither necessary nor expected that you will feel ovaries on every patient. Keep the patient's comfort in mind. Even experienced, competent physicians do not *always* feel the ovaries. Inability to feel the adnexa is often just as important as feeling the adnexa. It is a significant negative for the skilled clinician, meaning that no pathology is evident.

way down the abdomen. The ovary should be felt trapped between your fingers. It normally feels about the size of an almond. It should be mobile and free of the side walls. The fallopian tubes will not be palpable unless they are pathologically enlarged. (Fig. 2–3).

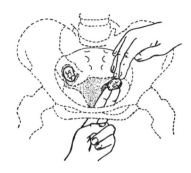

Figure 2–3. Palpation of the adnexae.

24. Tell the patient that the final part of the examination is the exam of the rectum. Repeat rectally the exam of the uterus and ovaries as in step 23. A rectal exam is quite uncomfortable for most people. It should, therefore, be completed as quickly and gently as possible. Tell the patient what you intend to do. Ask her to bear down as if she were going to move her bowels. Besides relaxing the patient, this helps you feel where to insert your finger. Keeping your index finger in the vagina, *slowly* insert your middle finger into the rectum as

The exam is important for three reasons: the information it gives about the rectum, the rectovaginal septum, and confirmation of your vaginal findings. Additionally, you can feel 1 to 2 cm higher into the pelvis than you can feel vaginally. Explaining these facts to a patient helps her to understand why such an uncomfortable procedure is necessary.

the sphincter relaxes. Place your rectovaginal fingers laterally with your abdominal hand on the same side. Move your hands together across the abdomen to the opposite side. Be sure your vaginal finger stays under the cervix.

Feel both uterosacral ligaments. They should be obvious, symmetrical, smooth, and nontender. Feel posteriorly across the uterus. It should feel smooth. The mucosas—or two peritoneal surfaces—should slide across each other. If not, suspect endometriosis. Feel for puckering, shortening, scarring—all suggestive of endometriosis.

25. Offer the woman a tissue to wipe off excess lubricant before she dresses. Ask her to move back on the table and then to sit up.

If she sits up first, she will fall on the floor.

26. Remove your glove(s) and wash your hands.

Remember to turn off the faucet with a paper towel to avoid contaminating your hands with anything (GC, trichomonas) that may be on the faucet.

Hints

1. Many women make extra effort to be clean prior to a pelvic examination by douching. You may want to inquire as to whether or not the patient douches and how often. Ask her not to douche for 48 hours prior to examination, so that you can observe the usual state of her vagina.

2. Clinicians' feelings about a one- or two-glove technique vary, as do their preferences for which hand to use for the examination. The use of two gloves protects the examiner from possible contact with disease organisms such as *Neisseria gonorrhoeae*. However, beginners using this technique often forget to keep one hand clean and, consequently, may contaminate the light and other objects.

3. Once you perform a pelvic exam, you will see that you can feel one side of the pelvis better than the other. The angle of your hand allows the right-handed examiner to examine the patient's right side better and vice versa. To compensate for the difference, some clinicians use their left hand to examine the left side and their right hand to examine the right side.

THE VAGINAL SPECULUM

The vaginal speculum (Fig. 2–4) is an instrument that facilitates visualization of the cervix and vaginal walls. Note the parts of the speculum:

A. Upper blade
B. Lower blade
C. Handle
D. Screw attaching the upper and lower blades
E. Lever separating the upper and lower blades
F. Screw to fix the blades in position

There are two types of specula: the Pederson and the Graves (Fig. 2–5 and 2–6). The Pederson speculum has flat and narrow blades that barely curve on the sides. The standard Pederson works well for most nulliparous women. Occasionally, it is necessary to use the Pederson for a multiparous woman who is sensitive to objects being placed in her vagina.The Graves speculum has blades that are wider, higher, and curved on the sides. Most women who have had a baby can accommodate the standard (medium) Graves speculum. Its wider, curved blades keep the looser vaginal walls of the multiparous woman separated for visualization.

Both specula are available in a pediatric size as well as the standard size (Fig. 2–7). The pediatric specula are usually reserved for young children. The length of the blades does not usually allow the examiner to reach the cervix of girls who are pubertal or older. A Pederson with extra narrow blades is also available (Fig. 2–8).

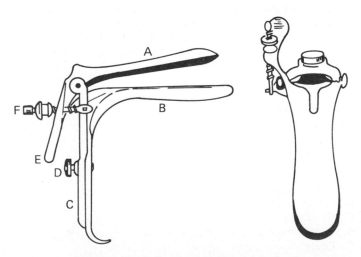

Figure 2–4. Parts of the vaginal speculum.

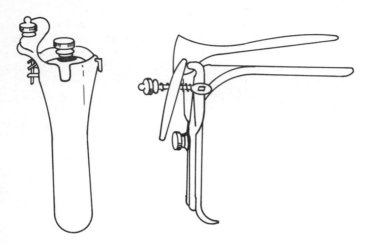

Figure 2–5. Medium Pederson speculum.

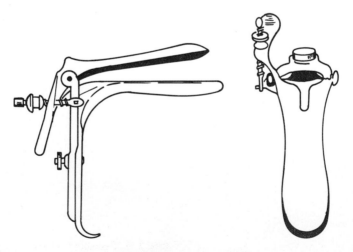

Figure 2–6. Medium Graves speculum.

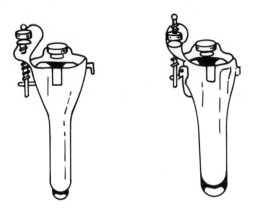

Figure 2–7. Pediatric specula: A. Pederson; B. Graves.

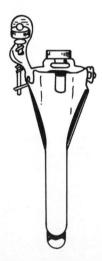

Figure 2–8. Pediatric Pederson speculum with extra-narrow blades.

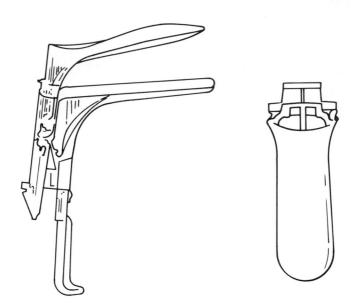

Figure 2–9. Disposable plastic speculum.

The disposable plastic speculum (Fig. 2–9) may be used in some institutions. It makes a loud "click" when the lower blade is disengaged for removal. Women should be alerted to the noise prior to disengaging to avoid startling the patient. Women who perform or plan to begin performing self-examination of the cervix and vagina appreciate being given the plastic speculum to take home. It should be washed after each use. Most women find that, for self-examination, insertion is most easily accomplished with the handle up rather than down.

3

Operative Management*

Jeffrey W. Ellis, M.D.

ROUTINE ADMITTING ORDERS

Admitting orders will vary according to the patient's condition and the planned operative procedure.

Orders should be specified in the following sequence:

1. Vital signs
2. Diet
3. Activity
4. Laboratory studies
5. Radiologic studies
6. Other special studies
7. Medications
8. Special care
9. Respiratory care

1. Vital Signs. In most patients admitted for elective procedures, vital signs (pulse, respirations, blood pressure, temperature) may be taken every 8 hours or every 12 hours (q8h, q12h). More frequent assessment may be required in acutely ill patients (q1h, q2h, q4h).

*This chapter appears in both *A Clinical Manual of Obstetrics* and *A Clinical Manual of Gynecology*.

2. Diet. A regular diet may be given to most patients up to the night before surgery. The patient should receive nothing by mouth (NPO) for at least 8 hours prior to surgery. A clear liquid diet may be required before certain radiographic studies and before some surgical procedures in which bowel surgery is a possibility.

3. Activity. Most patients are allowed unrestricted activity prior to surgery (up ad lib). Special bed positions should be specified if necessary (Trendelenburg position, semi-Fowler's position, etc.).

4. Laboratory Studies. Most hospitals require the following laboratory studies prior to surgery: complete blood count, urinalysis, prothrombin time (PT), partial thromboplastin time (PTT), platelet count, electrolytes, blood urea nitrogen (BUN), creatinine, direct and indirect bilirubin, alkaline phosphatase, SGOT, SGPT. Other studies may be necessary according to significant history and physical examination.

5. Radiologic Studies. Most hospitals require a chest x-ray prior to surgery. Additional diagnostic studies may be required for complete preoperative evaluation: intravenous pyelogram (IVP), lower gastrointestinal series (LGI), voiding cystourethrogram, and so on.

6. Other Special Studies. An electrocardiogram should be obtained on all patients over the age of 35 years and on all patients with a history of cardiac or pulmonary disease. Additional studies that may be required include: pulmonary function studies (PFT), ultrasound, and computed axial tomography (CAT scan).

7. Medications. Patient comfort medications (analgesics, hypnotics, laxatives) and therapeutic medications should be specified. Some physicians suggest a "non-PRN" sleeping medication the night before surgery to allow the patient adequate sleep prior to surgery (example: secobarbital, 100 mg at 11 P.M.).

8. Special Care. Specify the following: wound care, catheter care, skin care, and colostomy care.

9. Respiratory Care. Patients who smoke should be vigorously encouraged to cease smoking two to four weeks before elective surgery. Upon admission, all patients should be provided with a voluntary respiratory exiciser (Uniflow, Triflow, etc.) with instructions for the nursing staff to teach the patient the proper use of the instrument and to verify that the patient has acquired facility with the device. This presurgical emphasis fixes in the patient's mind the importance of good respiratory effort in the postoperative period, thus increasing patient compliance in these matters.

PREOPERATIVE ORDERS

Preoperative orders will vary according to the type and site of surgery and the general condition of the patient.

Orders should be specified in the following sequence:

	Example
1. *Diet*	Nothing by mouth after midnight
2. *Patient preparation*	
Abdomen–perineum	Shave abdomen from umbilicus to symphysis
Bowel	Tap water enema until clear two hours before surgery
Vagina	Betadine douche the evening before surgery
Skin	Scrub abdomen with soap and water one hour before surgery
Bladder	Void on call to operating room
3. *Medications*	
Preoperative sedation (to be given IM on call to operating room)	Meperidine (Demerol), 50 mg; hydroxyzine (Vistaril), 25 mg; atropine, 0.4 mg
Antibiotics	If prophylactic antibiotics are

given, the first dose should be administered parenterally within two hours before surgery.

4. *Blood bank* (Every hospital has its own protocol about the availability of blood for surgery.)

Type and crossmatch two units of whole blood.

PREOPERATIVE NOTES
Prior to any operative procedure, the following note should be recorded in the medical record.

	Example
1. *Preoperative diagnosis*	Uterine myomata
2. *Planned procedure*	Vaginal hysterectomy
3. *Surgeons*	Drs. _____
4. *Preoperative laboratory*	Summary of pertinent laboratory studies
5. *Blood bank*	Whole blood, 2 units, available

POSTOPERATIVE NOTES
The postoperative note provides a summary of the surgical procedure.

	Example
1. *Preoperative diagnosis*	Uterine myomata
2. *Postoperative diagnosis*	Same
3. *Procedure*	Vaginal hysterectomy
4. *Surgeon*	Dr. _____
5. *Assistant*	Dr. _____
6. *Anesthesia*	General endotracheal, halothane and thiopental
7. *Anesthesiologist*	Dr. _____
8. *Fluids administered*	2000 mL lactated Ringer's so-

	lution; 2 units of packed red blood cells.
9. *Estimated blood loss*	300 ml
10. *Urinary output*	600 ml
11. *Findings* (The careful and detailed description of operative findings and procedures is one of the *most crucial* roles of the operative note, yet it is also the most often neglected aspect of the note.)	Uterus: 12-week size, multi-nodular; tubes and ovaries: normal
12. *Complications*	None
13. *Tubes and drains*	Foley catheter, nasogastric tube
14. *Condition of patient*	Tolerated procedure well, brought to recovery room awake and extubated

POSTOPERATIVE ORDERS

Minor Procedures. During minor gynecologic procedures, blood loss is usually minimal and the abdominal cavity is not entered. Examples include dilatation and curettage, cone biopsy, Bartholin cystectomy. Postoperatively, the patient should rapidly regain normal preoperative status.

	Example
1. *Vital signs*	Every 15 minutes until stable, then every four hours.
2. *Diet*	Regular diet when fully recovered from anesthesia.
3. *Activity*	Unrestricted activity when fully recovered from anesthesia.
4. *Intravenous fluids*	Dextrose, 5%, in Ringer's lactate at a rate of 125 ml/hour.

	Discontinue when the patient is fully awake and tolerating a diet.
5. *Special observations*	Inform the service of heavy vaginal bleeding or inability to void.
6. *Medications*	Specify analgesics, hypnotics, antibiotics; resume other necessary medications.

Major Procedures. Examples include abdominal hysterectomy, vaginal hysterectomy, salpingectomy. Major procedures usually involve the following:

1. Bowel manipulation with resulting paralytic ileus.
2. Operative blood loss of 100 to 1000 mL or more.
3. Longer anesthesia time with resulting pulmonary atelectasis and accumulation of pulmonary secretions.

Postoperative management is thus aimed at:

1. Careful and frequent monitoring of vital signs.
2. Maintenance of adequate intravascular volume through careful monitoring of intake and output.
3. "Bowel rest" until peristaltic function resumes.
4. Pulmonary therapy.

An example of immediate postoperative orders after an abdominal hysterectomy follows:

	Example
1. *Vital signs*	q 15 minutes until stable, then q1h × 2, then q2h × 2, then q4h.
2. *Diet*	Nothing by mouth (NPO)
3. *Activity*	Complete bed rest for 8 hours, then ambulate with assistance for 10 minutes q4h.

4. *Intravenous fluids*	Dextrose, 5% in Ringer's lactate to run at 125 mL/hour
5. *Tubes and drains*	Foley catheter to closed drainage bag, nasogastric tube to low, intermittent suction.
6. *Intake and output*	Record q2h.
7. *Medications*	Meperidine, 75 mg IM q3h PRN.
8. *Respiratory care* (Whatever respiratory care is selected, it should be ordered "around-the-clock" in the immediate postoperative period, and *not* "while awake.")	Turn, cough, and hyperventilate q2h, ultrasonic nebulizer for 10 minutes q2h.
9. *Laboratory*	CBC at 10:00 P.M. and 7:00 A.M.
10. *Notify service*	Pulse greater than 120; systolic BP less than 90; diastolic BP less than 60; temperature greater than 101F; urine output less than 60 ml in any two-hour interval.

POSTOPERATIVE ROUNDS

During daily postoperative rounds, the following areas should be evaluated and entered into the medical record:

Postoperative Day Number (POD#)

1. *Review of chart*	Vital signs; intake and output; nursing notes.
2. *Patient complaints and observations*	Location and degree of pain; vaginal drainage or bleeding; bowel movement or passage of flatus; nausea or vomiting; difficulty with urination; expectoration.

3. *Physical examination* — Auscultate chest; auscultate abdomen for bowel sounds; palpate abdomen; examine incision; examine lower extremities and IV sites for evidence of phlebitis; evaluate vaginal drainage or bleeding.

4. *Treatment plan* — Re-evaluate diet, activity, frequency of vital signs; intravenous fluids; necessity of tubes and drains; medications; special care. Order new laboratory studies as indicated.

4

Diagnosis of Pregnancy*
Jeffrey W. Ellis, M.D.

PRACTICE PRINCIPLES

The diagnosis of pregnancy can often be made on the basis of history and physical examination. Sensitive laboratory studies may be necessary to confirm an early gestation. The use of potentially teratogenic drugs or radiographic studies in women in the reproductive age range requires testing in any case where pregnancy is suspected. Pregnancy complicated by serious maternal disease, such as diabetes, is best managed when the diagnosis is made early.

SIGNS AND SYMPTOMS OF PREGNANCY

A. *Presumptive signs and symptoms*
   1. Cessation of menstruation
   2. Nausea and vomiting
   3. Breast changes: tenderness, enlargement, increased pigmentation
   4. Cyanosis of the vagina and cervix
   5. Frequent urination
   6. Easy fatigability
   7. Increased pigmentation of the skin
   8. Abdominal striae

*This chapter appears in both *A Clinical Manual of Obstetrics* and *A Clinical Manual of Gynecology*.

B. *Probable signs and symptoms*
  1. Abdominal enlargement
  2. Changes in the size, shape, and consistency of the uterus (enlarged, globular, soft)
  3. Softening of the cervix
  4. Painless uterine contractions
  5. Ballottement of the abdomen revealing a discrete mass (fetus)
  6. Palpation of fetal parts
C. *Positive signs of pregnancy*
  1. Auscultation of fetal heart sounds
  2. Active fetal movements perceived by an examiner
  3. Radiographic or ultrasound demonstration of a fetus

BIOLOGIC TESTS OF PREGNANCY

Biologic tests are no longer used in clinical practice. They are all based on the observation that chorionic gonadotropin in the urine of pregnant women will, when injected subcutaneously into a variety of test animals, induce ovulatory phenomena.

CLINICAL TESTS OF PREGNANCY

High doses of oral or parenteral progesterone will often induce withdrawal bleeding if pregnancy is not the cause of amenorrhea. Progesterone is no longer approved for this use, as it is implicated in teratogenicity.

RADIOLOGIC TESTS OF PREGNANCY

1. *Abdominal x-ray films* should not be used to diagnose pregnancy because of the potential hazards to the fetus.
2. *Ultrasound* can demonstrate a gestational sac 21 ± 3 days after ovulation. Fetal cardiac activity can be detected reliably 5 weeks after ovulation.

ENDOCRINE TESTS OF PREGNANCY

These tests are based on the detection of human chorionic gonadotropin (hCG) in either urine or serum. The β- subunit of hCG confers biologic and immunologic specificity.

A. *Urinary tests.* Detection of hCG is based on various immunologic reactions. The first urine voided in the morning should be used for evaluation since it is usually the most concentrated urine produced during the day. Table 4–1 summarizes currently available urine pregnancy tests. In performing the pregnancy test, instructions for use of the specific product must be followed carefully. Sensitivities of the individual tests must be noted.

TABLE 4–1. QUALITATIVE IMMUNOLOGIC (URINE) TESTS FOR PREGNANCY

Test	Source	Sensitivity* (IU)
SLIDE TESTS		
Latex Aglutination Inhibition†		
Gravindex 90	Ortho Diagnostics	3.5
Pregna β-slide	International Diagnostics	2.0
Pregnate	Fisher Scientific	2.0–4.0
Pregnosis	Roche Diagnostics	1.5–2.5
Prognosticon Dri-dot	Organon Diagnostics	1.0–2.0
Prognosticon Slide Test	Organon Diagnostics	1.0–2.0
UCG Slide Test	Wampole Laboratories	2.0
Direct Latex Agglutination‡		
Dap Test Macro	Wampole Laboratories	2.0

(*Continued*)

TABLE 4-1. QUALITATIVE IMMUNOLOGIC (URINE) TESTS FOR PREGNANCY (Cont.)

Test	Source	Sensitivity* (IU)
TUBE TESTS		
Hemagglutination Inhibition§		
Gravindex 90	Ortho Diagnostics	0.5
Neocept	Organon Diagnostics	0.2
Pregna-β	International Diagnostics	0.4–0.8
Prognosticon Accuspheres	Organon Diagnostics	0.75–0.85
UCG-Lyphotest	Wampole Laboratories	0.5–1.0
UCG-Quik-Tube	Wampole Laboratories	1.0
UCG-Test	Wampole Laboratories	0.5–1.3
Indirect Agglutination Inhibition‖		
Placentex	Roche Diagnostics	1.0
Sensi-Tex	Roche Diagnostics	0.25

*Minimal detectable levels of hCG/ml urine.
†End points: *positive,* no agglutination; *negative,* agglutination.
‡End points: *positive,* agglutination; *negative,* no agglutination.
§End points: *positive,* red blood cells settle to the bottom of the tube and form a ring; *negative,* red blood cells agglutinate but remain in suspension.
‖End points: *positive,* milky white solution; *negative,* flocculation.

1. *False-negative results.* hCG is present in the urine but is not detected.
   a) Dilute urine (low specific gravity)
   b) The amount of hCG in the urine is below the minimum sensitivity level of the test.

    c) Damaged reagents
    d) Excessive vibration (tube tests)
  2. *False-positive results*
    a) *hCG is present but the patient is not pregnant*
      (1) Trophoblastic diseases
      (2) hCG-producing ovarian tumors (choriocarcinoma)
      (3) Nontrophoblastic tumors that produce hCG (colon, pancreas, breast, lung, thyroid)
      (4) After injection of hCG to induce ovulation
    b) *Cross reactivity with high levels of LH*
      (1) Perimenopausal and postmenopausal women
      (2) After injection of substances to induce ovulation that contain LH
      (3) Normal preovulatory LH surge
    c) *Substances that interfere with the immunologic reaction*
      (1) Proteinuria
      (2) Nonspecific agglutinins in the urine
      (3) Drugs (chlorpromazine, thioridazine, trifluoperazine)
      (4) Soaps and detergents in the urine specimen containers
      (5) Blood
      (6) Bacteria
B. *Serum tests.* Detection of hCG is based on radioassay techniques. These tests may be used when greater sensitivity is required than may be obtained with urine tests. Numerous tests are currently marketed with differing sensitivities. The physician should be aware of the sensitivities of the test used in his institution. Table 4–2 summarizes several currently available radioassays.
  1. *Radioreceptor assay* (RRA)
    a) *Principle.* A bovine corpus luteum membrane is the receptor site for binding hCG.
    b) *False-negative results*
      (1) The amount of hCG in the serum is below the minimum sensitivity of the test.
      (2) Defective materials

TABLE 4–2. RADIOASSAY (SERUM/PLASMA) TESTS FOR PREGNANCY

Test	Source	Sensitivity* (mIU)
Beta-Tec	Wampole Laboratories	3–50
β-hCG Radioimmuno-assay Kit†	Becton Dickinson	30 (serum) 100 (urine)
Biocept-G‡	Wampole Laboratories	200
Chorio-Shure	NML Laboratories	40
Concept-7-BHCG†	Leeco Diagnostics	30 (serum) 100 (urine)
HCG-β Radioimmuno-assay Kit	BIO-RIA	<6
Preg-CG Assay	Cambridge Nuclear	40
Preg-Stat	Sereno Laboratories	25
Roche β-hCG RIA	Roche Diagnostics	6

*Minimum detectable levels of hCG/ml.
†Tests which may detect hCG in urine
‡Radioreceptor Assay

    c) *False-positive results*
       (1) High levels of LH may bind receptor sites
       (2) hCG may be detected from sources other than pregnancy
 2. *Radioimmunoassay* (RIA)
    a) *Principle.* Antibody specifically detects the presence of the β-subunit of hCG
    b) *False-negative results*
       (1) The amount of hCG in the serum is below the minimum sensitivity of the test
       (2) Defective materials

c) *False-positive results*
   (1) At lower levels of sensitivity, LH may be detected
   (2) hCG may be detected from sources other than pregnancy

BIBLIOGRAPHY

Arkin C, Noto T: A false positive immunologic pregnancy test with tubo-ovarian abscess. Am J Clin Pathol 58:314, 1972

Derman R, et al.: Early diagnosis of pregnancy. J. Reprod Med 26:149, 1981

Gailani S, et al.: HCG in non-trophoblastic neoplasms. Cancer 38:1684, 1976

Hogan W, Price J: Proteinuria as a cause of false positive results in pregnancy tests. Obstet Gynecol 29:585, 1967

Marshall J, et al.: Plasma and urinary chorionic gonadotropin during early human pregnancy. Obstet Gynecol 32:760, 1968

Ravel R, et al.: Effects of certain psychotropic drugs on immunologic pregnancy tests. Am J Obstet Gynecol 105:1222, 1969

5

Maternal Adaptations to Pregnancy

Jeffrey W. Ellis, M.D.

PRACTICE PRINCIPLES

Numerous anatomic and physiologic changes occur in the mother in response to the developing conceptus. Many of these changes would be considered pathologic in the absence of pregnancy. A thorough knowledge of these normal changes is necessary when evaluating possible maternal diseases.

REPRODUCTIVE SYSTEM

A. *Uterine corpus*
  1. *Anatomic changes*
     a) *Intrauterine capacity.* Increased 500 to 1000 times at term
     b) *Weight.* Increased from 70 to 1000 gm at term due to hypertrophy of myometrial fibers
     c) *Blood vessels.* Increased diameter of arteries and veins
     d) *Blood supply.* Progressively increases to 10 percent of cardiac output at term
     e) *Lymphatics.* Increase in size
     f) *Nerve supply.* Increased fiber size; 50 percent size increase in the cervical ganglia

2. *Functional changes*

    Contractility: painless, irregular contractions occur during the first trimester, continuing until the onset of labor (Braxton-Hicks contractions)

B. *Cervix*

  1. *Anatomic changes*

    a) *Size.* Increased due to edema, increased vascularity, and hypertrophy of endocervical glands

    b) *Blood supply.* Progressive increase leading to bluish color and softening

  2. *Functional changes. Mucus secretion* increased due to hypertrophy and hyperplasia of endocervical glands

C. *Vagina*

  1. *Anatomic changes*

    a) *Size (capacity).* Increased due to relaxation of connective tissue support and hypertrophy of smooth muscle cells

    b) *Mucosa.* Increased thickness with hypertrophy of papillae

    c) *Blood supply.* Increased leading to bluish color

  2. *Functional changes. Mucus secretion.* Increased, probably due to increased vascularity

D. *Vulva*

  1. *Anatomic changes*

    a) Increased *pigmentation*

    b) *Relaxation* of support

    c) *Varicosities* may develop as a result of venous compression by the enlarging uterus

E. *Ovaries*

  1. *Anatomic changes*

    a) Increased vascularity

    b) Decidual reaction may occur on the surface

    c) The corpus luteum of pregnancy reaches a maximum size 60 to 70 days after ovulation, then begins to regress until nearly total obliteration occurs at midgestation. Progesterone production parallels size changes

  2. *Functional changes*

    a) Ovulation ceases due to low levels of FSH and LH

   b) Lack of follicle maturation leads to low levels of
      estrogen and progesterone excretion
F. *Fallopian tubes*
   1. *Anatomic changes*
      a) Flattening of epithclium
      b) Irregular areas of decidual reaction
      c) Increased vascularity
   2. *Functional changes.* Normal peristaltic activity stops due
      to high levels of progesterone

ABDOMINAL WALL AND SKIN

Anatomic Changes	Etiology
1. *Striae* over abdomen, breasts, thighs	Stretching of underlying connective tissue; possibly a direct estrogen or cortisol effect
2. *Diastasis recti,* a separation of the rectus muscles	Increased intraabdominal volume
3. *Linea nigra,* increased pigmentation in abdominal midline	Increased MSH or ACTH (a direct estrogen effect?)
4. *Chloasma,* irregular facial pigmentation	Increased MSH or ACTH? (a direct estrogen effect?)
5. *Vascular spiders*	A direct estrogen effect?
6. *Palmar erythema*	A direct estrogen effect?

Functional Changes	Etiology
Increased activity of sweat and sebaceous glands	Elevated androgens

BREASTS

Anatomic Changes	Etiology
1. *Size* increased	Estrogen and progesterone stimulate acinar and ductal growth

Anatomic Changes

Etiology

2. *Nipples and areolae* enlarge

3. *Nipples and areolae* darken

A direct estrogen effect

Increased MSH or ACTH?; A direct estrogen effect?

4. *Blood supply* increases

5. *Montgomery's follicles* prominent (hypertrophic sebaceous glands)

Unknown

Functional Changes

Colostrum secreted after the second month of gestation

Combined effect of estrogen, prolactin, insulin, and thyroid hormones

HEMATOLOGIC SYSTEM

Blood Component Changes

Etiology

1. *Red blood cell mass* increased about 33 percent at term

Erythropoietin increased, erythroid hyperplasia

2. *Reticulocytes* slightly increased

Erythropoietin increased, erythroid hyperplasia

3. *White blood cell count* slightly increased (range 5000–12,000 mm^3)

Unknown

4. *Total plasma volume* increased 40 to 50 percent; maximum at 36 weeks, then slightly declines to term

5. *Total blood volume* increased 40 to 50 percent at term

Increased plasma and red blood cell volume

6. *Hematocrit* decreased up to 7 percent, *hemoglobin* concentration decreased up to 1.5 gm/100 ml

Increase in plasma volume is greater than the increase in RBC volume

7. *Sedimentation rate* increased up to 40 mm/hour

Hemodilution; increased fibrinogen

Coagulation System Changes	Etiology
1. *Factors II, VII, VIII, IX, X* increased; *fibrinogen* increased 50 percent	Increased liver production
2. *Factors XI, XIII,* decreased	Hemodilution
3. *Prothrombin time (PT)* shortened slightly; *partial thromboplastic time* shortened slightly	Increased coagulation factors
4. *Platelet count* unchanged	Unknown
5. *Plasminogen* increased with no evidence of increased fibrinolytic activity	Unknown

CARDIOVASCULAR SYSTEM

Anatomic Changes	Etiology	Result
1. Heart displaced upward and to the left	Enlarging uterus	a. PMI moves laterally b. *Apparent* cardiomegaly on chest x-ray c. Left axis deviation on ECG
2. Cardiac dilatation of 10 to 15 percent	Increased filling	Slight cardiomegaly

Functional Changes	Etiology
1. *Pulse* increased 10 to 15 beats/minute	Baroceptor effect
2. *Stroke volume* increased 20 to 40 percent	Starling effect
3. *Cardiac output* increased 30 percent beginning at 12	Starling effect

Functional Changes	**Etiology**
weeks, reaching plateau at 30 weeks	
4. *Blood pressure* unchanged in first and third trimesters	
5. *Blood pressure* decreased in second trimester	Decreased peripheral vascular resistance
6. *Femoral venous pressure* increased	Inferior vena cava (IVC) compression

Additional Changes in Physical Examination	**Etiology**
1. Split first heart sound (S_1) present	Unknown
2. Third heart sound (S_3) occasionally present	Unknown
3. Systolic ejection murmur at second left intercostal space in 95 percent of patients	Increased flow through pulmonic valve; increased compliance at pulmonary outflow tract producing turbulence

RESPIRATORY SYSTEM

Anatomic Changes	**Etiology**
1. Elevation of diaphragms	Enlarging uterus
2. Thoracic cage circumference increased 5 to 10 cm	Relaxation of ligamentous supports of ribs
3. Engorgement of mucous membranes of sinuses and nasopharynx	Increased vascularity

Functional Changes	**Etiology**
1. *Respiratory rate* increased 2 to 4 respirations/minute	Stimulation of CNS respiratory center by progesterone
2. *Tidal volume* increased 40 percent	
3. *Minute volume* increased 40 percent	

Functional Changes	Etiology
4. *Functional residual capacity* decreased 20 percent	Elevation of diaphragms
5. *Vital capacity* unchanged	
6. *Compliance unchanged*	
7. *Total pulmonary resistance* decreased	Progesterone decreases bronchomotor tone?
8. P_{CO_2} decreased P_{O_2} unchanged	Increased ventilation
9. Effective alveolar ventilation increased 70 percent	

ALIMENTARY SYSTEM

Anatomic Changes	Etiology	Result
1. *Stomach* displaced upward	Enlarging uterus	Esophageal reflux
2. *Appendix* displaced upward towards right upper quandrant	Enlarging uterus	Acute appendicitis may present with pain above usual location
3. *Hemorrhoids* develop	Enlarging uterus compresses venous return	Rectal pain; bleeding
4. *Gingival* swelling	Increased vascularity	Gingival bleeding

Functional Changes	Etiology	Result
1. *Gastric emptying* decreased	Progesterone relaxes smooth muscle	Reflux, belching, bloating
2. *Intestinal motility* decreased	Progesterone relaxes smooth muscle	Bloating, constipation

Functional Changes	Etiology	Result
3. *Gastric hypochlorhydria*	Unknown	Decreased absorption of certain substances
4. *Salivary secretions* increased (ptyalism)	Unknown	

HEPATIC SYSTEM

Anatomic changes · · · · · · · · · · · · None

Functional Changes	Etiology
1. *Alkaline phosphates* increased 50 percent	Placenta produces heat-stable alkaline phosphatase; heat-labile liver alkaline phosphatase unchanged
2. *Serum albumin* decreased 25 percent to 2.5 to 3.0 mg/100 ml	Dilution effect; production unchanged
3. *Globulins* increased	Unknown
4. *Total serum proteins* decreased by 1 gm/100 ml	Dilution effect
5. *Direct bilirubin* may be increased slightly	Cholestasis (progesterone relaxes smooth muscle activity of the collecting system)
6. *SGOT and SGPT* unchanged	
7. *Leucine aminopeptidase* increased	Unknown

URINARY SYSTEM

Anatomic changes	Etiology	Result
1. *Bladder capacity* decreased	Compression of bladder by enlarging uterus	Urinary frequency and urgency

Anatomic changes	Etiology	Result
	or by descent of the presenting part of the fetus	
2. *Hydroureter, hydronephrosis*	Compression of ureter by enlarging uterus or by descent of the presenting part of the fetus	Urine stasis may predispose to ascending infection or acute hydronephrotic change

Functional Changes	Etiology
1. *Renal plasma flow* increased 30 to 50 percent	Increased cardiac output
2. *Glomerular filtration rate* increased 30 to 50 percent	Increased cardiac output
3. *Creatinine clearance* increased up to 150 ml/minute	Increased glomerular filtration rate
4. *Blood urea nitrogen (BUN)* decreased to 5 to 10 mg/100 ml	Hemodilution; increased glomerular filtration rate
5. *Glycosuria, aminoaciduria*	Increased glomerular filtration rate; decreased tubular resorption
6. *Urine pH increased*	Increased serum bicarbonate
7. *Renin increased, angiotension increased*	Unknown

ENDOCRINE SYSTEM

A. *Parathyroid*

Anatomic Changes	Etiology
Slight size increase (hyperplasia and hypertrophy)	Increased fetal calcium demands?

Functional Changes

Parathormone increases progressively beginning in midtrimester	Increased fetal calcium demands

B. *Pituitary*

Anatomic Changes **Etiology**

Slight enlargement of anterior lobe	Hypertrophy of acidophilic cells

Functional Changes **Etiology**

1. *FSH and LH* decreased — Negative feedback of elevated estrogen levels
2. *Growth hormone* decreased — Negative feedback of elevated levels of human placental lactogen (HPL)
3. *Prolactin* increased — Estrogen effect
4. *ACTH* unchanged
5. *TSH* unchanged

C. *Thyroid*

Anatomic Changes **Etiology**

Size increased up to 50 percent	Increased vascularity; glandular hyperplasia; total body iodine decreased due to increased GFR

Functional Changes

1. *Thyroid binding globulin (TBG)* increased 30 percent — Estrogen effect
2. *Total thyroxin (T_4)* increased 10 to 15 percent — Increased TBG
3. *T_3 uptake* decreased 30 percent — Increased TBG

Functional Changes

4. *Unbound (free) thyroxin* unchanged	Increased TBG
5. *Protein-bound iodine* increased	Increased TBG
6. *Basal metabolic rate* increased to +15 to +25 percent	Oxygen consumption of fetus

D. *Adrenal*

Anatomic Changes	**Etiology**
Slight enlargement of cortex	Hypertrophy of zona fasciculata

Functional Changes	**Etiology**
1. *Transcortin* (cortisol binding protein) increased	Estrogen effect
2. *Plasma cortisol* increased	Increased transcortin
3. *Catecholamines* unchanged	
4. *Aldosterone* increased	Production stimulated by natiuresis caused by progesterone

MUSCULOSKELETAL SYSTEMS

Anatomic changes	Etiology	Result
1. *Lordosis*	Compensation in center of gravity as abdomen enlarges	Backache; calf and thigh pain
2. *Mobility* increased at sacroiliac and sacrococcygeal joints		Low back pain

Anatomic changes	Etiology	Result
3. *Symphysis pubis* separates		Pain over pubis
4. *Demineralization*	Inadequate maternal intake of calcium; increased fetal demand	

GENERAL METABOLIC CHANGES

A. *Water.* No change in metabolism
B. *Protein.* No change in metabolism
C. *Fat.* Factors increased probably secondary to lipolytic effects of HPL.
  1. Total lipids increased 40 to 50 percent
  2. Total serum cholesterol increased 40 percent
  3. Serum phospholipids increased 30 to 40 percent
  4. Free fatty acids increased 50 to 60 percent
D. *Carbohydrates*
  1. *Circulating insulin increased* as a result of hypertrophy of β-cells of islets of Langerhans, HPL-induced gluconeogenesis
  2. *Fasting blood sugar* decreased (upper limit of normal 90 mg%)
E. *Minerals.* No change in metabolism, but increased retention for growth requirements of fetal and maternal tissues
F. *Electrolytes and acid-base* balance

Functional Change	Etiology
1. *Potassium* decreased to 3.0 to 3.5 mEq/liter	Respiratory alkalosis
2. *Sodium* unchanged	
3. *Chloride* unchanged	
4. *Calcium* slightly decreased	Decreased serum albumin
5. *Magnesium* slightly decreased	Decreased serum albumin

Functional Change	Etiology
6. *pH unchanged*	
7. *Bicarbonate* decreased to 22 m moles	Respiratory alkalosis
8. *Serum osmolality* decreased 7 percent	Dilution effect

BIBLIOGRAPHY

General

Hytten FE, Leitch I: The Physiology of Human Pregnancy. Oxford, Blackwell, 1971

Hytten FE, Thomson AM: Maternal physiologic adjustments. In Assali NS (ed): Biology of Gestation, Vol 1. New York, Academic Press, 1968

Endocrine System

Aboul-Khair S, et al.: The physiological changes in thyroid function during pregnancy. Clin Sci 27:195, 1964

Fuchs F, Klopper A: Endocrinology of Pregnancy. London, Harper & Row, 1971

Cardiovascular System

Andros GJ: Blood pressure in normal pregnancy. Am J Obstet Gynecol 50:300, 1945

Canton WL, et al.: Plasma volume and extravascular fluid volume during pregnancy and the puerperium. Am J Obstet Gynecol 57:471, 1949

Lee MM: A study of cardiac output at rest throughout pregnancy. J Obstet Gynecol Br Commonw 74:319, 1967

Little B: Water and electrolyte balance during pregnancy. Anesthesiology 26:400, 1965

Pritchard JA: Changes in blood volume during pregnancy and delivery. Anesthesiology 26:393, 1965

Coagulation

Talbert LM, Langdell RD: Normal values of certain factors in the blood clotting mechanism in pregnancy. Am J Obstet Gynecol 90:44, 1964

Pulmonary System
Gee JB, et al.: Pulmonary mechanics during pregnancy. J. Clin Invest 46:945, 1967

Gastrointestinal System
Gryboski WA, Spiro HM: The effect of pregnancy on gastric secretion. N Engl J Med 225:351, 1958

Urinary System
Sims E, Krantz K: Serial studies of renal function during pregnancy and the puerperium in normal women. J Clin Invest 37:1764, 1958

Cutaneous System
Bean WB: Vascular changes in the skin in pregnancy: vascular spiders and palmar erythema. Surg Gynecol Obstet 88:739, 1949

Wade TR, et al.: Skin changes and diseases associated with pregnancy. Obstet Gynecol 52:233, 1978

6

Prenatal Care
Jeffrey W. Ellis, M.D.

PRACTICE PRINCIPLES
The care of the pregnant patient prior to labor and delivery is aimed at assuring optimum health of the mother and the fetus.

INITIAL OFFICE VISIT
During the first prenatal office visit a detailed past medical history is obtained and a thorough physical examination is performed.

A. *History of present pregnancy*
  1. *Menstrual history.* On the basis of the patient's recent menstrual history, the estimated date of delivery may be calculated. The following data should be obtained.
     a) The date of the beginning of the *last normal menstrual* period. *The "normality" of this period must be carefully ascertained by detailed comparison between the timing, duration, and severity of the last period and those preceding it. Care with this step will greatly*

reduce the most common cause of size-dates disparity: faulty dating because of careless history.

b) The dates of any bleeding episodes *after* the last normal menstrual period.

c) The dates and results of pregnancy tests.

d) Factors that may have affected recent ovulation
   (1) A history of menstrual irregularity suggestive of anovulation
   (2) A history of recent oral contraceptive use
   (3) A history of induced ovulation

2. *Calculation of the estimated date of delivery.* The estimated date of delivery (estimated date of confinement, EDC) may be calculated in the following ways
   a) Add 9 months and 7 days to the first day of the last normal menstrual period.
   b) Add 280 days to the first day of the last normal menstrual period.
   c) Add 267 days to the date of the last ovulation if known.
   d) Use of various "dating nomograms" ("dating wheels") is also common and acceptable.

3. *History of previous pregnancies.* The following information is obtained regarding previous pregnancies
   a) *Dates* of deliveries
   b) *Length* of gestations
   c) *Antepartum complications*
      (1) Diagnosis
      (2) Medications required
      (3) Details of antepartum hospitalizations
   d) *Labor*
      (1) Spontaneous or induced
      (2) Length of labors
      (3) Requirement for augmentation with oxytocin
   e) *Intrapartum complications*
      (1) Bleeding
      (2) Elevated blood pressure
      (3) Seizure

         (4) Protracted labor
         (5) Fetal heart rate abnormality
    f) *Delivery*
         (1) Method of delivery
             (a) Spontaneous
             (b) Forceps—low, mid, high
             (c) Vacuum extraction
             (d) Cesarean section (lower segment or classical)
             (e) Version or extraction
         (2) Fetal presentation
         (3) Lacerations
         (4) Anesthesia
         (5) Episotomy
    g) *Condition of infant*
         (1) Weight
         (2) Sex
         (3) Condition at birth (Apgar score)
         (4) Neonatal complications
         (5) Present health
    h) *Postpartum complications*
         (1) Infection
         (2) Bleeding
         (3) Elevated blood pressure
         (4) Seizure

4. *Past medical history*
5. *Past surgical history*
6. *Social history* — The general outline discussed in Chapter 2 should be followed.
7. *Family history*
8. *Review of systems*
9. *Current medications.* Obtain details regarding names of drugs, dosage, length of use, and indications for use. Include nonprescription drugs.
10. *Current symptoms.* The patient should be allowed to relate any physical or psychologic problems. The patient should be specifically questioned regarding the following symptoms.

a) Nausea and vomiting
b) Headache
c) Edema
d) Abdominal pain
e) Bleeding
f) Discharge
g) Urinary symptoms

B. *Physical examination.* A thorough general physical examination should be performed with specific documentation of the following.

1. *Height of the uterine fundus.* Measured with a centimeter tape from the top of the symphysis pubis to the top of the fundus
2. Identification of the fetal lie and presentation
3. *Auscultation of fetal heart tones.* Usually with a Doppler device before 18 weeks gestation and with the stethoscope (fetoscope) after 18 weeks gestation
4. *Clinical pelvimetry*
5. *Identification of any specific abnormalities of the pelvic organs*

C. *Routine laboratory studies on all patients*

1. Complete blood count (CBC) with red blood cells indices
2. Urinalysis
3. Serologic screening for syphilis (RPR, VDRL)
4. ABO blood type, RH factor, indirect Coombs test
5. Rubella titer
6. Pap smear
7. Cervical culture for gonorrhea
8. Qualatitive hemoglobin determination (sickledex) in black patients
9. A postprandial blood glucose, usually the one-hour value

D. *Additional Laboratory Studies.* The following laboratory studies are indicated on the basis of abnormal routine studies, abnormal physical examination, significant past history, significant family history, and current symptoms.

Abnormal Screening Studies	Evaluation
1. *Hemoglobin concentration less than 10 gm/100 ml*	Serum iron, total iron binding capacity (TIBC), serum folate, hemoglobin electrophoresis, stool guaiac
2. *Bactiuria*	Urine culture
3. *Hematuria*	Urine culture, microscopic examination of urine sediment
4. *Glycosuria*	Oral glucose tolerance test
5. *Proteinuria*	Twenty-four-hour urine for total protein; microscopic examination of urine sediment
6. *Positive RPR or VDRL*	Fluorescent treponemal antibody (FTA), Dark-field examination of lesions
7. *Positive indirect Coombs test*	Antibody identification, antibody titer
8. *Abnormal Pap smear*	Identify and treat cervicitis; repeat Pap; colposcopy if abnormalities persist
9. *Hemoglobin other than AA*	Quantitative hemoglobin electrophoresis

Abnormal Physical Examination	Evaluation
1. *Enlarged thyroid, tachycardia*	T_4, T_3 resin uptake, T_7
2. *Diastolic murmur*	ECG, echocardiogram, chest x-ray
3. *Irregular pulse*	ECG
4. *Other appropriate laboratory testing as indicated*	

Family History	Evaluation
1. *Diabetes*	Oral glucose tolerance test
2. *Congenital anomalies*	Consider amniocentesis with chromosome and biochemical

Family History   **Evaluation**
                            studies if appropriate, ul-
                            trasound
3. *Multiple gestation*   Ultrasound of abdomen if a
                            uterine size-date discrepancy
                            develops, HPL

4. *Other appropriate labora-*
   tory testing as indicated

Past History   **Evaluation**
1. *Seizure disorder*   Electroencephalogram (EEG)
2. *Diabetes*   Oral glucose tolerance test
3. *Cardiac Disease*   Chest x-ray, ECG, echocar-
                            diogram
4. *Pulmonary Disease*   Chest x-ray, TB skin test,
                            sputum culture and stain
5. *Hepatic disease*   Bilirubin (direct, indirect),
                            SGOT, SGPT, alkaline phos-
                            phatase, hepatitis antigen
6. *Urinary tract infection* Urine culture and sensitivity
7. *Unexplained intrauterine* Oral glucose tolerance test
   demise, recurrent spontane-
   ous abortion, previous in-
   fant greater than 4000 gm
8. *Infant with congenital* Amniocentesis, ultrasound,
   anomaly   TORCH viral titers; refer for
                            genetic counseling

E. *Medications.* In view of the increased requirements for
   vitamins and certain minerals during pregnancy, patients
   should receive oral iron and multivitamin-mineral sup-
   plements.
   1. *Iron.* One to three 325-mg tablets of *ferrous sulfate* per
      day after meals depending on the patient's hemoglobin
      concentration. If gastric intolerance develops with fer-
      rous sulfate, *ferrous gluconate* may be used in the same
      dosage. The patient should be instructed that mild
      constipation may develop and the stools will become dark

green to black in color. Parenteral iron may be necessary if the patient is unable to tolerate oral preparations.

2. *Multivitamin-mineral* preparations should be given once a day. Folic acid is given only if a specific deficiency is identified.

3. *Additional medications* (see *Current symptoms*).

4. All other prescribed medications should be reviewed for possible adverse effects on the fetus.

5. The patient should report to the physician before any non-prescription, over-the-counter drugs are used.

F. *Counseling and patient education.* During the first prenatal visit, the patient should be counseled in the following areas. Prenatal booklets and audiovisual aids are also helpful to the new patient. The patient and father should be encouraged to attend organized prenatal classes or prepared childbirth classes.

1. *Diet.* The increased nutritional requirements of pregnancy are usually met with a well-balanced diet of approximately 2000 to 2500 calories per day. The specific caloric requirement is calculated as 30 calories per kilogram of body weight plus 300 calories. The diet should include at least 60 to 80 gm of protein per day. Specific daily requirements of other required dietary components may be found in most obstetric textbooks.

2. *Weight gain.* The optimal weight gain during pregnancy with a single fetus is approximately 24 to 30 pounds. The usual distribution is: first trimester, 2 pounds; second trimester, 11 to 12 pounds, third trimester, 11 to 12 pounds. A total weight gain of less than 15 pounds may be associated with intrauterine fetal growth retardation. Excessive weight gain of over 40 pounds will *in itself* have no significant affect on the pregnancy.

3. *Activity.* Normal activity and exercise should be encouraged throughout pregnancy, unless contraindicated by complications.

a) *Exercise.* Contact sports and activities that may result in abdominal injury should be avoided. Swimming, bicycling, tennis, etc., are permitted.

b) *Occupational activities.* Most patients may be allowed to continue work to the end of pregnancy. The patient should not be allowed to work in a setting associated with strenuous physical activity, chemical hazards, radiation hazards, or potential for abdominal injury.

4. *Hygiene*
   a) *Tub baths and showers* are permitted.
   b) *Douching* should normally not be performed. In cases where douching is prescribed as an adjunct to the treatment of vaginal discharge, the fluid should not be allowed to enter the vagina under high pressure.
   c) *Dental care* may be undertaken at any time.

5. *Clothing.* Comfortable, nonconstricting clothing should be worn. As the breasts enlarge, most patients will be comfortable with a well-supporting brassiere. Clothing that constricts the lower extremities and inhibits venous return should be avoided.

6. *Travel.* No restrictions should be placed on travel until the last month of pregnancy when labor may be likely. When traveling, the patient should remain close to competent obstetric care.

7. *Smoking, alcohol, and drug use.* Patients should be counseled regarding the potential affects of tobacco, alcohol, and drugs.

8. *Sexual intercourse.* Normally, sexual intercourse is permitted throughout pregnancy. It should be prohibited in cases of placenta previa, threatened abortion, ruptured membranes, and premature labor.

9. *Antepartum complications.* The patient should be instructed to immediately report the following symptoms:

   • Bleeding
   • Ruptured membranes
   • Severe continuous headaches
   • Abdominal pain

- Visual disturbances
- Fever or chills
- Recurrent vomiting
- Edema of the face or hands
- Significant decrease in fetal movement

10. *Hospital entry*. Signs of labor and ruptured membranes should be explained. The patient should be instructed as to the appropriate time to enter the hospital.

   a) *Rupture of membranes*. The patient should report to the hospital immediately if she suspects membrane rupture.

   b) *Labor*. Unless a rapid delivery is suspected, the patient with a term gestation should enter the hospital when contractions are six to eight minutes apart, having been present for at least one hour. In the following circumstances, the patient should report to the hospital *immediately* if contractions begin:

      (1) Gestation less than 37 weeks
      (2) Multiple gestation
      (3) Abnormal presentation: breech, transverse lie
      (4) A cerclage suture in place

   c) *Location of obstetric department*. The patient should be given clear instructions about the location of the labor and delivery area. A tour of the obstetric department should be given prior to labor.

11. *Physician contact*. The patient should be provided with telephone numbers to reach the physician or the hospital 24 hours per day.

FOLLOWUP OFFICE VISITS

A. *Schedule* of appointments
   1. *Normal pregnancy*
      Up to 28 weeks gestation—every 4 weeks
      28 to 36 weeks gestation—every 2 weeks
      36 weeks gestation to delivery—every week

    2. *Complicated pregnancy*
       As needed for appropriate followup
B. *Evaluation*
    1. *Complaints.* Inquire if any problems have developed
    2. *Patient observations*
       a) Note the date that fetal movements were first felt by
         the patient (quickening)
       b) Note the patient's perception of the frequency of fetal
         activity
    3. *Physical examination*
       a) Weight
       b) Blood pressure
       c) Fundal height
       d) Fetal heart rate
       e) Fetal lie
       f) A vaginal examination may be performed weekly
         beginning at the 36th week to determine cervical
         dilatation and effacement, station and presenting
         part. The cervix, vagina, and vulva should be ex-
         amined for evidence of herpes.
    4. *Laboratory studies*
       a) Urine for protein and glucose at each visit
       b) CBC once during each trimester
       c) For all patients, repeat indirect Coombs test at the
         28th and 36th week
       d) Cervical culture for gonococcus at the 38th week
       e) For patients with a history of genital herpes virus
         infections or in cases of genital lesions suspicious for
         herpes virus, obtain a PAP smear or viral culture of
         the cervix and vagina for identification of intranuclear
         inclusion bodies.
C. *Counseling*
    1. Re-emphasize as necessary the points discussed under
       Counseling and patient education.
    2. Discuss the various types of anesthesia and analgesia and
       note patient choices.

D. *Treatment of Common Disorders*

	Treatment
1. *Headache*	Rule out toxemia, sinusitis, occular disorders *Rx:* Acetaminophen, 650 mg, orally q4h Codeine, 30 mg, orally q4h Neurology consultation if severe and persistent
2. *Heartburn* (reflux esophagitis)	*Rx:* Maalox or Mylanta, 30 cc orally, after meals and at bedtime Avoid the supine position after meals Sleep with the back elevated on pillows
3. *Indigestion*	*Rx:* Maalox or Mylanta, 30 cc orally, after meals and at bedtime Avoid fatty and spicy foods Avoid sodium bicarbonate antacids due to high salt content
4. *Nausea and vomiting*	*Rx:* Bendectin, 2 tablets at bedtime, 1 additional tablet in midafternoon as needed Phenergan rectal suppository, 25 mg 4 times a day Bland diet Frequent small feedings May require hospitalization if severe

5. *Abdominal pain*   Evaluation as indicated
6. *Constipation*   *Rx: Laxatives:* milk of magnesia, metamucil (avoid mineral oil, which may interfere with absorptions of fat-soluble vitamins)
                             Stool softeners: Colace
                             Increase fiber in diet
                             Include laxative fruits in the diet, e.g., prunes
7. *Hemorrhoids*   Treat constipation
                             Administer stool softeners
                             Rx: Tucks, Anusol, Proctofoam
                             Sitz baths
8. *Urinary frequency, urgency, incontinence*   Reassurance (due to compression of bladder); rule out urinary tract infection
9. *Dysuria*   Urine culture; treat after antibiotic sensitivities are obtained
10. *Backache*   *Rx:* acetaminophen, codeine
                             Local heat
                             Massage
                             Avoid heavy lifting and pushing
                             Avoid high-heeled shoes
11. *Varicose veins of lower extremities*   Nonconstricting support stockings
12. *Ptyalism* (excessive salivation)   Reassurance; anticholinergic drugs are usually unsuccessful
13. *Vaginal discharge*   Wetmount examination or culture; treat specific organism
14. *Vulvar varicosities*   T-Binder
15. *Breast tenderness*   Well-supporting brassierre; cold packs, rule out mastitis
16. *Syncope, dizziness*   Usually due to orthostatic hypotension; avoid the supine

position; advise the patient to
stand up or sit up slowly
Rule out cardiac and ear,
nose, and throat (ENT) disorders

BIBLIOGRAPHY

Amstey M, Schwarz R: Immunization during pregnancy. Contemp
Obstet/Gynecol 18:121, 1981

Browne JC, Dixon G: Antepartum Care. London, Churchill Living-
stone, 1978 (a thorough review of all aspects of antepartum care)

Niswander KR, et al.: Weight gain during pregnancy and prepregnancy
weight. Obstet Gynecol 33:482, 1969

7

Drugs and Toxic Agents in Pregnancy

Sandra A. Carson, M.D.

PRACTICE PRINCIPLES

A pregnant woman in today's rapidly expanding pharmaceutical market inevitably exposes her fetus to one or more drugs. In one study, the average antenatal patient ingested 3.4 drugs during her pregnancy.[1] Fortunately, most drugs exert no harmful effects. A few drugs, however, do affect mother or fetus adversely, and no drugs can be considered absolutely safe. The drugs that alter embryonic development and result in congenital anomalies may be called teratogens. It is the responsibility of the obstetrician-gynecologist to recognize teratogens.

PRINCIPLES OF TERATOLOGY

A. The teratogenic effects of any agent depend on several factors
   1. *The agent itself.* Some agents cause abnormal development in all cases, whereas other agents are less consistently, if at all, teratogenic.
   2. *The pharmacogenetics of mother and fetus.* Not all embryos exposed to a teratogen will be affected. The effect will be influenced by relative rates of absorption,

maternal metabolism, placental transfer, and fetal metabolism.

3. *Exposure during a particular time in gestation.* The time during embryogenesis when cells of a given organ system divide most rapidly is the period of greatest teratogenic susceptibility. Once developed, the system becomes relatively resistant to teratogens. Table 7–1 lists the time in which major organ systems develop.

4. *Dose.* Low doses of teratogens may have no effect;

TABLE 7–1. DEVELOPMENT OF FETAL ORGAN SYSTEMS

Embryonic Age (weeks from conception)	Embryonic Development
1	Implantation. Embryo relatively resistant to teratogenic effects except embryocides.
2–3	Craniofacial development; musculoskeletal and central nervous system differentiation
4	Limb buds; cardiovascular system enlarges
5	Limb buds segment; nose, eyes, ears become prominent
	Urinary system begins to differentiate; gonadal differentiation
6	Fingers and toes formed
7–8	Maxilla fused; eyelids formed
9–10	External and internal genitalia differentiate; most other major organ systems formed. Embryo relatively resistant to teratogens.
11	Genitourinary system complete

intermediate doses cause a specific malformation pattern; high doses may lead to death of the embryo. Moreover, doses required to produce malformation may differ at various times during gestation.

B. *Drugs*

These principles of teratology should be considered whenever assessing potential effects of a drug. Unfortunately, such considerations have not always been raised. Even formal studies often show flaws in experimental design. Not surprisingly, the literature consists of many confusing and incomplete reports condemning certain agents. Often only one or two cases exist to illustrate a teratogenic effect, and negative evidence is unlikely to be reported. Frequently, it is difficult to differentiate an anomaly that occurs as a result of a chronic disease process (e.g., epilepsy) from a result of the drug used to treat that disease (e.g., diphenylhydantoin). Many drugs are used in combination, and their teratogenic effects may be additive and individually indistinguishable (e.g., antineoplastic drugs).

Teratogenicity of an agent is thus difficult to prove or disprove. Decisions based on less than ideal scientific evidence were necessary in order to construct Table 7–2, which lists commonly used drugs and their purported teratogenic effects. Inclusion of a drug in Table 7–2 is somewhat arbitrary and includes agents only in general use. Exclusion of a drug from this list does not confirm its safety. For example, thalidomide, a well-known confirmed teratogen, is not included because of its market unavailability. For each drug, evidence is categorized as *confirmed, strong, suggestive,* or *poor. There are few confirmed teratogens. However, in advising patients it is wise to emphasize that no drug can be verified as absolutely safe to all fetuses. Thus, drugs should be administered only if benefit to mother or fetus outweighs potential risk.* When counseling a patient about the teratogenic risk of drugs, one must also remember the overall incidence of congenital anomalies in an unexposed population is 2 to 3 percent.

TABLE 7-2. TERATOGENIC (T) / NEONATAL (N) EFFECTS OF VARIOUS AGENTS

Agent	Effect	Evidence	Ref.
ANTICOAGULANTS			
Heparin	N: increased intrauterine death	Poor	17
Warfarin	T: nasal hypoplasia, retardation, chondrodysplasia punctata in first trimester; retardation, optic atrophy, microcephaly in second trimester	Confirmed	17,18
		Strong	17
	N: fatal fetal hemorrhage	Confirmed	19
ANTICONVULSANTS			
Diphenylhydantoin	T: digital hypoplasia; nail dysplasia; intrauterine growth retardation; microcephaly, broad, depressed nasal bridge; hernias	Confirmed	20, 21
Magnesium sulfate	N: respiratory and motor depression	Strong	11
Phenobarbital	T: no known effects N: withdrawal not usual at anticonvulsant doses		11

Trimethadione	T: developmental delay; V-shaped eyebrows; epicanthal folds; low set ears; irregular teeth; cardiovascular and visceral anomalies	Confirmed	22, 23
ANTIEMETICS			
Chlorpromazine	N: repiratory depression	Suggestive	12, 24
Doxylamine dicyclomine	T, N: no known effects		25, 26
Meclizine	T, N: no known effects		27
Meclizine and pyridoxine (Benedictin)	T, N: no known effects		26
Prochlorperazine	T, N: no known effects		27
ANTIHYPERTENSIVES			
α-Methyldopa	T, N: no known effects	Confirmed	111
Hexamethonium	N: fetal ganglionic blockade resulting in paralytic ileus		28
Hydralazine	T, N: no known effects in humans T: possible skeletal defects in animals		29
Propranolol	N: hypoglycemia, bradycardia T: intrauterine growth retardation	Suggestive Poor	30 31

(Continued)

TABLE 7-2. TERATOGENIC (T) / NEONATAL (N) EFFECTS OF VARIOUS AGENTS (Cont.)

Agent	Effect	Evidence	Ref.
ANTIHYPERTENSIVES (CONT.)			
Reserpine	N: nasal discharge T: no known effects	Confirmed	32
ANTIMICROBIALS			
Cephalosporins	T, N: no known effects		12
Chloramphenicol	T: no known effects N: bone marrow depression; abdominal distention; cyanosis; vascular collapse (gray baby syndrome)	Confirmed Confirmed	11
Chloroquine	T: sensineural deafness in two case reports	Poor	33
Eyrthromycin	T, N: no known effects		111
Ethambutol	T, N: no known effects		34, 35
Ethionamide	T: CNS defects	Strong	36
Gentamicin	T, N: no known effects		111
Isoniazid	T, N: no known effects		37
Kanamycin	T: hearing deficit	Suggestive	38

Lincomycin	T, N: no known effects		10
Metronidazole	T, N: no known effects in humans T: mutagenic in bacteria	Poor	12, 39, 40 111
Neomycin	T, N: no known effects		11
Nitrofurantoin	N: hemolytic anemia in G–6–PD–deficient fetus	Confirmed	11
Para-aminosalicylic acid (PAS)	T, N: no known effects		37
Penicillin	T, N: no known effects		10, 12
Primaquine	N: hemolytic anemia in G–6–PD–deficient fetus	Confirmed	11
Pyrimethamine	T: cleft lip and cleft palate	Suggestive	12, 41
Quinacrine	T: one case reported of multiple anomalies	Poor	42
Rifampin	T, N: no known effects		34
Streptomycin	T: hearing deficit	Strong	43, 44
Sulfonamides	T: no known effects N: hemolytic anemia in G–6–PD–deficient fetus; displaces bilirubin from albumin binding sites possibly leading to kernicterus	Confirmed Strong	45

(Continued)

TABLE 7-2. TERATOGENIC (T) / NEONATAL (N) EFFECTS OF VARIOUS AGENTS (Cont.)

Agent	Effect	Evidence	Ref.
ANTIMICROBIALS (CONT.)			
Tetracycline	T: incorporated in deciduous teeth and bones in 2nd–5th months of gestation.	Confirmed	46
Tobramycin	T, N: no known effects		12
Trimethoprin and sulfamethoxazole	T: limb defects, cleft palate and microagnathia in rats	Poor	12,47
ANTINEOPLASTICS			
Actinomycin-D	T: cranial anomalies in rats	Suggestive	12
Aminopterin	T: triangular facies; intrauterine growth retardation; arched palate; abortifacient		48, 49, 50
Azathioprine	T: adrenal insufficiency; intrauterine growth retardation; leukopenia	Poor	12, 51
Busulfan	T: intrauterine growth retardation; gonadal dysgenesis; various malformations	Strong	52, 53
Chlorambucil	T: one reported case of unilateral renal agenesis	Poor	54

84

Cyclophosphamide	T: limb defects; craniofacial anomalies; germ cell aplasia	Confirmed	55, 56
5–Fluorouracil	T: radial aplasia, absent digits, hypoplastic aorta, gastrointestinal aplasias, urinary tract dysplasia in one case report	Poor	57
6–Mercaptopurine	T, N: no known effects		24
Methotrexate	T: skeletal defects	Confirmed	58
Nitrogen mustard	N: intrauterine death T: spontaneous abortion	Suggestive Suggestive	59, 60
Procarbazine	T: possible renal anomalies	Poor	61, 62
Triethylenemelamine	T, N: no known effects		63
Thio-TEPA	T: growth retardation and skeletal defects in rats T, N: no known effect in humans		12 63
Vinblastine Vincristine	T, N: no known effects in humans; ocular and facial anomalies in rats		64, 65

(Continued)

TABLE 7-2. TERATOGENIC (T) / NEONATAL (N) EFFECTS OF VARIOUS AGENTS (Cont.)

Agent	Effect	Evidence	Ref.
DIURETICS			
Furosemide	T, N: no known effects		
Spironolactone	T, N: no known effects		12
Thiazides	N: Thrombocytopenia	Confirmed	66
ENVIRONMENTAL AGENTS			
Chlorobiphenyls	T: dark brown skin stains, intrauterine growth retardation	Strong	67
Mercury (organic)	T: cerebral palsy; chorea; ataxia, seizures, mental retardation, blindness	Confirmed	68
Naphthalene (moth balls)	T: hemolytic anemia in G–6–PD–deficient fetus	Confirmed	69
HORMONES AND ANTAGONISTS			
Androgens	T: masculinization of female fetus; little effect in male fetus	Confirmed	10
Bromocryptine	T, N: no known effects		
Clomiphene citrate	T: aneuploidy; neural tube defects	Poor	71, 72

Corticosteroids	T: no known effects in humans; cleft palate in rodents	Strong	73, 74
	N: acute adrenal insufficiency		
Cyproterone acetate	T: feminization of male fetus	Strong	75
Diethylstilbesterol (DES)	T: anomalies of the genital tract—vaginal adenosis and adenocarcinoma in females; epididymal cysts, hypotrophic testes, abnormal semen analysis in males	Strong	76, 77
Estrogens (other than DES)	T: no known effects in humans; feminization of male rats		78
Human menopausal gonadotropin (Pergonal)	T: aneuploidy	Poor	79
Iodine—131 Millicurie dose	T: cretinism	Confirmed	12
Microcurie dose	T: no known effect		
Iodides (inorganic)	T: fetal goiter; cretinism	Confirmed	80

(Continued)

TABLE 7–2. TERATOGENIC (T) / NEONATAL (N) EFFECTS OF VARIOUS AGENTS (Cont.)

Agent	Effect	Evidence	Ref.
HORMONES AND ANTAGONISTS (CONT.)			
Insulin (and oral hypoglycemics)	T: unable to differentiate teratogenic effects from those related to diabetes mellitus		
Methimazole	T: ulcerlike midline scalp defect	Suggestive	81
Oxytocin	N: hyperbilirubinemia	Suggestive	82
Progestins	T: masculinization of female fetus (large doses of 19-nor derivatives except norethyndrel)	Confirmed	83, 84, 85
	N: vertebral, anal, tracheo-esophageal, renal, limb, cardio-vascular anomalies	Suggestive	86, 87
Thiourea agents (other than methimazole)	T: hypothyroidism; compensatory hypertrophic goiter; no cretinism	Confirmed	88
Thyroid hormone	T, N: no known effects		

PSYCHOTROPIC DRUGS

Drug		Confidence	Reference
Alcohol	T: intrauterine growth retardation; ocular, joint, and cardiac anomalies (strongly dose related) N: alcohol withdrawal	Confirmed	89, 90
Amphetamines	T: biliary atresia, Oral clefts	Poor Poor	91 92
Chlordiazepoxide	T: sporadic cases with no pattern of anomalies	Poor	27, 93
Diazepam	T: cleft lip; cleft palate	Strong	13, 94
Haloperidol	T: two case reports of limb malformations	Poor	95
Lithium	T: Ebstein's anomaly and other cardiovascular defects	Suggestive	96
Lysergic acid diethylamide (LSD)	T: limb bud defects; nervous system anomalies	Suggestive	97
Marijuana	T: sporadic cases with no pattern of anomalies	Poor	12
Meprobamate	T: sporadic cases with no pattern of anomalies	Poor	27

(Continued)

TABLE 7–2. TERATOGENIC (T) / NEONATAL (N) EFFECTS OF VARIOUS AGENTS (Cont.)

Agent	Effect	Evidence	Ref.
PSYCHOTROPIC DRUGS (CONT.)			
Narcotic addiction	T: intrauterine growth retardation	Strong	11
	N: withdrawal; premature labor	Confirmed	
Phenothiazines	T: cardiovascular anomalies	Poor	98
Tricyclic anti-depressants	T: no known effects		99
VAGINAL PREPARATIONS			
Miconazole	T: no known effects		12
Nonoxynol–9	T: no known effects		10
Providine-iodine	T, N: iodine may be absorbed (see iodides)		
Podophyllum	T: peripheral neuropathy if absorbed	Suggestive	
Triple sulfa cream	T, N: drug may be absorbed (see sulfonamides)		

MISCELLANEOUS

Aminophylline	T, N: no known effects		10
Caffeine	T, N.: no known effects		111
Dextromethorphan	T, N: no known effects		10
Digitalis	T, N: no known effects		100
D-Penicillinase	T: generalized connective tissue defects	Suggestive	101, 102
Diphenhydramine	T: cleft palate	Poor	103
Expectorants	T, N: no known effects		10
Lead	T: mental impairment; growth retardation	Suggestive	11
Smoking (nicotine)	T: intrauterine growth retardation N: intrauterine death	Strong	104, 105
Theophylline	T, N: no known effects		10
Vitamin A (pharmacologic doses)	T: CNS, urinary tract, and ocular anomalies	Strong	106, 107, 108
Vitamin D (pharmacologic doses)	N: infantile hypercalcemia T: supravalvular aortic stenosis	Strong	109

C. *Physical Agents*

  1. Physical agents can also be teratogenic. Such agents include radiation, ultrasound, hyperthermia, and microwaves. Exposure may occur in the home, workplace, medical or dental facility, or in the general environment. Effects on the fetus vary with dose, exposure rate, and stage of gestation, in accordance with principles of teratology noted above. Microwave, hyperthermia, and ultrasound have not been shown to exert deleterious effects in humans at doses normally incurred.[4,5] However, ionizing radiation is a well-established cause of congenital anomalies in humans.

  2. The average American citizen receives 125 mrads per year of "background" radiation and another 55 mrads from medical x-rays.[4] Only if exposures are much higher does the potential for teratogenic effect exist. In addition to dose, several major considerations are apparent.

    a) *Ionizing radiation* early in gestation (one or two weeks after conception) usually results in an "all-or-none" phenomenon, i.e., the embryo is either killed or the radiation damage is corrected by cell repair. During this stage the embryo consists of undifferentiated cells, all of which have the potential of developing into many different organ systems.

    b) Exposure during the 3rd to 10th embryonic weeks, the period of major organogenesis, may result in gross malformations.

    c) The central nervous system is particularly sensitive throughout the first trimester, because radiation preferentially affects CNS. Claims that malformations of other systems were caused by irradiation can be dismissed if such defects are not accompanied by CNS defect.

    d) The human fetus becomes more resistant to radiation damage each gestational week.

    e) Radiation given over a period of time (chronic) is less likely to produce damage than a comparable dose given acutely.

TABLE 7–3. EFFECTS OF RADIATION

Dose	Effect
Less than 5 rads	No evidence of induced malformations
Greater than 10 rads	Fetus considered at significant risk
Greater than 25 rads	Microcephaly, mental retardation; CNS most sensitive[4]
Greater than 100 rads	Radiation sickness; growth retardation
450 rads	Fifty percent of exposed persons die; survivors may be predisposed to malignancy[110]

f) Fetal germ cell exposure may result in genetic mutations that become manifest only in offspring of the fetus.

g) Radiation exposure may predispose to later development of malignancy,[6] presumably also as result of mutations.

3. It is evident that accurate counseling following exposure during pregnancy requires knowledge of many factors: nature of radiation, dose, exposure time, and, of course, stage of gestation in which exposure occurred. Consultation with a radiation physicist may be necessary to calculate the exact radiation exposure. Table 7–3 summarizes current opinions concerning the relationship of exposure to teratogenic effects.

REFERENCES

1. Forfar J, Nelson M: Epidemiology of drugs taken by pregnant women: drugs that may affect the fetus adversely. Clin Pharmacol Ther 14:633, 1973
2. Simpson JL, Golbus MS, Martin A, Sarto GE: Genetics in Obstetrics and Gynecology. New York, Grune & Stratton, 1982

3. Wilson JG, Fraser FC (eds): Handbook of Teratology. New York, Plenum Press, 1977

4. Brent RL: Radiation and other physical agents. In Wilson JG, Fraser FC (eds): Handbook of Teratology. New York, Plenum Press, 1977, p 153

5. Edwards MJ, Wanner RA: Extremes of temperature. General principles and etiology. In Wilson JN, Fraser FC (eds): Handbook of Teratology. New York, Plenum Press, 1977, p 421

6. United Nations (1977): A report of the United Nation's Scientific Committee on the Effects of Atomic Radiation to the General Assembly, with Annexes. United Nations Publication No. E. 77 IX 1

7. Lewis RB, Schulman JD: Influence of acetylsalicylic acid, an inhibitor of prostaglandin synthesis, on the duration of human gestation and labor. Lancet 2:1159, 1973

8. Bleyer WA, Breckenridge RT: Studies on the detection of adverse drug reactions in the newborn. II. The effect of prenatal aspirin on newborn hemostasis. JAMA 213:2049, 1970

9. Corby DG: Aspirin in pregnancy: malunal and fetal effects. Pediatrics 62:930, 1978

10. Heinonen OP, Slone D, Shapiro S: Birth Defects and Drugs in Pregnancy. Littleton, Mass., Publ. Sciences Group, 1977

11. Stevenson RE: The Fetus and Newly Born Infant, 2nd ed. St. Louis, C.V. Mosby, 1977

12. Shepard TH: Catalog of Teratogenic Agents, 3rd ed. Baltimore, Johns Hopkins University Press, 1980

13. Aarskog D: Association between maternal intake of diazepam and oral clefts. Lancet 2:921, 1975

14. Cohen EN, Belville JW, Brown BW: Anesthesia, pregnancy, and miscarriage: a study of operating room nurses and anesthetics. Anesthesiology 35:343, 1971

15. Knill-Jones RP, Rodrigues LV, Moir DD, Spence AA: Anesthetic practice and pregnancy. Lancet 1:1326, 1972

16. Basford, AB, Fink BR: The teratogenicity of halothane in the rat. Anesthesiology 29:1167, 1968

17. Hall JG, Pauli RM, Wilson KM: Maternal and fetal sequelae of anticoagulation during pregnancy. Am J Med 68:122, 1980

18. Holzgreve W, Cary JC, Hall BD: Warfarin-induced fetal abnormalities. Lancet 2:914, 1976

19. Von Sydow G: Hypoprothrombinemia and cerebral injury in a newborn infant after dicoumarin treatment of the mother. Nord Med 34:1171, 1947

20. Barr M Jr, Poznanski AK, Schmickel RD: Digital hypoplasia and anticonvulsants during gestation: a teratogenic syndrome? J Pediatr 84:254, 1974
21. Hanson JW, Smith DW: The fetal hydantoin syndrome. J Pediatr 87:285, 1975
22. Zackai EH, Mellman WJ, Neiderer B, Hanson JW: The fetal trimethadione syndrome. J Pediatr 87:280, 1975
23. Feldman GL, Weaver DD, Lovrien EW: The fetal trimethadione syndrome. The American Society of Human Genetics 28th Annual Meeting, Program and Abstracts, San Diego, California, 1977, 41A
24. Sokal JE, Lessmans EM: Effects of cancer chemotherapeutic agents on the human fetus. JAMA 172:1765, 1960
25. Shapiro S, Heinonen OP, Siskind V, et al.: Antenatal exposure to doxylamine succinate and dicyclomine hydrochloride (Bendectin) in relation to congenital malformations, perinatal mortality rate, birth weight, and intelligence quotient score. Am J Obstet Gynecol 128:480, 1977
26. Smithells RW, Sheppard S: Teratogenicity testing in humans: a method demonstrating safety of Bendectin. Teratology 17:31, 1976
27. Milkovich L, Van Den Berg BJ: Effects of prenatal meprobamate and chlordiazepoxide hydrochloride on human embryonic and fetal development. N Engl J Med 291:1268, 1974
28. Morris N: Hexamethonium compounds in the treatment of preeclampsia and essential hypertension during pregnancy. Lancet 1:322, 1953
29. Rapalea RS, Parr RN, Lin TZ, Bhatnagam RS: Biochemical basis of skeletal defects induced by hydralazine. Teratology 15:185, 1977
30. Habib A, McCarthy JS: Effects on the neonate of propranolol administered during pregnancy. J Pediatr 91:808, 1977
31. Gladstone GC, Hordof A, Gersony WM: Propranolol administration during pregnancy; effects on the fetus. J Pediatr 86:962, 1974
32. Desmond MM, Rogers SF, Lindley JE, Moyer JH: Management of toxemia of pregnancy wth reserpine. Obstet Gynecol 10:140, 1957
33. Hart CW, Nauton RF: The ototoxiation of chloroquine phosphate. Arch Otolaryngol 80:407, 1964
34. Jentgens H: Antituberculise chemotherapre and Schwagerschaftsabbusch. Prax Pneumol 27:479, 1973
35. Bobrowitz ID: Ethambutol in pregnancy. Chest 66:20, 1974
36. Potwprpwslo M, Sianozecka E, Szufladowicz R: Ethionamide treatment and pregnancy. Pol Med J 5:1152, 1966
37. Marynowski A, Sianoazecka E: Comparison of the incidence of

congenital malformations in neonates from healthy mothers and from patients treated for tuberculosis. Ginekol Pol 43:713, 1972

38. Fujimori H: Influence of kanamycin on hearing acuity in the neonate and suckling. Presented at the 10th Anniversary of the Kanamycin Conference, Tokyo, 1967

39. Legator MS, Gonner TH, Stoeckel M: Detection of mutagenic activity of metronidazole and niradazole in body fluids of humans and mice. Science 188:1118, 1975

40. Peterson F: Mecloizine and congenital abnormalities. Lancet 1:675, 1964

41. Sullivan GE, Takacs E: Comparative teratogenicity of pyrimethamine in rats and hamsters. Teratology 4:205, 1971

42. Vevera J, Zatloukal F: Pfipad urozenych malformaet zpusobenyck pravdepodobne atetrinem, podavan-ym uranem tehotenstvi. Cs Pediatr 19:211, 1964

43. Rasmussen F: The oto-toxic effect of streptomycin and dihydrostreptomycin on the foetus. Scand J 43:521, 1974

44. Ganguin G, Rempt E: Streptomycinbehandlung in der Schwangerschaft und ihre Ansirkung auf des Gehor des Kindes. Z Laryngol Rhinol Otol Ihre Grenzgeb 49:496, 1970

45. Richards IDG: A retrospective inquiry into possible teratogenic effects of drugs in pregnancy. In Klingberg MA, Abramovici A, Chenuke J (eds): Drugs and Fetal Development. New York, Plenum Press, 1972, p 441

46. Wallman IS, Hilton HB: Teeth pigmented by tetracycline. Lancet 1:827, 1962

47. Udall V: Toxicology of sulphonamide-trimethoprim combinations. Postgrad Med J 45:42, 1969

48. Thiersch JB: Therapeutic abortions with a folic acid antagonist, 4-aminopteroyglutamic acid (4-amino P.G.A.) administered by the oral route. Am J Obstet Gynecol 63:1298, 1952

49. Thiersch JB: The control of reproduction in rats with the aid of antimetabolites. Early experience with antimetabolites as abortifacient agents in man. Acta Endocrinol (Suppl) 28:37, 1956

50. Goetsch C: An evaluation of aminopterin as an abortifacient. Am J Obstet Gynecol 83:1474, 1962

51. Nolan GH, et al.: Renal cadaver transplantation followed by successful pregnancies. Obstet Gynecol 43:732, 1974

52. Diamond I, Anderson MM, McCreadie SR: Transplacental transmission of busulfan (myleran) in a mother with leukemia. Pediatrics 25:85, 1960

53. De Rezende J, Coslovsky S, De Aguiar PB: Leucemia et gravidez. Rev Ginecol Obstet 117:46, 1965
54. Shotton D, Monie IW: Possible teratogenic effect of chlorambucil on a human fetus. JAMA 186:74, 1963
55. Greenberg LH, Tanaka KR: Cogenital anomalies probably induced by cyclophosphamide. JAMA 188:423, 1964
56. Toledo TM, Harper RC, Moses RH: Fetal effects during cyclophosphamide and irradiation therapy. Ann Intern Med 74:87, 1971
57. Stephens JD, et al.: Multiple congenital anomalies in a fetus exposed to 5-fluorouracil during the first trimester. Am J Obstet Gynecol 137:747, 1980
58. Milunsky A, Graef JW, Gaynor MF Jr: Methotrexate-induced congenital malformations, with a review of the literature. J Pediatr 72:790, 1968
59. Nicholson HO: Cytoxic drugs in pregnancy. Review of reported cases. J Obstet Gynecol Br Commonw 75:307, 1968
60. Garrett MJ: Teratogenic effects of combination chemotherapy. Ann Int Med 80:667, 1974
61. Mennuti MT, Sheppard TH, Mellman WJ: Fetal renal malformation following treatment of Hodgkins disease during pregnancy. Obstet Gynecol 46:194, 1975
62. Wells JH, Marshall JR, Carbone PP: Procarbazine therapy for Hodgkins' disease in early pregnancy. JAMA 205:935, 1968
63. Nishimura H, Tanimura T: Information in prenatal hazards of drugs. In Clinical Aspects of the Teratogenicity of Drugs. Amsterdam, Excerpta Medica, 1976, p 106
64. Armstrong JG: Dyke RW, Fonts PJ: Vinblastine sulfate treatment of Hodgkins disease during pregnancy. Science 143:703, 1964
65. Demyer W: Cleft lip and jaw induced in fetal rats by vincristine. Arch Anat 48:181, 1965
66. Rodriguez SU, Leiken SL, Hiller MC: Neonatal thrombocytopenia associated with ante-partum administration of thiazide drugs. N Engl J Med 270:881, 1964
67. Miller RW: Cola-colored babies: chlorobiphenyl poisoning in Japan. Teratology 4:211, 1971
68. Nelson MM, Forfar JO: Association between drugs administered during pregnancy and congenital abnormalities of the fetus. Br Med J 1:523, 1971
69. Anzieulewics JA, Dick HJ, Chairulli EE: Transplacental naphthalene poisoning. Am J Obstet Gynecol 78:518, 1959

70. Grumbach MM, Ducharme Jr: The effects of androgens on fetal sexual development. Fertil Steril 11:157, 1960

71. Asch RH, Greenblatt RB: Update on the safety and efficacy of clomiphene citrate as a therapeutic agent. J Repro Med 17:175, 1976

72. Oakley GP, Flynt JW: Hormonal pregnancy tests and congenital malformations. Lancet 2:256, 1973

73. Bongiovanni AM, McPaddan AJ: Steroids during pregnancy and possible fetal consequences. Fertil Steril 11:181, 1960

74. Serment H, Ruf H: Les dangers pour le product de conception de medicaments admistres a la femme enciente. Bull Fed Soc Gynecol Obstet Lang Fr 20:69, 1968

75. Steinbeck H, Neuman F: Aspects of steroidal influence on fetal development. In Klingberg MA, Abramovici A, Chemke J (eds): Drugs and Fetal Development. New York, Plenum Press, 1972, p 227

76. Herbst AL, Ulfelder H, Poskanzer DC: Adenocarcinoma of the vagina. Association of maternal stilbesterol therapy with tumor appearance in young women. N Engl J Med 284:878, 1971

77. Gill WB, Schumacher GFB, Bibbo M: Pathological semen and anatomical abnormalities of the genital tract in human male subjects exposed to diethylstilbestrol in utero. J Urol 117:477, 1977

78. Greene RR, Burrill MW, Ivy AC: Experimental intersexuality: the effects of estrogens on the antenatal sexual development of the rat. Am J Anat 67:305, 1940

79. Boue J, Boue A, Lazar P: Retrospective and prospective epidemiological studies of 1500 karyotyped spontaneous human abortions. Teratology 12:11, 1975

80. Wolff J: Iodide goiter and the pharmacologic effects of excess iodide. Am J Med 47:101, 1969

81. Milham S Jr, Elledge W: Maternal methimazole and congenital defects in children. Teratology 5:125, 1972

82. Davies DP, et al.: Neonatal jaundice and maternal oxytocin infusion. Br Med J 3:476, 1973

83. Jacobson, BD: Hazards of norethindrone therapy during pregnancy. Am J Obstet Gynecol 84:962, 1962

84. Nora JJ, Nora AH, Perinchief AG, Ingram JW, et al.: Congenital abnormalities and first-trimester exposure to progestaten/oestrogen. Lancet 1:313, 1976

85. Heinonen OP, et al.: Cardiovascular birth defects and antenatal exposure to female sex hormones. N Engl J Med 296:67, 1977

86. Nora JJ, Nora AH: Birth defects and oral contraceptives. Lancet 1:941, 1973

87. Nora AH, Nora JJ: A syndrome of multiple congenital anomalies associated with teratogenic exposure. Arch Environ Health 30:17, 1975

88. Burrow GN, Bartsocas C, Klatskin EH, Grunt JA: Children exposed in utero to propylthiouracil. Am J Dis Child 116:161, 1968.

89. Jones KL, Smith DW, Ulleland CN, Streissguth AP: Pattern of malformation in offspring of chronic alcoholic mothers. Lancet 1:1267, 1973

90. Jones KL, Smith DW, Streissguth AP, Myrianthopolous NC: Outcome in offspring of chronic alcoholic women. Lancet 1:1076, 1974

91. Levin JN: Amphetamine ingestion with biliary atresia. J Pediatr 79:130, 1971

92. Milkovich L, Van Den Berg BJ: Effects of antenatal exposure to anorectic drugs. Am J Obstet 129:637, 1977

93. Hartz SC, Heinonen OP, Shapiro S, Siskind V, Slone D: Antenatal exposure to meprobamate and chlordiagepoxide in relation to malformations, mental development and childhood mortality. N Engl J Med 292:726, 1975

94. Saxen I, Saxen L: Association between maternal intake of diazepam and oral clefts. Lancet 2:498, 1975

95. Kopelman AE, McCullar FW, Heggeness L: Limb malformations following maternal use of haloperidol. JAMA 231:62, 1975

96. Weller RO: Lithium, Ebstein's anomaly, and other congenital heart defects. Lancet 2:594, 1974

97. Jacobson CB, Berlin CM: Possible reproductive detriment in LSD users. JAMA 222:1367, 1972

98. Slone D, Siskind V, Heinonen OP, et al.: Antenatal exposure to the phenothiazines in relation to congenital malformations, perinatal mortality rate, birth weight, and intelligence quotient score. Am J Obstet Gynecol 128:486, 1977

99. Banister P, Dafoe C, Smith ESO, Miller J: Possible teratogenicity of tricyclic antidepressants. Lancet 1:838, 1972

100. Laros RK, Hage ML, Hayashi RH: Pregnancy and heart valve prosthesis. Obstet Gynecol 35:241, 1970

101. Mjolnerod OK, Rasmussen K, Dommerud SA, Gjeruldsen ST: Congenital connective-tissue defect probably due to D-penicillamine treatment in pregnancy. Lancet 1:673, 1971

102. Solomon L, Abrams G, Dinner M, Berman L: Neonatal abnormalities associated with D-penicillamine treatment during pregnancy. N Engl J Med 296:54, 1977

103. Saxen I: Cleft palate and maternal diphenhydramine intake. Lancet 1:407, 1974

104. Simpson WJA: A preliminary report on cigarette smoking and the incidence of prematurity. Am J Obstet Gynecol 73:808, 1957

105. Rush D, Kass EH: Maternal smoking: a reassessment of the association with perinatal mortality. Am J Epidemiol 96:183, 1972

106. Bernhardt IB, Dorsey DJ: Hypervitaminosis A and congenital renal anomalies in a human infant. Obstet Gynecol 43:750, 1974

107. Gal I, Sharman IM, Pryse-Davies J: Vitamin A in relation to human congenital malformations. Adv Teratol 5:143, 1972

108. Lamba PA, Sood NN: Congenital microphthalmus and colobomata in maternal vitamin A deficiency. J Pediatr Ophthalmol 5:115, 1968

109. Friedman WF: Vitamin D and the supravalvular aortic stenosis syndrome. Adv Teratol 3:85, 1968

110. Oppenheim BE, Griem ML, Meier P: The effect of diagnostic x-ray exposure on the human fetus; an examination of the evidence. Radiology 114:529

111. Berkowitz, R, Coustan D, Mochizuki T: Handbook for Prescribing Medications During Pregnancy. Little Brown & Co., Boston, 1981

8

Antenatal Diagnosis

Maureen Bocian, M.D.

PRACTICE PRINCIPLES

The ability to detect severe fetal abnormality in time to allow the
option of selective pregnancy termination is a relatively recent
achievement that has enabled thousands of couples at risk, who
would formerly have been too anxious to attempt or complete a
pregnancy, to have healthy children. Because the great majority
(over 95 percent) of fetuses tested prenatally are normal, it is
important to recognize that prenatal diagnosis, rather than being
an avenue to termination of pregnancy, often allows the birth of
children who might never have been conceived or carried to
term.

In the first obstetrical interview the obstetrician should obtain
a history — including age, race, ethnic background, and previous
genetic conditions in the family — in order to ascertain the need
for counseling and for tests which would be useful in case of
potential genetic disease in the fetus. The investigation of
possible genetic conditions should include questions regarding
congenital abnormalities, mental retardation, unusual health
problems, multiple family members affected with the same or
similar disorders, and a history of two or more first trimester
miscarriages. These questions should concern not only the
patient but also the father of the pregnancy and any other
appropriate family members. If the history is relevant, the
patient must be informed of the recurrence risks and of the

existence and availability of any appropriate tests. This frequently requires consultation with a geneticist. Once the patient understands the risks of occurrence of the condition and the tests, she should be given the opportunity to decline to participate in testing if she so desires.

PRIOR CONSIDERATIONS

A. Confirm the diagnosis for which the pregnancy is at risk. In many cases this is best done by the geneticist, who will take a family history and pedigree and review the history, records, x-rays, and photographs of the proband and of any other affected individuals.
B. Has prenatal diagnosis been accomplished in this disorder? By what method? Can diagnosis be accomplished in the midtrimester?
C. Work with experts in each area related to the prenatal diagnosis of the specific disorder
   1. An obstetrician with experience in *midtrimester* genetic amniocentesis
   2. A skilled genetic counselor
   3. An ultrasonographer with experience in diagnosing specific abnormalities in utero, preferably using a real-time scanner
   4. Laboratories with expertise in α-fetoprotein assay in amniotic fluid and serum and in culturing amniotic fluid cells and interpreting banded karyotypes (fetal karyotypes should be done using modern banding methods).
   5. Special biochemical analyses or other studies may only be available in one or a few centers in the country; arrangements should be made before prenatal diagnosis is attempted.
D. The patient must understand the risk of occurrence of the condition and its variability in affected individuals versus the risks and limitations of prenatal diagnosis.

INDICATIONS FOR MIDTRIMESTER AMNIOCENTESIS

A. *Advanced maternal age (Table 8–1)*

1. The risk of the birth of an offsprng with an autosomal trisomy (+21, +18, +13) or with certain X-chromosome polysomies (XXX, XXY) gradually increases with maternal age. The risk of *trisomy 21* (+21, Down's syndrome), which is nearly 1 in 1660 at age 20 years, is 1 in 885 at age 30, 1 in 365 at age 35, 1 in 109 at age 40, and 1 in 32 at age 45. The *combined* risk for an offspring with trisomy 21 *or*

TABLE 8–1. RISKS OF CYTOGENETIC ABNORMALITIES AT BIRTH ACCORDING TO MATERNAL AGE*

Maternal Age (yr)	Trisomy 21 Only (Down's Syndrome)	All Clinically Significant Cytogenetic Abnormalities†
<15	1:1000	1:435
15	1:1000	1:435
16	1:1111	1:455
17	1:1250	1:476
18	1:1429	1:500
19	1:1667	1:526
20	1:1667	1:526
21	1:1667	1:526
22	1:1667	1:526
23	1:1429	1:500
24	1:1250	1:476
25	1:1250	1:476
26	1:1111	1:455
27	1:1000	1:435
28	1:1000	1:435
29	1:909	1:400
30	1:909	1:400
31	1:833	1:370

(Continued)

**TABLE 8–1. RISKS OF CYTOGENETIC ABNOR-
MALITIES (Cont.)**

32	1:714	1:333
33	1:588	1:294
34	1:455	1:250
35	1:370	1:204
36	1:286	1:169
37	1:222	1:137
38	1:175	1:112
39	1:139	1:92
40	1:109	1:73
41	1:85	1:58
42	1:67	1:47
43	1:53	1:37
44	1:41	1:29
45	1:32	1:23
46	1:25	1:18
47	1:20	1:14
48	1:16	1:11
49	1:12	1:9
>50	>1:11	> 1:8

*Note that there are wide confidence intervals for these esti-
mates, irrespective of age.

†Includes trisomy 13 and 18, XXY, XYY, and other abnormalities
(including a variety of rare conditions, most of which have no
significant parental age association).
(Adapted from the presentation "Estimated rates of clinically
significant cytogenetic abnormalities in livebirths by one year
maternal age interval," Hook ED and Cross PK, American
Society of Human Genetics annual meeting, Minneapolis, Octo-
ber 1979.)

any other clinically significant chromosome abormality is
1 in 530 at age 20, 1 in 400 at age 30, 1 in 200 at age 35, 1
in 70 at age 40, and 1 in 23 at age 45. It is generally
considered that the diagnostic benefits outweigh the risks
of amniocentesis only for women 35 and older. This age

limit is arbitrary and is not based on any sudden biologic change in women at this age.

B. *Previous chromosomally abnormal offspring*

1. *Autosomal trisomy or X-chromosome polysomy.* Following the birth of a child with autosomol trisomy or X-chromosome polysomy, the risk of subsequent offspring with a chromosomal abnormality may be increased in all subsequent pregnancies. The couples at highest risk (above that associated with maternal age alone) are those with a child with trisomy 21 born at or below the maternal age of 29 years (1 percent recurrence risk). Above this age, the recurrence risk is essentially the same as that for maternal age alone.

2. *Structural chromosomal abnormalities.* The parents of all children with structural chromosomal rearrangements (translocations, inversions, duplications, deficiencies, etc.) should be karyotyped. In cases in which one of the parents carries the rearrangement, the couple will have an increased risk for chromosomal abnormalities in subsequent pregnancies. Although recurrence risk presumably is not increased for those couples whose karyotypes are normal, amniocentesis usually is offered since such potential factors as undetected parental mosaicism involving the gonads cannot be ruled out.

3. *Mosaicism.* Chromosomal mosaicism is generally considered to be a postconceptual event and does not increase the risk of subsequent chromosomal abnormality.

4. If one prospective parent gives a history of a relative with a chromosomal abnormality and the affected individual's karyotype results are not known, peripheral blood karyotype on the prospective parent can be done and, if normal, will obviate the need for amniocentesis. This would not be practical after the 16th week of pregnancy, and in such cases amniocentesis can be offered after appropriate counseling.

C. *Presence of a chromosomal rearrangement in either parent*
   1. *Translocations.* About 1 in 500 individuals is a balanced translocation carrier. Such people generally have higher risks of having chromosomally abnormal offspring than do those with advanced maternal age.
      a) *Robertsonian translocations* involve the acrocentric chromosomes (Nos. D-13, 14, 15; G-21, 22). Three to 5 percent of patients with Down's syndrome have an unbalanced translocation, which most commonly is between Nos. 14 and 21, but may also be between 13;21, 15;21, 21;21, or 21;22. In about half of patients with Down's due to a D/G translocation and in most due to a G/G translocation, the abnormality originated *de novo* in the child and is not present in either parent. In such cases the recurrence risk for Down's in subsequent offspring of the parents is not increased; however, amniocentesis can be offered for reassurance in future pregnancies, especially since gonadal mosaicism cannot be ruled out. In about half of patients with Down's due to a D/G translocation and in some due to a G/G translocation, one parent will carry the translocation chromosome in "balanced" form. *Theoretically,* the risk that a parent with a balanced D/G or 21;22 translocation will have a child with Down's is 33 percent. However, based on *empirical* data, the *actual* risks are lower (Table 8–2). A parent who carries a 21;21 or a 13;13 translocation has a 100 percent risk of having a chromosomally abnormal child.
      b) *Reciprocal translocations* involve a break in each of two chromosomes, with exchange of terminal segments. In *de novo* cases with normal parental karyotypes, recurrence risk is not increased. If a parent carries a balanced translocation, the specific recurrence risk is different for each individual rearrangement. Counseling frequently cannot be based on the particular translocation present because of lack of

TABLE 8–2. RISKS OF UNBALANCED TRANSLOCA-TIONS IN OFFSPRING OF CARRIERS OF BALANCED ROBERTSONIAN TRANSLOCATIONS

Translocation	Carrier	Risk (%)
t(Dq;21q)	Maternal	10
t(Dq;21q)	Paternal	2–3
t(21q;22q)	Maternal or paternal	5
t(21q;21q)	Maternal or paternal	100
t(13q;14q) or t(13q;15q)	Maternal	2
t(13q;14q) or t(13q;15q)	Paternal	No increase
t(13q;13q)	Maternal or paternal	100

empirical data. In such cases the following general principles may be used.

(1) If a woman with a balanced reciprocal transloca-tion has previously produced a chromosomally abnormal child, the risk for chromosomal abnor-malities in her offspring is approximately 10 percent.

(2) If a man with a balanced reciprocal translocation has previously produced a chromosomally abnor-mal child, the risk is approximately 2 to 3 percent.

(3) Translocation carriers who have no abnormal offspring and no family history of abnormal individuals probably have a lower risk; however, amniocentesis is still offered.

2. *Inversions.* Individuals with chromosomal inversions are at increased risk of producing offspring with partial duplications and/or deficiencies of chromosomal mate-rial. As with reciprocal translocations, the risk is different in each case and depends not only on the chromosome

involved, but also on the length of the involved segment: the longer the inverted segment the higher the risk. In general, a female carrier has a risk of 10 to 15 percent and a male carrier 2 to 5 percent if these individuals have produced or have a family history of a chromosomally abnormal child. If there are no previous abnormal individuals the risk may be less. (Some normal chromosomal variants — "polymorphisms" or "heteromorphisms" — involve inversions, such as the small pericentric inversion of chromosome 9. These are not associated with phenotypic abnormality in the parent or the fetus. One should discuss such cases with the geneticist before counseling the patient.)

3. *Other abnormal parental karyotypes*

   a) Males with XYY and females with X chromosome abnormalities such as XXX, isochromosomes (X_i) or partial deletions (X_{del}) of X, and XO (the latter have been reported in a few instances to reproduce) are theoretically at risk for offspring with abnormal karyotypes:

Parental Karyotype	Theoretically At Risk For
XYY	XXY, XYY
XXX	XXY, XXX
XO	XO
X_i or X_{del}	X_i or X_{del}

   b) Parents with chromosomal mosaicism usually appear phenotypically normal. Parental mosaicism for trisomy 21 (most often maternal, less often paternal) has been well described and usually is detected after the birth of more than one affected child. The magnitude of the increased risk for abnormal offspring depends on the proportion of abnormal cells in the gonad and, therefore, cannot be stated specifically.

D. *Couples at increased risk for fetal neural tube defects (NTD) and other open defects*
  1. *Assessment of risk*
     a) History of a previous child with a NTD
        (1) For a couple with one affected child with isolated spina bifida or isolated anencephaly, the risk of recurrence is 3 to 5 percent (closer to 3 percent in the United States). After two affected children, the risk is 12 to 15 percent. If the NTD was associated with a syndrome, e.g., Meckel's syndrome (autosomal recessive, with a 25 percent recurrence risk) or a chromosomal abnormality, the risk is that of recurrence of the syndrome itself.
        (2) A history of spina bifida *occulta* does not increase the risk for a NTD.
     b) Prospective parent with a NTD. A couple in which one parent has a NTD has a 3 to 4 percent risk for offspring with a NTD. (Parental spina bifida *occulta* does not carry an increased risk for offspring with a NTD.)
     c) If a second-degree relative of the fetus (grandparent, uncle, aunt, half-sib, nephew, niece) has a NTD, the risk to the fetus is approximately 1 to 2 percent.
     d) First cousin (of the fetus) with a NTD. If the affected individual is a maternal relative the risk is 0.9 percent; an affected paternal relative indicates a 0.5 percent risk.
     e) A history or suspicion of other open or thinwalled defects that may cause elevated α-fetoprotein (AFP).
     f) It has been suggested that there may be a two- to eight-fold increase of NTD over population frequencies following the birth of a child with isolated hydrocephalus and, therefore, that AFP determination and ultrasound examination of the fetal spine should be offered in addition to serial ultrasound examinations of the fetal skull and ventricles. Con-

versely, because of the association of NTD with hydrocephalus, AFP should be determined whenever hydrocephalus is suspected on a routine ultrasound examination.

Couples at increased risk for NTD should be offered expert ultrasound and amniocentesis for AFP. Maternal serum AFP (MS-AFP), a less reliable but acceptable alternative to amniotic fluid AFP (AF-AFP), can be offered and also should be done in conjunction with ultrasound.

2. *Use of AFP for prenatal diagnosis*

α-Fetoprotein is the major serum protein of the human fetus. Levels in fetal serum are always at least 100 times greater than in the amniotic fluid. AFP is elevated in amniotic fluid samples from pregnancies with open NTD, including both anencephaly and spina bifida, as well as in pregnancies with other kinds of open or thinwalled defects.

AFP is also present in maternal serum. The AFP in the amniotic fluid is derived from fetal serum AFP filtered by the fetal kidney, whereas the majority of AFP in maternal serum probably originates from transplacental diffusion. Therefore, although fetal and amniotic fluid levels decrease with advancing gestation, maternal serum levels increase. Maternal serum AFP (*MS-AFP*) is difficult to detect during the first trimester but rises sharply during the second trimester. The steep rise in normal MS-AFP values and the changes in AF-AFP levels during the second trimester means that accurate determination of gestational age is crucial in interpreting AF-AFP and MS-AFP levels.

a) Open fetal defects result in increased amounts of AFP in the amniotic fluid compartment, and subsequent transfer to the maternal circulation results in increased MS-AFP as well. All anencephalic fetuses and 85 to 90 percent of fetuses with spina bifida have open lesions. The 10 to 15 percent of spina bifida with closed (skin-covered) lesions cannot be detected by prenatal AFP assay. (However, many can be visualized by ultrasound.) The severity of an open lesion cannot be predicted from the concentration of AFP.

b) *False-negative* results are rare when the test is performed in laboratories with developed expertise in AFP measurements. As noted above, closed NTDs may not be diagnosed. If the patient does not void between the ultrasound and the amniocentesis, inadvertent aspiration of maternal urine may occur and result in a false-negative result.

c) *False-positive* elevations may be due to contamination of the amniotic fluid specimen with fetal blood or to the presence of other open fetal defects (such as omphalocele, gastroschisis, open skin defects, teratomas, cystic hygroma), fetal demise with maceration, decreased fetal swallowing (as in gastrointestinal obstruction or severe CNS abnormalities), or massive fetal proteinuria (as in the Finnish form of congenital nephrosis). Reports of elevated AFP in pregnancies with Turner's syndrome are probably due to the presence of associated cystic hygroma. When bloody amniotic fluid is obtained, some method of estimating fetal serum contamination such as Kleihauer-Betke, HbF electrophoresis, or immunoelectrophoresis is essential in the event an elevation (+ 3 SD) is found. Therefore, a MS-AFP sample may be obtained immediately before doing amniocentesis for AF-AFP, since it will be helpful in the interpretation of bloody amniotic fluid with an elevated AFP level.

d) Only laboratories with established expertise in AF-AFP and MS-AFP should be used. Most laboratories use 5 standard deviations above the normal mean as a cutoff point for AF-AFP. Values between 3 and 5 standard deviations above the normal mean may require the use of ultrasound and/or amniography for confirmation. When elevated AF-AFP is found, it is recommended that a decision or diagnosis not be made without a second sonogram and repeat amniocentesis that may also include amniography. Amniography should be considered in the case of borderline elevation of AF-AFP and normal results on real-time ultrasound . The family must be counseled concerning the risk of an abnormality and the possibility of a false-positive (estimated to occur in less than 0.1 percent of normal pregnancies), especially when there is an elevated AFP level with no corroborating evidence from the sonogram or amniogram.

e) Patients at risk for NTD can be placed within three general groups:

 (1) *High risk*. Those whose risk is 3 percent or greater (a couple with a previous child with a NTD; a prospective parent with a NTD).

 (2) *Moderate risk*. Those whose risk lies between that of the high-risk group and that of the general population in their geographic area.

 (3) *Low risk*. Patients at the population risk (varies from 1 to 8/1000 depending on the geographic location: 1.4 to 3.1/1000 in the United States).

Patients in the high-risk group should be offered ultrasound and amniocentesis for AF-AFP, with MS-AFP drawn immediately before the amniocentesis procedure. High-risk patients who refuse amniocentesis should be offered ultrasound and MS-AFP as an alternative. Patients in the moderate-risk group are more distantly related to an index case (e.g., half-siblings, first cousins, nieces/nephews), and the risks vary, both for degree of relatedness and for population incidences. Overall, the risk for NTD in relatives of affected individuals is approximately 1 to 2 percent. If careful examination by ultrasonography *and* MS-AFP are normal, the risk for an undiagnosed NTD becomes about 1 in 1000, and amniocentesis is then generally considered not to be indicated.

3. *Maternal serum screening for AFP*. Ninety-five percent of all affected children with NTD are born to parents not known to be at high risk. Screening programs are being developed to identify those women in the general population with a high enough risk of producing a fetus with an open NTD to justify amniocentesis. The best time to screen is in the 17th menstrual week of pregnancy; the test is much less effective before 16 weeks and for practical reasons should be done before 19 to 20 weeks. At 16 to 18 weeks' gestation, 88 percent of anencephalic fetuses and 79 percent of fetuses with spina bifida can be detected by elevated MS-AFP. However, between 1.7 and 7.4 percent of *all* pregnant women have elevated levels at this gestational date, depending on the upper limit of normal used by each laboratory. To avoid unnecessary amniocentesis, screening schemes have been developed to exclude the most common causes of elevated MS-AFP before specific diagnostic tests are offered:

a) *Initial serum sample* at 16 to 18 menstrual weeks
   (1) Normal: stop.
   (2) Elevated: obtain a second serum sample within 1 to 2 weeks.

b) *Second serum sample*
   (1) Normal: stop. Reassure patient that she is not at increased risk for NTD.
   (2) Elevated: obtain sonogram.

c) *Sonogram*
   (1) Additional studies are *not* indicated if the sonogram shows:
      (a) Multiple pregnancy: stop. (Very high MS-AFP values in multiple pregnancy are not insignificant, but cases of NTD-affected twin pregnancy are rare.)
      (b) Gestational age was previously underestimated; MS-AFP values are normal for corrected gestational age: stop.
      (c) Fetal demise: stop. (MS-AFP levels in such cases may be much higher than in NTD-

affected pregnancies and may reach 1000
ng/ml or more.)

   (d) Anencephaly: advise parents; obtain decision on termination.

(2) If the sonogram shows no explanation for the
elevated MS-AFP, proceed with counseling and
offer amniocentesis for AF-AFP and fetal karyotype. (The average risk of NTD in patients with
unexplained sustained elevation of MS-AFP in
the United States is 1 in 12. Patients whose
original risk was high are more likely to have an
affected pregnancy; those who originally were in a
low-risk group may have a pregnancy with one of
the other defects discussed above or may have a
false-positive elevation of AF-AFP.)

d) *Amniocentesis*

(1) If AF-AFP is normal, stop. Follow as high-risk
pregnancy (various complications of pregnancy
such as fetal distress, premature labor, preeclampsia, hypertension, and Rh-
isoimmunization have been associated with
elevated MS-AFP.)

(2) If AF-AFP is elevated:

   (a) Reevaluate with ultrasound including real-
time scanning.

   (b) Test amniotic fluid specimen for fetal serum
contamination.

   (c) Amniography may be considered as noted
above.

Low levels of MS-AFP (less than 0.3 times the
median) also may be significant. Preliminary data
suggest that although the majority of these low
levels are found in normal pregnancies (either
with correct dates or where gestational dates have
been underestimated), there is an increased likelihood of fetal demise, molar pregnancy, or non-

pregnancy. Therefore, ultrasound and close follow-up are indicated in women with low MS-AFP levels.

Routine maternal serum screening should be done only with proper information for the patient, who should understand the possible outcomes, risks of additional tests, and that compliance is voluntary. Results must be communicated to patient and obstetrician promptly (immediately in case of abnormal results). Proper facilities for follow-up of abnormal results must be readily available.

New methods of prenatal diagnosis of NTD, e.g., amniotic fluid acetylcholinesterase analysis, rapidly adhering cell assay, and determination of AFP isoprotein proportions by differential binding to concanavalin A are under investigation and show promise of becoming useful adjuncts to AF-AFP assay.

E. *Couples with previous offspring with multiple congenital anomalies*
   1. Amniocentesis is indicated if the previous child had a chromosomal abnormality or open defect. In cases in which no cytogenetic studies were done and the spectrum of abnormalities is not consistent with a recognizable nonchromosomal syndrome, amniocentesis can be offered. Consultation with a geneticist is advisable in such cases.

F. *History of multiple spontaneous abortions*
   1. Couples with a history of two or more spontaneous abortions have at least a 3 to 5 percent likelihood of an abnormal karyotype (usually a balanced rearrangement) in one parent. Such couples should be offered peripheral blood karyotyping with banding to rule out the presence of subtle chromosomal changes. Parental karyotyping is best done prior to pregnancy and in any case must be

completed by the 16th week of gestation so that amniocentesis, if indicated, can be offered.

2. In couples with a history of two or more spontaneous
abortions in a previous mating of one spouse, blood
karyotyping is indicated only for that individual.

G. *Intrauterine growth retardation*

1. If intrauterine growth retardation (IUGR) is diagnosed
and confirmed by ultrasound before 20 weeks' gestation,
fetal karyotype analysis is indicated. When IUGR is
noted after this time, fetal karyotype analysis still may be
considered, since knowledge of a fetal chromosomal
abnormality may affect delivery management.

H. *Couples at risk for inborn errors of metabolism*

1. The great majority of these disorders, characterized by an
abnormality or absence of a protein (usually an enzyme),
are inherited as autosomal recessive traits. Some are X-
linked or, rarely, autosomal dominant.

2. When both members of a couple are known to be
heterozygous (carriers) for an autosomal recessive
metabolic disorder, either through the birth of an affected child or through carrier screening for such disorders as Tay-Sachs disease, there is a 25 percent risk in
each subsequent pregnancy.

3. Nearly 100 disorders can be diagnosed in utero by assay
for a missing enzyme or by using appropriate metabolic
reactions in cultured amniotic fluid fibroblasts. Most of
these are rare disorders in which diagnosis has been
attempted only a few times. The diagnostic problems are
different for each disorder and for many have only been
perfected in a few specialized laboratories. The following
considerations are essential before prenatal diagnosis of
metabolic disorders can be attempted:

a) The abnormality must be expressed in cells commonly
grown from amniotic fluid.

b) The abnormality must be expressed in the midtrimester.

c) One must be able to differentiate clearly between
normal or carrier and affected fetuses.

d) The assay must be able to be accomplished within a time limit (usually not more than four to six weeks).

e) The family under study must be investigated for their specific phenotypic expression of the metabolic abnormality before attempting biochemical analysis of amniotic fluid cells.

The numbers of disorders meeting the criteria for prenatal diagnosis has been expanding rapidly, and diagnostic methods for specific inborn errors change frequently. Information about a disorder must be obtained from a specialist active in the field before prenatal diagnosis is attempted. When attempting prenatal diagnosis of an X-linked disorder (e.g., Hunter syndrome, hemophilia, Lesch-Nyhan syndrome, etc.), karyotyping for fetal sex determination should also be performed. In the case of elective abortion following a prediction of fetal abnormality, appropriate fetal tissues should be collected for biochemical confirmation.

I. *Couples at risk for X-linked disorders.* Accurate midtrimester prenatal diagnosis can be made in only a few of the more than 200 recognized X-linked disorders. For the remainder, couples can avoid having affected offspring only by aborting all male fetuses. Since only 50 percent of male offspring of a carrier mother will be affected, prospective parents in this situation must consider whether to abort a fetus which may be normal. Therefore, it is especially important that the diagnosis and recurrence risk figures provided to such couples are accurate.

1. Since the mutant gene for X-linked disorders is on the X chromosome, males affected with *X-linked recessive* disorders cannot have affected sons (a son receives the Y chromosome, not the X, from the father). Since the father transmits his X chromosome to every daughter, however, all daughters will be carriers of the mutant gene. A carrier mother gives one of her two X chromosomes to each offspring. Therefore, half her sons will receive the X with the mutant gene and will be affected,

and half will be normal. Similarly, half the daughters of a carrier mother will be carriers and half will not.

Although counseling for X-linked recessive disorders appears relatively straightforward if the father is affected or the mother is a *proven* carrier, in many instances accurate determination of risk may require special statistical analysis. For this reason, it is advisable that all recurrence risks for such disorders be provided with the assistance of a genetic counselor.

2. In *X-linked dominant* disorders, which are extremely rare, females also are affected, but males are much more severely affected. All daughters of an affected male — but none of his sons — will be affected. Half the sons and half the daughters of an affected female will also have the disorder. Some of these conditions are early lethals in affected males; in such cases the majority of males who survive past midtrimester are normal, and some parents may elect to limit live-born offspring to males. It is advisable that all couples at risk for X-linked dominant disorders be counseled with the assistance of a genetic counselor.

Although there are three approaches to prenatal sex determination (fetal karyotyping, X- and Y-body analysis, and amniotic fluid testosterone assay), only fetal karyotyping is sufficiently reliable and informative. Although simple and rapid, both the X- and Y-body assays have appreciable drawbacks, especially false-positive and false-negative results, and these methods are *not* recommended for prenatal diagnosis. Similarly, amniotic fluid testosterone levels in midtrimester, while reasonably accurate, should be considered only as an adjunct to fetal karyotyping, ultimately becoming useful in cases where cell culture fails or maternal cell contamination occurs. (Testosterone levels are much greater in fetal and maternal serum than in amniotic fluid; therefore, contamination with fetal *or* maternal blood must be avoided.)

3. *Sex-limited* disorders are autosomal traits that are expressed in only one sex. Counseling for these depends on

the specific condition involved. Fetal sex determination for social reasons alone should not be considered an indication for prenatal diagnosis (Table 8–3).

TABLE 8–3. INBORN ERRORS OF METABOLISM FOR WHICH MIDTRIMESTER PRENATAL DIAGNOSIS HAS BEEN ACHIEVED (A) OR IS CONSIDERED POSSIBLE BUT HAS NOT YET BEEN ACHIEVED (P)

Acatalasemia	(P)
Adenosine deaminase deficiency	(A)
Adrenogenital syndrome (21-hydroxylase deficiency)	(A)
α-1-Antitrypsin deficiency	(A)
Arginase deficiency	(A)
Argininosuccinic aciduria	(A)
Aspartylglycosaminuria	(P)
Cholesteryl ester storage disease	(P)
*Chronic granulomatous disease	(A)
Citrullinemia	(A)
Cystathionuria	(P)
Cystinosis	(A)
Dihydropteridine reductase deficiency (hyperphenylalanemia type V)	(P)
*Fabry's disease	(A)
Farber's disease	(A)
Fucosidosis	(A)
Galactokinase deficiency	(P)
Galactosemia	(A)
Gaucher disease	
Type I (adult)	(P)
Type II (infantile)	(A)
Type III (juvenile)	(P)
*Glucose-6-phosphate dehydrogenase deficiency	(P)
Glutaric acidemia	(A)
Glycogen storage disease	
Type II (Pompe's disease)	(A)
Type III (debrancher deficiency)	(P)
Type IV (branching enzyme deficiency)	(A)
Type VIII (phosphorylase kinase deficiency)	(P)

(Continued)

TABLE 8–3. INBORN ERRORS OF METABOLISM (Cont.)

GM$_1$ gangliosidosis
   Type I (infantile; generalized
   gangliosidosis)   (A)
   Type II (juvenile)   (A)
   Type III (adult)   (P)
GM$_2$ gangliosidosis
   Type I (Tay-Sachs disease)   (A)
   Type II (Sandhoff's disease)   (A)
   Type III (juvenile Tay-Sachs)   (P)
   Type IV (juvenile Sandhoff's)   (P)
   Type V (adult)   (P)
*Hemophilia A   (A)
Histidinemia   (P)
Homocystinuria   (A)
†Hypercholesterolemia, familial
(homozygous)   (A)
Hyperlysinemia   (P)
Hyperornithinemia
   Type I   (P)
   Type II   (P)
Hypophosphatasia   (A)
Hypothyroidism (reverse T$_3$ deficiency)   (P)
Hypervalinemia   (P)
*Ichthyosis (steroid sulfatase deficiency)   (A)
Isovaleric acidemia   (P)
Krabbe disease (globoid cell
leukodystrophy)
   Infantile   (A)
   Juvenile   (P)
   Adult   (P)
Lactosyl ceramidosis   (P)
*Lesch-Nyhan syndrome   (A)
Lysosomal acid phosphatase deficiency   (A)
Mannosidosis   (A)
Maple syrup urine disease
   Severe infantile form   (A)
   Intermittent form   (P)
*Menkes' disease   (A)

(Continued)

TABLE 8–3. INBORN ERRORS OF METABOLISM (Cont.)

Metachromatic leukodystrophy	
Infantile	(A)
Juvenile	(P)
Adult	(P)
β-Methylocrotonic aciduria	(P)
Methylenetetrahydrofolate reductase deficiency	(A)
Methylmalonic acidemia;	
B_{12}-responsive	(A)
B_{12}-unresponsive	(A)
Mucolipidosis	
Type I (sialidosis)	(P)
Type II (I-cell disease)	(A)
Type III (pseudo-Hurler polydystrophy)	(A)
Type IV	(A)
Mucopolysaccharidosis	
Type IH (Hurler)	(A)
Type IS (Scheie)	(A)
Type IH/S (Hurler-Scheie)	(P)
*Type II (Hunter)	(A)
Type IIIa (Sanfilippo-A)	(A)
Type IIIb (Sanfilippo-B)	(A)
Type IIIc (Sanfilippo-C)	(P)
Type IV (Morquio)	(P)
Type VI (Marateaux-Lamy)	(A)
Type VII (α-glucuronidase deficiency)	(P)
Type VIII (glucosamine-6-sulfate)	(P)
Multiple sulfatase deficiency	
(mucosulfatidosis)	(P)
Myotonic dystrophy	(A)
Nephrosis (congenital)	(A)
Niemann-Pick disease	
Type A	(A)
Type B	(A)
Type C	(P)
Orotic aciduria	(P)
Phosphohexose isomerase deficiency	(P)

(Continued)

TABLE 8–3. INBORN ERRORS OF METABOLISM (Cont.)

Porphyrias	
Acute intermittent	(A)
Congenital erythropoietic	(A)
Coproporphyria	(P)
Protoporphyria	(P)
Prolidase deficiency	(A)
Propionic acidemia (ketotic hyper-glycinemia)	(A)
Pyruvate decarboxylase deficiency	(P)
Pyruvate dehydrogenase deficiency	(P)
Refsum disease (phytanic acid storage disease)	(A)
Saccharopinuria	(P)
Sickle cell anemia	(A)
Sulfite oxidase deficiency	(A)
α-Thalassemia (homozygous)	(A)
β-Thalassemia (homozygous)	(A)
$\beta°\delta°$-Thalassemia	(A)
Wolman's disease	(A)
Xeroderma pigmentosum	(A)

X-linked inheritance (*) or autosomal dominant inheritance (†) are indicated—*all others are autosomal recessive.*

POSSIBLE INCREASED RISK

Conditions for which there is insufficient evidence regarding the advisability of offering amniocentesis for prenatal diagnosis are discussed below. *Each case should be judged individually.*

A. *History of radiation therapy and/or exposure to chemotherapeutic agents prior to pregnancy.* Whereas some data indicate that prior history of multiple x-rays, irradiation therapy, or chemotherapy may predispose to chromosomal anomalies in future offspring, other studies have shown no correlation. At present, there is insufficient data to justify routine amniocentesis based solely on such a history in either parent.

B. *History of infertility*. Couples with prolonged infertility without apparent anatomic or metabolic etiology should have blood chromosome analysis. In those who have normal karyotypes with no evidence of chromosomal rearrangement, there is insufficient evidence to indicate that prenatal diagnosis should be offered routinely. This is especially important in that such pregnancies are particularly valuable to these couples and should not be exposed to unnecessary risk.

C. *Pregnancies occurring after induced ovulation*. Preliminary data suggest that women who conceive with the use of clomiphene citrate may be at increased risk for offspring with chromosomal abnormalities. It is not clear whether the increased risk, if any, is due to clomiphene citrate itself or to the primary condition for which the drug was given. Since these pregnancies are also "premium," couples must understand the evidence in terms of the possible benefits versus risks and expense of the procedure.

D. *Maternal thyroid disease*. Although some data suggest an association between parental antithyroid antibodies or women with hypo- or hyperthyroidism and an increased risk of offspring with Downs' syndrome or gonadal dysgenesis, there is insufficient evidence to justify amniocentesis.

E. *Advanced paternal age*. Preliminary data indicate that a paternal age of 55 or more may increase the risk of Down's syndrome twofold. Amniocentesis is unjustified in couples with advanced paternal age and a maternal age less than 30, but it may be considered when the maternal age is approaching 35.

F. *Parental anxiety*. When prospective parents who are at no increased risk seek prenatal genetic studies because of concern about birth defects or mental retardation, they should be counseled about the risks, limitations, pitfalls, and cost of prenatal diagnosis and helped to balance these against the chance of occurrence of disorders detectable by midtrimester amniocentesis. If they continue to show undue anxiety, amniocentesis may be offered.

WHEN AMNIOCENTESIS IS NOT INDICATED

A. *X-irradiation during pregnancy*. Patients receiving irradiation during pregnancy should be counseled that there is no evidence of increased risk for fetal abnormality with fetal exposures of less than 5 rads (the exposure should be calculated by fetal or gonadal dose, not overall dose). Also, there is no evidence of increased chromosomal abnormalities in such fetuses. Chromosomal breakage may be seen in cultured amniotic fluid cells but has not been shown to be related to actual abnormalities in the fetus. Therefore, amniocentesis in such a case may only confuse the issue and lead to unnecessary anxiety or unwarranted termination of pregnancy.

B. *Exposure to drugs or chemicals during pregnancy*. There is no evidence that exposure to medications, illicit drugs, or anesthetics during pregnancy causes detectable chromosomal damage. Although some industrial chemicals such as vinyl chloride may cause nonspecific chromosomal changes in the peripheral blood of exposed workers and their children, none has been related to clinical abnormality. Prenatal diagnosis is not indicated in view of such nonspecific findings.

C. *Viral infections during pregnancy*. Amniocentesis for karyotype analysis or for virus isolation is not indicated routinely even in pregnant women with serologic evidence of acute infection. Isolation of virus from amniotic fluid does not necessarily indicate infection of fetal tissues or the presence of resulting abnormality. Conversely, failure to find virus in the amniotic fluid may occur in the presence of virus in fetal tissues.

UNUSUAL RESULTS ON FETAL KARYOTYPING

All cases in which there are unusual results on fetal karyotyping must be discussed with the geneticist before counseling the patient.

A. *Apparently balanced chromosomal translocation.* First, obtain blood karyotypes on both parents as soon as possible. If one normal parent carries the same translocation, the fetus is at no increased risk for clinical abnormality. For fetuses with *de novo,* apparently balanced translocations, there is some evidence of increased risk for mental retardation, although specific risk figures cannot be given. (In pregnancies conceived with artificial insemination, the donor should also be karyotyped to uncover the translocation.)

B. *Chromosomal mosaicism.* The analysis of amniotic cells from multiple separate culture vessels or from individual colonies allows the cytogeneticist to decide with reasonable — but not absolute — accuracy whether the abnormal cell line arose in vitro or whether it accurately reflects an abnormality in the fetus. Generally, if the abnormal line is found in only one culture vessel or in only one clone, the greatest likelihood is that it arose as an in vitro artifact and does not reflect an abnormality in the fetus. Additional evidence of in vitro artifact is an abnormality that is seen frequently as an artifact in amniotic fluid culture but that rarely has been confirmed in the newborn — examples are tetraploidy, trisomy 2, trisomy 20. However, if the abnormal cell line is one known to occur relatively frequently in the live-born (e.g., trisomy 21, 13, and 18, X-polysomy, triploidy), greater caution must be taken in counseling the prospective parents, even if the abnormal line was found in only a single flask or clone.

Mosaicism found in an amniotic fluid sample cannot be invalidated by subsequent normal findings in a second amniocentesis, since true mosaicism may not manifest itself in any one amniotic fluid sample. Conversely, in some cases in which moasaicism appeared in more than one sample, the fetus or newborn was normal.

C. *Unusual abnormal karyotypes.* Multiple translocations in the same cell, marker chromosomes, extra small chromosomes, ring chromosomes, double trisomy, etc., should be discussed with the geneticist before the patient is counseled.

In all cases of suspected fetal chromosomal abnormality, blood or other appropriate tissues should be obtained for confirmation of karyotype from either the live-born or the abortus.

AMNIOCENTESIS METHODS

A. *Technique.* Midtrimester genetic amniocentesis requires greater skill and expertise than midtrimester amniocentesis for therapeutic abortion or third trimester diagnostic amniocentesis. This procedure should be performed only by those who have had supervised training and experience in *midtrimester diagnostic* amniocentesis and who maintain expertise by performing at least 100 procedures a year.

B. *Patient.* She must understand the procedure and its risks, benefits, and limitations.

C. *Physician.* He or she must work closely with the cytogenetics laboratory so that samples are obtained properly and transported safely. Any special tests, such as enzyme assays, should be planned in advance with the laboratory.

D. *Ultrasound* is strongly recommended before amniocentesis to (1) estimate gestational age, (2) locate the placenta, (3) rule out multiple pregnancy, and (4) look for gross fetal, uterine, or adnexal abnormalities, fetal demise, missed abortion, hydatid mole, etc.

E. *Amniocentesis* is an outpatient procedure best performed at 15 to 16 weeks' gestation. At this time the uterus is accessible by the transcutaneous abdominal approach, and there is 180 to 200 ml of amniotic fluid present, a good ratio of viable to nonviable cells in the fluid, and enough time remains in the midtrimester to grow cells and perform chromosomal or biochemical analyses and to repeat the test if necessary.

F. The patient should sign an *informed consent* form that includes all aspects of the amniocentesis procedure and of the laboratory studies (see below "Counseling Issues in

Prenatal Diagnoses" p 136). The patient should be informed of the tests to be performed on the amniotic fluid sample. When the indication for amniocentesis is either a previous open defect or a biochemical disorder, cytogenetic studies should also be offered. The overall frequency of chromosomal abnormalities and the fact that there are reports of incidental diagnosis of chromosomal abnormalities in fluid obtained for biochemical studies or α-fetoprotein assay indicate that once fluid has been obtained, routine karyotype analysis is advisable. Similarly, α-fetoprotein should be considered for every amniotic fluid specimen. Patients who may refuse additional studies because of cost or other factors should be required to sign a release form.

G. *Midtrimester amniocentesis procedure*

1. Before beginning the procedure, draw maternal blood if needed for serum α-fetoprotein, maternal karyotype, etc. If the mother is Rh-negative, draw blood for antibody titer and for Kleihauer-Betke test.

2. The patient should void immediately before the procedure to avoid inadvertent aspiration of urine.

3. One percent lidocaine may be used for local anesthesia if there is no history of sensitivity.

4. Make sure that the syringes and tubes used are sterile and nontoxic to amniotic cells (check with the cytogenetics laboratory).

5. Use percutaneous insertion of a 22-gauge, 3½-inch spinal needle in the midline of the abdomen, perpendicular to the center of the uterine cavity. Do not remove the stylet until the needle has been inserted. Clear the needle into the first syringe (2 to 3 ml) and change syringes (this will minimize maternal cell contamination and bloody fluid samples). Aspirate approximately 10 ml into each of three to four syringes. Reinsert the stylet and remove the needle. (No more than two insertions should be carried out in any single amniocentesis.)

6. Make sure all tubes are clearly labeled. Transport specimens as quickly as possible to the laboratory at ambient

temperature. If specimens are to be shipped, obtain transport instructions from the laboratory before the procedure is performed.

7. Inadvertent culture of urine will delay fetal diagnosis and may result in mistaken analysis of maternal cells. To confirm that the specimen is amniotic fluid, use the crystalline arborization test ("fern test"): place several drops of amniotic fluid on an acid-cleaned slide, air dry, and examine without a coverslip under low power ($\times 100$) for the characteristic fernlike, crystalline arborization pattern of amniotic fluid. A dipstick for glucose and protein can also be used but is unreliable if the patient has diabetes, renal disease, or polyhydramnios.

8. If pre-amniocentesis ultrasound examination shows the presence of twins, the prospective parents must be counseled.

   a) Two gestational sacs can be tapped separately; but if the twins are contained in a common sac, they cannot be studied individually.

   b) In a case in which one fetus is abnormal and the other normal, it is unlikely that selective termination can be performed on the abnormal fetus without harm to the normal one.

   c) When two gestational sacs are seen, amniocentesis can be performed under ultrasonographic guidance. The first sac is tapped; amniotic fluid is removed; and before removing the needle, 1 to 3 ml of sterile indigo carmine (0.8 percent diluted with sterile water to give a final concentration of 0.08 percent) is instilled. The needle is removed and the patient is ambulated for five minutes. The second fetus is then located ultrasonographically and a second amniocentesis performed. Aspiration of clear fluid indicates that the second sac has been entered, whereas aspiration of bluish fluid indicates that the first sac has been re-entered.

9. In the Rh-negative woman, a Kleihauer-Betke test should be obtained before and after the amniocentesis.

Whether or not amniocentesis disrupts the fetomaternal circulation and thereby causes isoimmunization is a controversial question, and some studies suggest that anti-D-immunoglobulin in midtrimester may itself be associated with fetal risk. There is no consensus concerning the advisability of routinely administering anti-D-immunoglobulin to Rh-negative unsensitized women following midtrimester amniocentesis.

FETAL VISUALIZATION

It is now possible to diagnose many internal and external fetal structural abnormalities by direct visualization of fetal anatomy. There are definite advantages and limitations associated with each method of fetal visualization (ultrasonography, radiography, amniography, fetography, fetoscopy). Careful consideration of the suspected abnormality and the expertise available allows the formulation of a suitable plan utilizing one or a combination of these modalities. Direct discussion between the referring physician and the radiologist, ultrasonographer, or fetoscopist is essential. (Computerized tomography delivers too much radiation and provides a poor image because of fetal movements; therefore, it is considered unsatisfactory for prenatal diagnosis.)

A. *Ultrasonography.* The ultrasonographer should be advised in advance of the possible diagnosis and should be cautious and experienced in midtrimester examination for fetal anomalies so as to avoid misdiagnosis. A combination of sonographic techniques can be used; B-mode gray-scale equipment produces high-resolution static images, whereas real-time machines allow visualization of fetal movements but with poorer resolution.
   1. *Benefits* of ultrasound for prenatal diagnosis
      a) There is no ionizing radiation.
      b) The procedure is noninvasive.
      c) Both internal and external fetal structures can be visualized.

2. No risk to the fetus at diagnostic dose levels is presently known (but long-term effects, if any, are unknown).

   Frequently, small structures such as digits, genitalia, and facies cannot be visualized, and limbs cannot always be visualized in their entirety.

3. Indications for midtrimester ultrasound
   a) As part of amniocentesis or fetoscopy procedures.
   b) When elevated AFP is found in amniotic fluid or maternal serum.
   c) When the uterus is large or small for dates (polyhydramnios, oligohydramnios, inaccurate dates, multiple pregnancy, intrauterine growth retardation, uterine fibromata, pelvic mass).
   d) In pregnancies at risk for a disorder associated with a structural abnormality that can be visualized ultrasonographically.
      (1) *Hydrocephalus.* If present, this condition can be diagnosed beginning at 17 weeks. The biparietal diameter (BPD) must be determined at the level of the lateral ventricles. Since it is believed that the BPD is a late indicator of hydrocephalus, the width and nature of the ventricles and the cephalothoracic ratio must also be considered. Serial examinations beginning at 16 weeks are suggested. It is important to counsel the patient that a fetus that appears normal in the midtrimester may develop hydrocephalus later and that a normal examination does not rule out the possibility that hydrocephalus will occur.
      (2) *Neural tube defects.* Anencephaly can be diagnosed by 14 weeks' gestation. Because of the grave consequences of making this diagnosis, it is generally accepted that confirmation of a sonographic diagnosis of anencephally in midtrimester should be confirmed by AF-AFP determination. In later gestation, an unusual fetal position may cause false-positive results by making the fetal

head inaccessible to ultrasound examination, and radiographs should be obtained for confirmation. To examine for spina bifida, the whole spine must be examined both in the longitudinal and, especially, in the transverse plane at right angles to the spinal axis at each level from the cervical to the caudal region. Small defects may be missed. Serial examinations (in combination with AFP determination) should be performed on women at high risk for NTD.

(3) *Microcephaly*. This requires serial examinations of BPD and head-body proportion to detect falling head-to-abdominal circumference ratio.

(4) *Spinal and intracranial tumors*. These have been noted on midtrimester ultrasound examination.

(5) *Cystic hygroma*. Although it may look like a meningocele or encephalocele, the experienced sonographer can frequently distinguish hygroma from these other conditions.

(6) *Cardiac abnormalities*. With new real-time scanners, a four-chamber view of the fetal heart is possible after 20 weeks, and such views have been used by experts late in the second trimester and in the third trimester to diagnose arrhythmias and gross abnormalities, including tricuspid atresia, hypoplastic ventricle, large VSD, and endocardial cushion defects.

(7) *Omphalocele and gastroschisis*. In the former, the viscera are enclosed in a fluid-filled sac, and there is an increased association with other structural defects and chomosomal abnormalities. In the latter, no sac is seen and there is no increased association with other malformations or chromosomal abnormalities. In differentiating between the two, the insertion of the cord frequently can be identified by the experienced sonographer.

(8) *Duodenal atresia*. This condition is suggested by

dilation of the stomach and proximal duodenum. Other intestinal atresias may result in dilated loops of bowel.

(9) *Hydrops, ascites.* Hydrops fetalis is identified by the findings of a double outline of the fetal scalp and/or trunk, the presence of fetal ascites and organomegaly, and placental enlargement and thickening.

(10) *Fetal subcutaneous edema.* This edema has been associated with chromosomal abnormalities in the midtrimester.

(11) *Diaphragmatic hernia.*

(12) *Renal agenesis or dysplasia.* The kidneys are visible late in the second trimester, and the size of the fetal kidneys can be determined in relation to the fetal abdomen. Multicystic or polycystic kidneys frequently can be diagnosed at this time. The fetal bladder can be visualized at 20 weeks. Since the fetal bladder fills and empties approximately every 90 minutes, it should be visualized by the end of a routine examination period. Examination should be repeated in an hour if the bladder is not seen during the first examination. Absence of the fetal bladder after 20 weeks, especially with oligohydramnios, strongly suggests renal agenesis. A dilated bladder suggests a urethral obstruction, and ureteropelvic junction obstructions have also been shown by ultrasound.

(13) *Skeletal dysplasias.* One should look for abnormalities, e.g., abnormal head-trunk ratio, thoracic abnormalities, abnormal limb lengths, etc. Radiographs are frequently useful.

(14) *Limb defects.* Limb length and length measurements should be done by experienced individuals. Tangential sections of a limb can produce artificially short measurements.

B. *Transabdominal, direct-vision fetoscopy.* Relatively new and highly specialized, this procedure is performed only by a limited number of skilled investigators in academic research centers. Through the use of endoscopic instruments in conjunction with expert ultrasound, this method allows not only direct fetal visualization, but also sampling of fetal blood and tissues for biochemical, hematologic, and histologic evaluation. The procedure is best done between the 15th and 18th weeks of gestation for visualization and between 18 and 20 weeks for fetal blood sampling. For a family contemplating the procedure, accurate diagnosis in a proband, recurrence risks, and feasibility of diagnosis by this method must be ascertained and discussed.

1. *Advantages.* Allows prenatal diagnosis of some conditions unable to be diagnosed by other methods.
2. *Disadvantages*
   a) The endoscopes in use today are inflexible; an anterior placenta cannot be approached for fetal blood sampling.
   b) Blood samples are rarely 100 percent fetal and are usually admixed with amniotic fluid or maternal blood. One must determine the percentage of fetal versus maternal blood in the sample by cell size distribution with an electronic cell sizer and/or by the Kleihauer-Betke stain for fetal hemoglobin.
   c) Only a small visual field is obtained (about a 70-degree angle of visualization and a 2-cm depth of focus); such complicating factors as fetal movement, fetal position, amniotic fluid clouded by blood or meconium, or a veil of amnion obstructing the lens may not allow the fetal part in question to be seen.
   d) Risks include blood loss (reduction of fetal blood volume is usually less than 3 percent), fetal injury or loss (10 percent loss), maternal or fetal infection (1 percent), damage to maternal abdominal or uterine vessel or to maternal bowel or bladder, chronic amniotic fluid leakage (2 to 3 percent), and possibility of Rh isoimmunization or placental damage.

Fetal blood sampling by fetoscopy has been applied to the

prenatal diagnosis of hemoglobinopathies (β-thalassemia and sickle cell anemia), hemophilia A, white cell disorders such as chronic granulomatous disease, platelet disorders, and certain enzyme deficiencies. (Duchenne muscular dystrophy diagnosis by elevation of fetal serum creatine phosphokinase levels has not proved to be reliable.) Skin biopsy has allowed diagnosis of certain ichthyosis and epidermolysis syndromes.

An alternate method of fetal blood sampling is direct placental aspiration without use of the fetoscope. Most samples [200 μl] are largely or totally maternal blood, but pure fetal samples can be obtained. This procedure is only appropriate for those diagnostic tests that can be done satisfactorily on fetal samples that may be admixed with maternal blood or placental interstitial fluid. Only skilled, experienced investigators should perform direct placental aspiration. Potential risks include fetal blood loss, fetal injury or loss, amnionitis, and Rh isoimmunization. A larger sampling needle is used than in fetoscopy, and the approach to the fetal vessels is blind. Advantages include the avoidance of fetoscopy with its larger-diameter fetoscope and longer periods of intrauterine manipulation.

C. *Fetal radiographic visualization*
   1. *Direct radiography.* By 16 weeks' gestation, fetal skeletal ossification is sufficiently well advanced to allow examination of most tubular bones (long and short bones of the limbs, clavicles, ribs). Conditions associated with such abnormalities as absence or dysplasia of these bones are theoretically diagnosable by this method. Fetal radiography should be employed when this seems to be the best method to obtain useful information. There are no data that indicate major fetal risks from one or a few roentgenograms, especially after the first trimester and when suitably modified to expose fetus to as little irradiation as possible. The procedure should be performed late enough to allow any fetal abnormality to become recognizable, but time also must be left for possible additional procedures to be utilized and diag-

nosis obtained before 24 weeks' gestation. Between 15 and 18 weeks the fetus is usually in a transverse lie, so that a film should be taken in the prone position. After 24 weeks (third-trimester diagnosis can be of benefit in guiding decisions about obstetrical and perinatal management), a 45-degree prone compression oblique is suggested to throw fetal shadows away from the maternal spine. Between 18 and 24 weeks the radiologist may choose the most suitable procedure. If located near the radiology suite, preliminary ultrasound may be used to determine fetal position to guide the radiologist. The x-ray should be reviewed immediately to determine whether it is acceptable, will require a different projection, or will be unlikely to give further information. Magnification views usually are unnecessary. Fetal movement can be minimized by maternal sedation with 10 mg IV morphine sulfate and films taken during the following 5 to 15 minutes.

2. *Contrast radiology.* These procedures require amniocentesis techniques and should be performed only by obstetricians skilled in midtrimester amniocentesis. They should be reserved for use in pregnancies at very high risk by virtue of ultrasonographic abnormalities or elevated AF-AFP.

Amniography utilizes a water-soluable contrast material to opacify the amniotic fluid and allow visualization of the fetal outline. At 18 to 19 weeks' gestation, 20 to 25 ml of amniotic fluid is removed (the fluid should be saved in the same way as for AFP and karyotype analysis in case it becomes evident that such studies are indicated). Then, 20 to 25 ml of sterile, 60 percent diatrizoate is injected into the amniotic sac. The patient is ambulated to distribute the contrast material evenly throughout the amniotic fluid. The radiologist should select the proper projection. For suspected neural tube defects, one must obtain true lateral views of the fetal back, since many such lesions are flat or scooped out and may be obscured by the slightest degree of rotation. Real-time ultrasonography may be used to determine the exact fetal position. (If appropriate, a film also can be taken 24 to 48 hours later to show the fetal digestive tract, outlined by fetal swallowing of amniotic fluid containing contrast material. However, since polyhydramnios dilutes the contrast material and renders amniography difficult to interpret, the use of amniography in gastrointestinal tract obstruction is limited.)

Fetography utilizes an oil-soluble contrast material injected into the amniotic fluid that then adheres to the vernix caseosa and clarifies fetal surface contours. About 9 ml of iophendylate, diiodostearate, or iodinated poppy-seed oil can be used. Absorption of the contrast material by the vernix is complete in about 24 hours. These oily iodinated materials may have minor effects on the fetal thyroid. The major risk of these procedures is an increase in spontaneous abortions, probably about 0.5 to 3.0 percent.

Informed consent should be obtained, including discussion of the limitations and risks of prenatal radiographic procedures — all of which usually require less than 1 rad of fetal exposure. Although potentially teratogenic or carcinogenic, there is no evidence that fetal exposures of less than 5 rads — especially after the first trimester — increase the risk for fetal abnormality. An in utero exposure of 1 rad carries an estimated absolute risk of 1 in 1700 for cancer during the first nine years of life. This must be compared with the risks for serious autosomal recessive (1 in 4), autosomal dominant (1 in 2), or multifactorial (1 in 20 to 1 in 100) conditions to occur.

COUNSELING ISSUES IN PRENATAL DIAGNOSIS

Prenatal counseling in routine cases can be provided by the obstetrician or by a qualified genetic counselor. Complex cases require consultation with a geneticist.

A. Counseling should involve both members of the couple.
B. Goals of prenatal counseling:
   1. To provide complete and correct information
   2. To help the couple make the best decision for themselves and their family
   3. To help them implement their decision
   4. To help them make the best possible adjustment to their decision
C. All patients seeking prenatal diagnosis should know that most birth defects cannot be diagnosed prenatally. There is a background risk in every pregnancy of about 2 to 3 percent for major congenital malformations; the majority of these do not increase with parental age and cannot be detected by amniocentesis or other diagnostic methods.
D. Specific counseling for the disorder in question should include:
   1. Mode of inheritance
   2. Recurrence risk
   3. Variability of expression of the disorder
   4. Quality of life associated with survival of an affected individual; complications and prognosis
   5. Treatment available
   6. Alternatives in case of a positive diagnosis (may include elective termination of pregnancy, raising the affected child at home, placing the child in foster care)
   7. Alternatives for reproduction in the case of autosomal recessive disorders (artificial insemination by a noncarrier of the disease)
   8. Possible burden of the disorder on the affected child, the parents, the siblings
E. Specific counseling for prenatal diagnostic procedures must include:
   1. Description of the amniocentesis and ultrasound procedures
   2. Potential risks of amniocentesis. Amniocentesis is considered a safe procedure with low risk (less than 1 percent) of complications *when done by an experienced*

individual who performs a minimum of 100 midtrimester genetic amniocenteses a year.

a) Potential risks to the fetus:
   (1) Needle injury or disruption of amniotic membranes
   (2) Infection, amnionitis (1/1000)
   (3) Abortion. There is no significant difference in midtrimester fetal loss between women who have had amniocentesis and those who have not; however, the risk of fetal loss may increase with the number of needle insertions required to obtain amniotic fluid
   (4) No clear evidence of abnormalities in delivery or subsequent development of infants exposed to amniocentesis in midtrimester now exists

b) Potential risks to the mother:
   (1) Amnionitis (1/1000)
   (2) Vaginal bleeding or vaginal amniotic fluid leakage occurs in about 1 percent and is usually inconsequential
   (3) Rh isoimmunization (see G.9. above under "Amniocentesis Methods") in an Rh-negative mother

3. The time required for diagnosis (usually about one week for AFP, two to four weeks for karyotypes, longer for biochemical studies) should be explained to the couple to reduce anxiety.

4. The following relatively uncommon but potential problems must be understood by the patient:
   a) Failure to obtain amniotic fluid; failure to obtain sufficient cells for analysis; slow growth or growth failure of the cultures (none of these indicates fetal abnormality); retap may be necessary
   b) Culture contamination and loss
   c) False-positive result (e.g., in vitro mosaicism or other artifact)
   d) False-negative result (e.g., failure to detect low levels of mosaicism, maternal cell contamination)

    e) Inability to obtain results

    f) Uninterpretable results (diagnostic accuracy of fetal karyotyping is in excess of 99.5 percent)

5. The couple should be advised of the informing procedure to be used in the case of a positive diagnosis.

6. The couple should be placed under no obligation to have a test or to act in a specific way on the results. The counselor provides information, and the patients base their decision on their own moral, ethical, religious, emotional, and financial considerations. The counselor should support their decision. Different couples will interpret the burdens of a chromosomally abnormal child and of a miscarriage differently. Given the same information, they may draw different conclusions about the advisability of amniocentesis or of elective termination of pregnancy.

BIBLIOGRAPHY

Gerbie AB: Antenatal diagnosis of genetic defects. Clin Obstet Gynecol 7:1, 1980

Kaback MM: Genetic Issues in Pediatric and Obstetric Practice. Chicago, Year Book Medical, 1981

Kaback MM (ed): Symposium on medical genetics. Pediatr Clin North Am 25:3, 1978

Karp LE: Genetic Engineering: Threat or Promise? Chicago, Nelson-Hall, 1976

Milunsky A (ed): Genetic Disorders and the Fetus: Diagnosis, prevention, and treatment. New York, Plenum Press, 1979

Schulman JD, Simpson JL (eds): Genetic Diseases in Pregnancy: Maternal Effects and Fetal Outcome. New York, Academic Press, 1981

Warshaw JB (ed): Symposium on fetal disease. Clin Perinatol 6:2, 1979

9

Antenatal Assessment of Fetal Well-Being

Jessica L. Thomason, M.D.

PRACTICE PRINCIPLES

While the conscientiously practicing physician is alert to physical signs indicating impending problems during gestation, these signs may be notoriously "soft," go unnoticed by the mother, or give no identifiable external clues. Neither biochemical nor biophysical changes can be easily identified by physical examination. At times the need for obstetrical intervention can be identified long before fetal demise. The need for physicians to identify fetuses at risk has culminated in a wide variety of tests for monitoring the high-risk pregnancy. The young clinician is often overwhelmed by the enormous number of available tests and frequently cannot discern which tests are best for evaluating different high-risk problems. Two general categories of tests include *biochemical* and *biophysical* testing.

A. *Biochemical tests*. These are most helpful if they include hormonal products reflecting only fetal metabolism; however, most of these tests include products of placental metabolism, and the combined maternal-fetoplacental unit. The length of the hormones' half-life is important since a sensitive test must reflect the rapid changes of the intrauterine environment. A discussion of the common biochemical tests follows with specific review of conditions most usefully monitored by each test.

B. *Biophysical testing.* Such testing is perhaps one of the most exciting obstetrical frontiers. With the advent of noninvasive sonographic and electronic techniques for examination of the fetus, a whole array of fetal assessment has become available to the physician. These tests often reflect the immediate fetal environment, and abnormalities preceding deterioration of the fetoplacental unit can readily be identified. The rich array of testing is discussed with specific reference given to which test is best for specific high-risk conditions.

BIOCHEMICAL TESTING

A. *Estriols.* Measurement of estrogens in humans has been studied since the 1920s. As technology has advanced, over 20 estrogens and their metabolites have been measured. Presently, measurement of estrogens in the plasma and serum is being compared to the more prevalent urinary estrogen in antenatal evaluation of the fetus.

1. *Metabolism.* The fetus, placenta, and maternal compartments must be functioning properly to obtain normal estriol (E_3) values during pregnancy. Over 90 percent of E_3 excreted by the mother during her gestation is produced by the fetoplacental unit. Intact normal functioning fetal adrenals are needed to convert C-21 precursors to dehydroepiandrosterone (DHEA) sulfate, which is then converted by the fetal liver rich in the 16α-hydroxylating enzyme to 16α-hydroxydehydroepiandrosterone sulfate (see Fig. 9–1). Placental sulfatase acts on

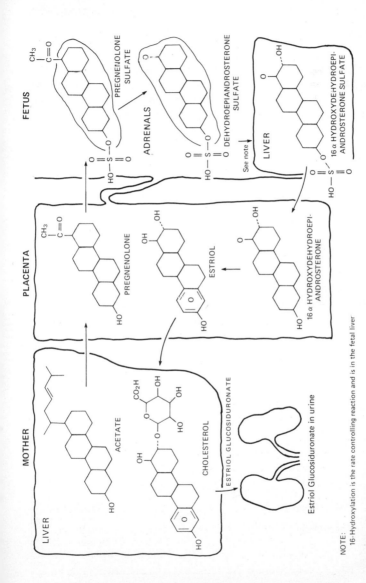

NOTE:
16-Hydroxylation is the rate controlling reaction and is in the fetal liver

Figure 9–1. Pathway of estriol biosynthesis in late pregnancy. (From Beischer NA: Obstet Gynecol Surv 24:320, 1969. Courtesy of Williams & Wilkins Co., Baltimore.)

this metabolite to form various 16α-hydroxylated androgens and by aromatase converts this to estriol (16α-hydroxyestradiol). Free or unconjugated E_3 enters the maternal circulation, where it undergoes conjugation by the liver with sufuric and glucuronic acid. Some of the conjugated E_3 is excreted in the urine, but a large portion enters the enterohepatic circulation. Secretion with the bile into the small intestine occurs, where bacteria unconjugate E_3. The unconjugated form is reabsorbed through gut mucosa to be reconjugated with glucuronic and sufuric acid, and the cycle is repeated.

At any point the sequence of events may be interrupted and cause spuriously low E_3 levels (Table 9-1). For example, steroids given to the mother will depress fetal corticotropin production and subsequently depress 16α-hydroxy metabolites from the fetus. Lack of functioning fetal adrenal tissue, as is seen in anencephaly, causes low E_3 levels. Placental sulfatase deficiency results in markedly reduced E_3 levels. Maternal antibiotics such as ampicillin and mandelamine interefere with the enterohepatic circulation, causing increased conjugated E_3

TABLE 9–1. FACTORS CAUSING INACCURATE ESTRIOL MEASUREMENT

Maternal Problems	Placental Problems
Medical diseases— hepatic, renal disease	Sulfatase deficiency
Habits—smoking	Abruption
Drug ingestion— antibiotics, aspirin, steroids	Infarction
Fetal Problems	**Collection Problems**
Anecephaly	Inadequate collections
	Position of mother
	Circadian rhythm

to be excreted in the feces rather than being unconjugated and reabsorbed as in the normal pathway. Severe
maternal hepatic or renal disease may also affect E_3
levels.

2. *Laboratory tests*

   a) Common laboratory tests include urinary "estriol,"
   plasma or serum "free" or "conjugated" estriol, and
   "spot" urinary E_3/creatinine ratios. Due to diurnal
   variation, inherent in both urinary E_3 and creatinine
   levels, as well as other confounding variables, the
   E_3/creatinine ratio has not been found to be accurate
   enough to correct for these fluctuations and is not
   routinely recommended when other tests are available.

   b) Most laboratories measure *24-hour urinary "estriols,"*
   but with the various methods of assay these reports
   may reflect urinary estrogen metabolites in addition to
   pure E_3 conjugates. This is not of grave importance,
   since over 90 percent of urinary estrogens are E_3-
   conjugates and decreasing E_3 — indicating fetal placental compromise — may still be recognized. Normal
   urinary estriols are shown for the duration of pregnancy in Fig. 9–2. Single urinary 24-hour collections
   are of less value clinically than are biweekly or daily
   collections. With more frequent collections a generalized trend in the pattern of secretion by the patient
   can be evaluated. *A drop of 35 percent from the mean
   of previous 24-hour collections is considered significant.*

   c) *Plasma or serum levels of estrogens* provide more
   rapid evaluation of the fetal placental unit and are
   more convenient for the patient; however, diurnal
   variation must be acknowledged. This can be
   minimized if the test is drawn with the patient in the
   same position at the same time each day. Unconjugated free plasma E_3 levels reflect the most recent
   changes in the functioning fetal placental unit with a

146

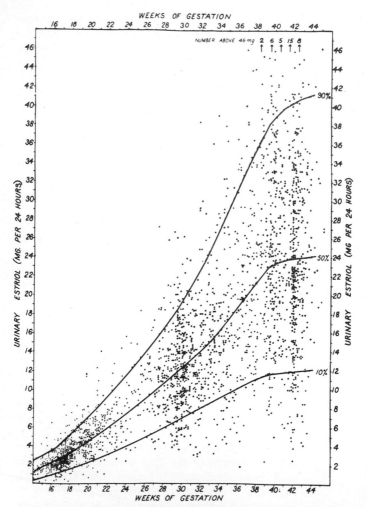

Figure 9–2. Estriol values from 14 weeks of gestation showing 10th, 50th, and 90th percentiles. (From Beischer, et al.: Am J Obstet Gynecol 103:485, 1969.)

half-life of 30 minutes. Conjugated E_3 has half-life of 4 hours. Normal plasma total estriol concentrations are shown in Figure 9–3.

d) E_4 (estetrol) has not been found to be of any greater value in assessing the fetus than estriols. For this reason most clinical laboratories do not offer measurement of this estrogen routinely.

3. *Clinical situations*

a) *Diabetes mellitus*. Daily or biweekly rising values can be reassuring. The measurement of E_3 is controversial due to the fact that antepartum impending fetal distress or demise can be missed due to rapid decrease in E_3.

b) *Intrauterine growth retardation*. IUGR pregnancies frequently are associated with *low E_3 values*. Rapid drops should alert the physician for the need to further evaluate this already compromised fetus.

c) *Postmaturity*. Estriol values normally fall after 40 weeks' gestation after having risen throughout pregnancy. When assessing *prolonged gestation* rising serial estriols have been associated with good fetal outcome. Dropping levels require close examination of the pregnancy and intervention if other parameters, such as the OCT, are also suspicious or indicate fetal distress.

d) *Hypertensive disorders of pregnancy*. Good correlation between fetal distress and dropping or low values.

e) *Limitations*. A number of disease states cause conditions that limit the usefulness of estriol measurements, namely, Rh disease, multiple gestation, trophoblastic diseases, and congential anomalies.

B. *Human chorionic gonadotropin*. Human chorionic gonadotropin (hCG) is a glycoprotein produced and secreted by the syncytiotrophoblast and has both α-and β-subunits. *The presence of hCG is the most accurate hormonal determination of viable trophoblastic tissue located somewhere in the body*. The α-subunit amino acid sequence is similar to human luteinizing hormone (hLH) and human follicle-stimulating

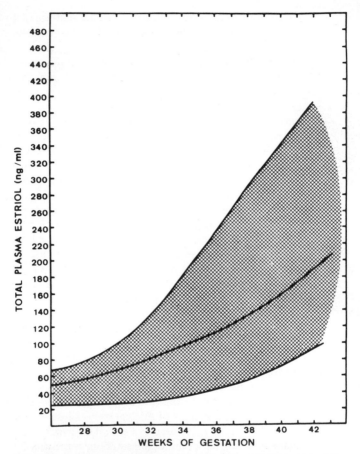

Figure 9-3. Plasma estriol concentration. The shaded area includes the 10th–90th percentiles. (From Gabbe SG: Clin Obstet Gynecol 21:359, 1978. Courtesy of Lippincott/Harper & Row.)

hormone (hFSH), and biologic activity between these hormones exists. The β-subunit is also similar to hLH but has some unique amino acid sequences, these constituting the basis for modern laboratory determination of hCG. However, some minimal cross reactivity with hLH exists in even the best of assays.

1. *Metabolism.* hCG is produced by the blastocyst, and although detection in maternal serum before implantation is controversial, it can be detected by the ninth or tenth day after ovulation. Thereafter, there is a steady rise in hCG through the first trimester to levels of 100,000 IU/ml or greater, with a slow decline in levels during the second trimester and persistent lower levels until after delivery. The *half-life* of hCG is 1.5 days, allowing one to calculate the clinical disappearance of the hormone if the original titer was known. A diurnal variation has little clinical significance, peak levels having been noted between 9:00 A.M. and noon. No variation in levels between male and female fetuses has been found, and clearance rates are unchanged throughout pregnancy.

2. *Function*
   a) hCG functions to maintain the corpus luteum early in pregnancy, after which the fetoplacental unit is able to shift to its own progesterone maintenance.
   b) hCG has been found to stimulate steroidogenesis in the fetoplacental unit, as well as stimulate testosterone production in male fetuses. Peak levels of hCG occur at the time of peak fetal serum testosterone levels.
   c) The function of hCG in ovarian development is less clear.
   d) An immunosuppressive effect has been noted with hCG, some authors suggesting that the hormone is necessary in allowing fetal tissue to be immunologically privileged.
   e) hCG has also been found to have some thyrotropic activity, presumably secondary to similar subunit amino acid sequences.

3. *Tests.* Laboratory tests for hCG may be divided into (1) biologic tests, (2) immunologic tests, and (3) radioimmunoassay (RIA).

   a) *Biologic tests* are not clinically useful because of their lack of sensitivity, specificity, and the time required for results.

   b) *Immunologic tests* are widely available commercially for both urine and serum. These tests work by classic antigen-antibody responses utilizing either direct agglutination or agglutination-inhibition reactions. Many of these tests are clinically useful, and rapid, reliable results can be obtained. However, sensitivity is a limiting factor, with 1 to 5 IU/ml being required before a positive test result is obtained with most test systems.

   c) *Radioimmunoassay* has a sensitivity of 5 to 10 mIU/ml. *Presently, this is the most sensitive and specific test available, and a negative test virtually rules out the chance of pregnancy anywhere within the body.* A positive test result indicates viable trophoblastic tissue; however, some neoplasms have been identified that produce hCG. These include melanomas, lymphomas, and some malignancies of the ovary, testis, and gastrointestinal tract, among others. High levels of hCG have been reported in some pregnancies complicated by multiple gestation, diabetes, Rh isoimmunization, and hypertension, although the significance of these is unknown.

4. *Clinical situations*

   a) *Early gestation* may be identified by most immunologic tests six weeks after the last missed period. Radioimmunoassays can detect pregnancy before the first missed period.

   b) Ectopic hormonal production can be confirmed if the uterus is devoid of a gestational sac and is helpful in the diagnosis of ectopic gestation or a tumor producing hCG.

      c) Low or falling levels are helpful in evaluating the threatened, incomplete, or missed abortion when combined with ultrasonographic examination of the uterus.

C. *Human placental lactogen (hPL)*. Other names for this same hormone include human chorionic somatomammotropin (hCS), chorionic growth-hormone prolactin (CGP), and purified placental lactogen (PPL). A large protein of 190 amino acids, it is the major placental product—more than 1 gm being produced at term.

  1. *Metabolism*

      a) Although having 60 to 80 percent amino acid sequences identical to human growth hormone and prolactin, hPL has been found to have minimal growth-promoting (somatotropic) activity, and evidence to support the lactogenic activity found in animal models is lacking in human studies. However, hPL has been studied extensively for its effect on carbohydrate metabolism during pregnancy. *hPL has both diabetogenic and insulinogenic properties,* yet studies presenting contradictory data abound and make total understanding of its function on glucose metabolism inexact. The most consistent finding is that maternal hypoglycemia causes an increase in plasma concentrations. This increase allows maternal mobilization of free fatty acids, facilitating hepatic glyconeogenesis with the resultant glucose substrate for fetal metabolism. As a result, the fetus is protected at all times, having available fuel for its metabolism regardless of maternal nutritional habits.

      b) hPL is synthesized by the syncytiotrophoblast with a half-life of approximately 30 minutes. It is detected by radioreceptor and radioimmunoassay, with the latter having higher specificity. As early as six to eight weeks from the last missed period, hPL can be detected in maternal blood. First-trimester values range from 0.1 to 1 μg/ml, while second-trimester values increase to 3 μg/ml (2–4), and third-trimester values of 5 to 10 μg/ml are normal. hPL secretion is constant and does not change due to maternal position, activity, or smoking habit. There is no circadian pattern to secretion nor is there any effect due to the onset of labor, of fetal sex, or fetal weight. Although increasing values of hPL during pregnancy seem to correlate with increasing placental mass, the finding is not a constant one.

c) hPL values increase throughout normal pregnancy until 37 weeks, at which time they reach a plateau or decline slightly. A value of 4 μg/ml or less in the third trimester is considered to be in the *fetal danger zone* and should alert the physician to examine the pregnancy for possible problems.

2. *Specific conditions*

   a) *Threatened abortion.* Attempts have been made to examine pregnancy outcomes and hPL values early in gestation. Although normal first-trimester values are reassuring, 20 percent of such women may proceed to abortion. An isolated low hPL value cannot be used as the sole criterion for terminating a threatened gestation.

   b) *Diabetes mellitus.* hPL values have been found to be of *limited value,* since large placentas (e.g., more syncytiotrophoblasts and higher hPL values) may occur in pregnancies with eventual poor fetal outcome.

   c) *Isoimmunization.* Normal or slightly elevated values are found and *cannot be used to predict fetal outcome.*

   d) *Multiple gestation.* Studies show *consistently higher values* than with normal singleton pregnancies regardless of fetal outcome.

   e) *Fetal anomalies.* Results *usually demonstrate normal values* regardless of major or minor congenital deformities, as could be expected with a normal, intact functioning placenta.

   f) *Postmaturity.* When dates are accurate, *low hPL*

values can be useful to alert the physician to an endangered fetus. Sonography and amniocentesis can also add information that in combination with falling hPL values, may dictate further evaluation and/or delivery.

g) *Intrauterine growth retardation* (IUGR). A *variable pattern* of hPL values may be seen. IUGR may be due to diseases of the placenta, fetus, or mother. IUGR on the basis of placental disease results in low values. In IUGR on the basis of fetal or maternal indications, however, hPL values are variable.

h) *Hypertension/toxemia.* In this complex group of diseases, if a low hPL value is found, careful examination of the gestation with other parameters seems warranted. It is in this group that low values have been associated most directly by some authors with fetal demise and/or compromise, especially in patients found to have small placentas associated with the disease process. *Pregnancies with hPL values in the "fetal danger zone" (less than 4 µg/ml in the third trimester) should be examined closely.*

D. α-*Fetoprotein.* (AFP) is a glycoprotein produced by the fetus from the yolk sac and liver beginning as early as eight days postconception. This is the major serum protein in fetal life, analogous to serum albumin in adult life, but its exact function to the fetus is unknown. During fetal life from early conception, AFP rises, peak production by the fetus is at 14 weeks' gestation, resulting in fetal serum levels of 2 to 3 mg/ml. Thereafter, fetal production falls during gestation and reaches adult levels by one to two years. Although fetal serum levels are measured in milligrams per milliliter, amniotic fluid levels are measured in micrograms per milliliter and maternal serum levels in nanograms per milliliter. A concentration gradient exists from fetal serum to maternal serum, and although fetal serum levels fall after 14 weeks, maternal serum levels rise progressively until 32 to 34 weeks, after which a decline is also noted. *Before 16 to 18 weeks' gestation, measurement of maternal serum levels is not reliably detectable, although measurement is theoretically possible as early as 12 to 13 weeks.* AFP is detected in laboratories by immunoelectrophoresis or radioimmunoassay. The half-life of AFP is measured in days. *Both high as well as low levels of AFP are of concern and should alert the physician to examine the pregnancy more carefully.* Gestational dating is possible with accurate amniotic fluid AFP levels, especially in late pregnancy when the standard deviation of levels is less.

1. *Low levels of AFP.* Low levels, especially in the early second trimester, have been found to indicate *impending fetal demise.* Likewise, pregnancies complicated by a blighted ovum have been found to have low levels in the first trimester.

2. *High levels of AFP*
   a) High levels have been found in association with various congenital defects, in conditions of placental separation, as an indicator of fetal distress or impending fetal demise, and in normal pregnancy conditions of multiple gestation. High levels have been found in pregnancies complicated by diabetes and Rh isoimmunization; however, low or normal levels in these high-risk situations are not always correlated with fetal distress or demise. Other tests used in combination with AFP are helpful to evaluate these complicated conditions.
   b) Elevated AFP levels have been found in the following congenital conditions:
      (1) Congenital nephrosis
      (2) Tetralogy of Fallot
      (3) Esophageal and/or duodenal atresia
      (4) Cervical hygroma
      (5) Omphalocele/gastroschisis
      (6) Some chromosomal abnormalities such as Down's syndrome
      (7) Ataxiatelangiectasia
      (8) Open neural tube defects (NTDs)
         (a) Anencephaly

(b) Myeloceles

(c) Some cases of hydrocephalus

(d) Closed NTDs are not associated with abnormal AFP levels

3. *Neural tube defects*

a) The *prevalence rate* of significant NTDs in the United States is approximately 1 per 1000 live births. The economic and social impact of such a child is enormous and would appear to easily offset the economic expense of mass screening programs initiated to identify such pregnancies at risk. The mother's serum must be screened between 15 and 19 weeks' gestation to avoid false-positive and false-negative results.

b) Six to eight percent of pregnancies screened in the United States in this manner will have AFP values three to five standard deviations from the mean. Significance is usually considered five standard deviations above the mean. A second maternal serum screen will eliminate 2 to 3 percent of the original 6 to 8 percent of high values, leaving 4 to 6 percent of mothers requiring further evaluation. With ultrasound elimination of multiple gestation and incorrect gestational age, 2 percent will require amniocentesis. This is easily performed at 16 to 19 weeks' gestation. Contamination of amniotic fluid with fetal red blood cells can falsely elevate AFP levels. Detection of this condition by the Kleihauer-Betke test eliminates any doubt. Should this occur, repeat amniocentesis can be carried out after 10 days. *Pregnancies with elevated amniotic AFP levels indicate a NTD and counseling of the parents should be instituted. Also, genetic counseling must be given for future pregnancies, since in 3 to 5 percent of these NTD will recur; a history of two previously affected pregnancies carries a 10 percent recurrence risk.*

E. *Pregnancy-specific β_1-glycoprotein*

1. This placental hormone was first characterized in the early 1970s and *has not gained wide acceptance as a useful*

test of the fetoplacental unit. It is produced by the syncytiotrophoblast as early as 7 days postovulation; levels increase generally until the 36th week of gestation, at which time they stabilize. One of the problems with its acceptance as an antenatal screening tool is its long half-life of 30 to 40 hours. Thus, the rapid changes that frequently occur in a high-risk pregnancy are not reflected by measurement of the hormone. Since it does not cross react with other glycoproteins having α- and β-subunits, detection in early pregnancy makes it a good candidate as an indicator of trophoblastic tissue. However, studies examining levels associated with gestational trophoblastic disease do not show any clear-cut advantage over conventional β-subunit hCG determinations.

2. The biologic function of β_1-glycoprotein is unknown.
3. At present, pregnancies complicated by IUGR give the most consistent β_1-glycoprotein measurement results, usually low or low normal levels. If low levels are found, further evaluation is indicated.

F. *Creatinine phosphokinase*
   1. Creatinine phosphokinase (CPK) is an enzyme that has been reported in many body tissues, but mainly in muscle. The enzyme functions in ATP-ADP reactions, liberating energy in the process. It is measured in amniotic fluid for the diagnosis of fetal demise. Prior to the availability of ultrasound to diagnose fetal demise, the methods in use could not detect positive signs of the death before several days or weeks had passed. A more accurage diagnosis was available with the measurement of amniotic CPK levels. Normal amniotic fluid levels are 0 to 30 ng/ml. Pregnancies complicated by fetal demise have a rapid daily rise of CPK well into the 100 ng/ml range at three to four days after death.
   2. *With the availability of ultrasonography, measurement of amniotic CPK levels for the diagnosis of fetal demise is only useful for research purposes.*

G. *Diamine oxidase*
   1. Diamine oxidase (DAO) is an enzyme whose origin is the

retroplacental maternal decidua. The enzyme destroys histamine, and although its exact function remains unknown, it is thought to be a maternal protector against the histamine and other diamines formed by the fetus. Its activity increases markedly into the 1000 unit range after pregnancy. Nonpregnant levels (3.4 ± 1.5 units) have been found in patients with gestational trophoblastic diseases. Unfortunately, levels of DAO appear only after four weeks of conception, and concentrations of this enzyme thus lag behind human chorionic gonadotropin levels by 7 to 10 days.

2. DAO has not been helpful in evaluating patients who are habitual aborters, have incompetent cervical os, or who have a poor obsetrical history. Its usefulness in evaluating pregnancies complicated by diabetes remains controversial. Perhaps its only use at this time has been the observation that in pregnancies doomed to abortion, low levels are usually seen, or the usual rise seen as the gestation advances is obliterated. *Its application as a useful, widespread antenatal screening tool for high-risk pregnancies has been unsuccessful.*

H. *Oxytocinase*

1. Oxytocinase (also known as *cystine aminopeptidase*) is a placental glycoprotein produced by the syncytiotrophoblast from the early first trimester until term. Demonstrating a sigmoid-shaped curve in normal pregnancy, with the steeper portion occurring at 32 weeks, its half-life of several days makes its usefulness somewhat limited. The function of oxytocinase is unknown.

2. The main usefulness of measuring oxytocinase may reside in the fact that it is a stable enzyme and can be easily assayed and that the results are easily reproducible. *However, its usefulness as an antepartum monitoring tool remains limited.* Values found in high-risk pregnancies have failed to show any correlation with fetal weights and correlation with placental weight is controversial. Its application in patients with IUGR has failed to be as useful as other monitoring techniques. While some multi-

ple gestations have high levels, others are found to be normal.

BIOPHYSICAL TESTING

A. *Fetal electronic monitoring.* A discussion of the advantages versus risks from electronic monitoring in antepartum and intrapartum pregnant patients is not germane to this chapter, and the reader is referred to the bibliographic listing for further information. Nor is a discussion of the various instruments available both in clinical and research situations relevant here. First, a description of fetal monitoring necessary for basic understanding of the method and the technical limiations of the various monitoring techniques are presented so that interpretation of electronic data can be performed accurately. This is followed by an explanation and evaluation of antepartum electronic fetal testing.

  1. *Terminology*
     a) Uterine irritability or contractions and frequency of contractions may be monitored by direct and indirect methods. External palpation of the intensity of uterine contractions may be grossly inaccurate, as has been proven in numerous studies. Contractions may be monitored electronically in an "indirect" way by placing a tocodynamometer on the mother's abdominal wall. The *frequency* and *duration* of the contraction are accurately monitored by this method. *Intensity* of the contraction is accurately reflected only by "direct" monitoring, e.g., placing a catheter filled with sterile water into the maternal uterus and attaching this to a pressure sensor, thus measuring intrauterine pressures (intrauterine pressure catheter, IUPC).
     b) *Uterine measurement terminology*
        (1) *Resting tone* of the uterus. Usually 10 mm Hg.
        (2) *Duration* of contraction. Values less than 45 seconds indicate slow labor.

    (3) *Length of time between contractions.* An *interval* of greater than 3 minutes indicates slow labor.

    (4) *Uterine amplitude.* Values greater than 75 mm Hg may indicate overstimulation. However, more accurate ways to discuss uterine activity include:

        (a) *Montevideo (M.) Units.* One unit is defined as the product of the average amplitude (mm Hg) multiplied by the frequency of uterine contractions in 10 minutes. Over 200 M. units per 10 minutes usually indicates uterine hyperstimulation.

        (b) *Alexandria (A.) units.* A unit is defined as the product of the average amplitude (mm Hg) × average duration (min) × average frequency (per 10 min). Average first-stage labor contractions, 225 A. units.

c) *Fetal heart rate (FHR) terminology*

    (1) *"Direct" or internal FHR* is more accurate and a fetal ECG is obtained by a direct electrode attached to the presenting part. The QRS complex is then amplified, filtered, counted, and finally converted to a printout for a continuous, permanent record.

    (2) *"Indirect" measurement of FHR* is by phonocardiogram, ultrasound, or abdominal electrocardiogram. Most currently available machines for clinical use employ the Doppler indirect technique. The signal undergoes the same process as the "direct" signal; however, the cardiotachometer is more accurate when the fetal wave is identified with the directly attached electrode rather than the indirect method of calculating beat-to-beat FHR.

    (3) By either method, *rate (beats/min, bpm)* is obtained by the formula: bpm = 60/interval (sec). For example, an FHR of 150 bpm recorded on the printout is obtained when the interval between beats is 0.4 seconds.

(4) *FHR Baseline Parameter.* The FHR between contractions on the area into which the FHR falls during 80 percent of a 10-minute interval.
   (a) *Normal:* 120 to 160 bpm
   (b) *Bradycardia.* Mild: 100 to 110 bpm; marked: ≤99 bpm
   (c) *Tachycardia.* Mild: 161 to 180 bpm; marked: > 180 bpm
   (d) *Variability*
      (i) *Short term.* Beat-to-beat or peak-to-peak amplitude changes in the FHR:

   0 Variability = 0 to 2 bpm
   +1 Variability = 3 to 5 bpm
   +2 Variability = 5 to 10 bpm (*normal*)
   +3 Variability = 11 to 25 bpm
   +4 Variability = >25 bpm

      (ii) *Long term.* Fluctuations of the FHR involving patterns of frequency (cycles/min) and amplitude of these cycles (range in bpm). Normal is considered 2 to 6 cycles/min with 6 to 10 bpm change.
(5) FHR *Periodic Parameter. The FHR related to uterine contractions.*
   (a) *No change.* Base line remains the same as the preceding FHR base line.
   (b) *Acceleration.* FHR increases 20 or more bpm with the uterine contraction.
   (c) *Deceleration.* FHR decreases with the uterine contraction. This is further divided into three patterns:
      (i) *Uniform pattern.* FHR patterns reflects the uterine contraction; these patterns tend to be repetitive.
      (ii) *"Early" decelerations.* FHR pattern ex-

actly mimics the uterine contraction in time of onset, maximal effect, and recovery. The pattern is indicative of head compression. Also known as type I (Caldeyro-Barcia).

(iii) *"Late" decelerations.* FHR pattern has the onset, maximal drop of FHR, and recovery lagging behind corresponding uterine contraction events. This pattern is associated with uteroplacental insufficiency. Also known as *type II (Caldeyro-Barcia)*

(d) *Variable pattern.* FHR pattern onset, maximal dip, and recovery are in a variable relationship to the uterine contraction. This is the most common pattern of FHR seen and indicates cord compression.

(e) *Mixed pattern.* Both variable and uniform patterns are present during the same uterine contraction.

2. *Pathologic correlation*

a) Base-line FHR other than normal should alert the physician to incipient or actual fetal distress.

b) *Tachycardias* may be associated with overt or occult chorioamnionitis, other causes of maternal fever, hyperthyroidism, fetal hypoxia, fetal arrhythmias, administration of various parasympathetic blocking drugs such as atropine, and administration of sympathomimetic drugs frequently used to inhibit labor such as terbutaline, ritodrine, etc.

c) *Bradycardias* may be the result of fetal arrhythmias, fetal distress, maternal hypokalemia, or administration of anesthetic agents with paracervical or epidural blocks.

d) *Decreased short-term variability* may simply reflect the sleeping cycle of the fetus or may indicate fetal hypoxia or distress, an immature or premature infant, or administration of depressant drugs to the mother.

e) *Increased short-term variability* may reflect a very active fetus or one just awakened. It can, however, indicate impending fetal distress.

f) *Accelerations* are often characteristic of an active healthy fetus and usually occur with fetal motion. However, there is some evidence that accelerations may represent fetal response to the cardiovascular compromise sometimes seen with cord compression and variable FHR decelerations.

g) *Decelerative FHR patterns* are clinically innocuous if of type I variety. Type II patterns, variable patterns, and mixed patterns are cause for close monitoring, especially since late, type II patterns have been associated with fetal hypoxia, acidosis, and distress, and can be associated with poor fetal outcome. Often, ominous patterns can be converted to more reassuring patterns by changing maternal position, avoiding portacaval-compression syndrome or deep Trendelenburg position, and by administering oxygen to the mother.

3. *Summary.* It is imperative that patterns be examined closely and conservative methods applied before considering cesarean section for fetal distress. Overall FHR patterns are correlated with the "window" or segment of FHR pattern being examined, and this is then correlated with physical exam (e.g., palpation of an umbilical cord), drugs administered to the mother, medical conditions affecting the pregnancy, and if necessary, fetal scalp blood pH before surgical intervention is entertained.

B. *Antepartum electronic monitoring*

1. *Nonstress test (NST)*

a) *Technique.* The patient is placed in the semi-Fowler position with a slight tilt to the left to avoid portacaval-compression syndrome and the electronic monitoring devices applied. After a satisfactory baseline FHR pattern has been obtained, the mother or an observer marks when fetal movement is felt, and the FHR is examined in relation to the movement. The test is generally run for a 20-minute period. If no accelerations are evident, some centers allow for a second 20-minute "window" of observation, since some fetuses have been documented to enter sleep cycles varying from 10 to 90 minutes.

b) *Test result classifications*
   - *Reactive.* FHR accelerations associated with fetal motion of 15 bpm lasting 15 seconds on two occasions during a 20-minute window.
   - *Nonreactive.* Any FHR pattern over 20 minutes not fulfilling "reactive" test criteria, e.g., accelerations not lasting 15 seconds; only one acceleration during 20 minutes.
   - *Unsatisfactory.* FHR patterns inadequate for interpretation due to technical failure or uncooperative fetus.

c) *Reliability*
   (1) *False-negatives* (test read a "reactive" when it was nonreactive). Reported less than 1 percent.
   (2) *False-positive* (test read as "nonreactive"). Has been reported as 60 to 80 percent. This is frequently due to a sleeping or "at rest" fetus, maternal drug intake, or maternal hypoglycemia.

d) *Frequency of testing.* Weekly from fetal viability.

e) *Reactive* NST's should be repeated weekly or biweekly as indicated by the clinical situation. *Nonreactive* NST's should be followed immediately by further fetal well-being studies, usually including a contraction stress test.

2. *Contraction stress test (CST; Oxytocin challenge test; OCT)*
   a) *Technique:* The patient is positioned as for the NST. Blood pressure is monitored every 10 minutes. After a

satisfactory base-line tracing is obtained, Oxytocin (Pitocin) is administered at a rate of 0.5 mUnits/min, doubling the infusion concentration every 15 minutes until three contractions lasting 40 to 60 seconds occur within a 10-minute "window."

b) *Test results*
   (1) Negative. No late decelerations occur at any point during the tracing prior to the test, during the OCT, and during the observation period after the oxytocin.
   (2) Positive. Late decelerations occurring in more than 50 percent of the uterine contractions, whether spontaneous or induced.
   (3) Suspicious. Late decelerations occurring in less than 50 percent of the uterine contractions.
   (4) Hyperstimulation. Decelerations occur due to excessive uterine stimulation, e.g., more than three contractions per 10 minutes or hypertonus of the base-line uterine tone.
   (5) Unsatisfactory. FHR pattern inadequate for interpretation due to technical failure or unresponsiveness of the uterus

c) *Reliability*
   (1) False-negative (defined as fetal death within one week of a negative OCT). Less than 1 percent.
   (2) False-positive (OCT positive but no evidence of fetal distress during labor). About 25 to 50 percent.
   (3) *Frequency of testing.* Weekly from fetal viability.

d) *Contraindications*
   (1) Patients at risk for uterine rupture such as previous cesarean section, severe polyhydramnios.
   (2) Patients at risk for premature labor, e.g., incompetent cervical os, previous premature labor.
   (3) Patients with vaginal bleeding of unknown etiology.
   (4) Placenta previa.

3. *Summary*. Since 75 percent of fetal deaths occur in the antepartum period, monitoring, whether biochemical or biophysical, is necessary to prevent these. Often biochemical testing is "inadequate" because of limitations of the test, patient noncompliance, or results "suggestive" of impending demise. Biophysical testing is helpful in these situations to confirm fetal jeopardy and dictate the need for intervention or to reassure the worried mother and obstetrician of fetal well-being. In conditions not easily monitored by the standard biochemical tests, NSTs and OCTs may be the only monitoring mechanism. For example, patients with poor obstetrical histories, including previous unexplained stillbirths, or patients with heart diseases, hemoglobinopathies, or poor nutritional status all present difficulties to management with biochemical assays. Other indications are pregnancies complicated by diabetes, Rh isoimmunization, multiple gestation, and disorders implicating placental abnormality such as the hypertensive disorders of pregnancy, postterm pregnancies, and intrauterine growth retardation.

At the point of fetal viability (28–30 weeks), all "at risk" pregnancies should be started on weekly NST examinations. The advantages of the NST are that large populations of high-risk pregnancies may be screened rapidly and relatively inexpensively in an outpatient setting; however, its lack of specificity (up to 80 percent false-negative) is a shortcoming. *If the NST is nonreactive, an OCT is indicated*. Retrospective analyses reveal lowest perinatal losses in pregnancies with serially obtained reactive NSTs and negative OCTs. Highest perinatal mortality rates are seen in pregnancies with nonreactive NSTs and positive OCTs.

C. *Ultrasound. Ultrasonography is a noninvasive technique of examining internal human structures, including the pregnant uterus and contents, by sound waves*. Because it has thus far proved safe for the fetus and mother and since it is a noninvasive technique, its clinical usefulness during gestation cannot be overemphasized. There are two basic types of ultrasonographic scanners available: static-image and dynamic-image. The *dynamic-image or "real-time" scanner* is clinically useful in outpatient settings for quick diagnosis and to detect fetal motion. *The static-image scanner* is necessary for some parameter measurements such as intrauterine volumes and has better resolution than dynamic-image machines. Both types of instruments have the technical ability to show structures in varying shades of gray and can also be termed *gray-scale* scanners. With either technique, tissue is examined in both the sagittal and transverse planes to the pelvis. A transducer is placed on the area to be studied. It produces preselected sound wave vibrations in a rapid manner with a frequency of 2 to 5 MHz (million vibrations per second) depending on the transducer selected. Echoes are produced as the sound waves bounce off the tissue they meet, and *images with the greatest resolution are produced when the sound waves are at precise right angles to the tissue being examined.* An oscilloscope displays the echoes and photographs of the display can be retained for the patient's record if desired.

1. *Structures examined*
   a) *Head size,* or *biparietal diameter (BPD),* has been studied in detail and related to fetal growth and gestational age. The measurement is made from the leading edges of the skull tables, which begin to appear around twelve weeks of gestation. Table 9-2 is a standard nomogram for determining gestational age from BPD measurements. However, it must be realized that populations in different areas of the country may have small differences in fetal skull growth, and it is generally best to obtain fetal growth curves developed from serial measurements made in the same area where one is practicing. The BPD grows at predictable rates: 4 mm/week at 16 to 28 weeks, 2 mm/week at 28 to 36 weeks, and 1.2 mm/week after 36 weeks. *Because of the parabolic*

nature of the growth curve and standard error of the method, *the worst time to attempt accurate dating of a pregnancy is in the last trimester of pregnancy. The best time is at 20 to 24 weeks of gestation, when growth is rapid.*

TABLE 9–2. YALE NOMOGRAM FOR BPD USING LEADING EDGE TO LEADING EDGE BASED ON B-MODE DOTS (GRATICULE)

(cm)	Weeks gestation	(cm)	Weeks gestation	(cm)	Weeks gestation
		4.2	18.9	6.9	28.1
		4.3	19.4	7.0	28.6
		4.4	19.4	7.1	29.1
		4.5	19.9	7.3	29.6
		4.6	20.4	7.4	30.0
		4.7	20.4	7.5	30.6
1.9	11.6	4.8	20.9	7.6	31.0
2.0	11.6	4.9	21.3	7.7	31.5
2.1	12.1	5.0	21.3	7.8	32.0
2.2	12.6	5.1	21.8	7.9	32.5
2.3	12.6	5.2	22.3	8.0	33.0
2.4	13.1	5.3	22.3	8.2	33.5
2.5	13.6	5.4	22.8	8.3	34.0
2.6	13.6	5.5	23.3	8.4	34.4
2.7	14.1	5.6	23.3	8.5	35.0
2.8	14.6	5.7	23.8	8.6	35.4
2.9	14.6	5.8	24.3	8.8	35.9
3.0	15.0	5.9	24.3	8.9	36.4
3.1	15.5	6.0	24.7	9.0*	36.9
3.2	15.5	6.1	25.2	9.1*	37.3
3.3	16.0	6.2	25.2	9.2*	37.8
3.4	16.5	6.3	25.7	9.3*	38.3
3.5	16.5	6.4	26.2	9.4*	38.8
3.6	17.0	6.5	26.2	9.6*	39.3
3.7	17.5	6.6	26.7	9.7*	39.8
3.8	17.9	6.7	27.2		
4.0	18.4	6.8	27.6		

*Indicates a fetus of 36 weeks or greater in a nondiabetic mother.
Courtesy of John C. Hobbins, M.D., Yale University School of Medicine.

b) Measurements of *abdominal circumference* at the level of the umbilical cord insertion, when utilized with BPD measurements, *allow easy calculation of fetal body weight*. Abdominal circumference should be read with the aid of a map reader. This is extremely helpful when accurate weight determination is critical in the management of premature labors. Before 32 weeks, the head of the fetus is always larger than the abdomen, allowing for a BPD: abdominal circumference ratio greater than 1. Between 32 and 36 weeks, the head and abdominal circumference are equal, giving a ratio equal to unity. However, after 36 weeks, the abdomen continues to grow rapidly, and the ratio decreases to less than 1. These values are helpful in evaluating adequate fetal growth and in determining if intrauterine growth retardation exists. (Table 9-3.)

c) *Crown-to-rump length* can be measured in the first trimester and can help to date pregnancies accurately. However, the fetus "tucks" its head after 12 weeks, making the measurement inaccurate thereafter. At this point, the parietal edges may begin to be measured for gestational dating.

d) *Ventricular size* may be measured and related to the *amount of cortex*. The distance between the *orbits* may be measured and related to *gestational age*.

e) Other structures that have commonly been examined closely include limb length, placental maturity, intrauterine volume and amniotic fluid. Other more sophisticated measurements have included the calculation of the cardiac postejection period, umbilical artery and vein size, kidney size and other structures.

2. *Utilization*

a) Perhaps the most common use of ultrasound is for *prediction of gestational age* whether by crown rump length, BPD measurements, or limb size measurements. Its use for accurate *prediction of fetal size,* especially when clinical determination is found to be

TABLE 9–3. ANTENATAL EVALUATION OF FETAL WEIGHT (IN GRAMS) USING ULTRASOUND MEASUREMENT OF BIPARIETAL DIAMETER AND ABDOMINAL CIRCUMFERENCE (16–21cm).

Biparietal diameters (in cm)	Abdominal Circumferences (in cm)					
	16.0	17.0	18.0	19.0	20.0	1.0
6.5	617	659	705	753	805	860
6.6	635	678	724	773	826	882
6.7	653	697	744	794	848	905
6.8	672	717	765	816	870	928
6.9	691	737	786	838	893	952
7.0	711	758	807	860	916	976
7.1	732	779	830	883	941	1,002
7.2	763	801	853	907	965	1,027
7.3	775	824	876	932	991	1,054
7.4	797	847	901	957	1,017	1,081
7.5	820	871	925	983	1,044	1,109
7.6	844	896	951	1,009	1,072	1,137
7.7	868	921	977	1,037	1,100	1,167
7.8	894	947	1,004	1,065	1,129	1,197
7.9	919	974	1,032	1,094	1,159	1,228
8.0	946	1,002	1,061	1,123	1,189	1,259
8.1	973	1,030	1,090	1,153	1,221	1,292
8.2	1,001	1,059	1,120	1,185	1,253	1,325
8.3	1,030	1,089	1,151	1,217	1,286	1,359
8.4	1,060	1,120	1,183	1,249	1,320	1,394
8.5	1,091	1,151	1,216	1,283	1,355	1,430
8.6	1,122	1,184	1,249	1,318	1,390	1,467
8.7	1,155	1,218	1,284	1,353	1,427	1.505
8.8	1,188	1,252	1,319	1,390	1,465	1,543
8.9	1,222	1,287	1,356	1,428	1,503	1,583
9.0	1,258	1,324	1,393	1,456	1,543	1,624
9.1	1,294	1,361	1,432	1,506	1,584	1,666
9.2	1,332	1,400	1,471	1,546	1,626	1,709
9.3	1,370	1,439	1,512	1,588	1,668	1,753
9.4	1,410	1,480	1,554	1,631	1,712	1,798
9.5	1,450	1,522	1,597	1,675	1,758	1,844

(Continued)

From Shepard MJ, et al.: An evaluation of two equations for predicting fetal weight by ultrasound. Am J Obstet/Gynecol 142:47, 1982.

TABLE 9–3 (Cont.). ANTENATAL EVALUATION OF FETAL WEIGHT (IN GRAMS) USING ULTRASOUND MEASUREMENT OF BIPARIETAL DIAMETER AND ABDOMINAL CIRCUMFERENCE (22–27 cm).

Biparietal diameters (in cm)	Abdominal circumferences (in cm)					
	22.0	23.0	24.0	25.0	26.0	27.0
6.5	919	982	1,049	1,121	1,198	1,280
6.6	942	1,006	1,074	1,147	1,225	1.308
6.7	965	1,030	1,100	1,174	1.253	1,337
6.8	990	1,056	1,126	1,201	1,281	1,367
6.9	1,015	1,082	1,153	1,229	1,310	1,397
7.0	1,040	1,108	1,181	1,258	1,340	1,427
7.1	1,066	1,135	1,209	1,287	1,370	1,459
7.2	1,093	1,163	1,238	1,317	1,401	1,491
7.3	1,121	1,192	1,267	1,348	1,433	1,524
7.4	1,149	1,221	1,297	1,379	1,465	1,557
7.5	1,178	1,251	1,328	1,411	1,499	1,592
7.6	1,207	1,281	1,360	1,444	1,533	1,627
7.7	1,238	1,313	1,393	1,477	1,567	1,663
7.8	1,269	1,345	1,426	1,512	1,603	1,699
7.9	1,301	1,378	1,460	1,547	1,639	1,737
8.0	1,333	1,412	1,495	1,583	1,676	1,775
8.1	1,367	1,446	1,531	1,620	1,714	1,814
8.2	1,401	1,482	1,567	1,657	1,753	1,854
8.3	1,436	1,518	1,605	1,696	1,793	1,895
8.4	1,473	1,555	1,643	1,735	1,833	1,936
8.5	1,510	1,594	1,682	1,776	1,875	1,979
8.6	1,548	1,633	1,722	1,817	1,917	2,022
8.7	1,586	1,673	1,764	1,859	1,960	2,067
8.8	1,626	1,714	1,806	1,903	2,005	2,113
8.9	1,667	1,756	1,849	1,947	2,050	2,159
9.0	1,709	1,799	1,893	1,992	2,097	2,207
9.1	1,752	1,843	1,938	2,039	2,144	2,255
9.2	1,796	1,888	1,984	2,086	2,193	2,305
9.3	1,841	1,934	2,032	2,135	2,242	2,356
9.4	1,887	1,982	2,080	2,184	2,293	2,407
9.5	1,935	2,030	2,130	2,235	2,345	2,460

(Continued)

TABLE 9–3 (Cont.). ANTENATAL EVALUATION OF FETAL WEIGHT (IN GRAMS) USING ULTRASOUND MEASUREMENT OF BIPARIETAL DIAMETER AND ABDOMINAL CIRCUMFERENCE (28–34 cm).

Biparietal diameters (in cm)	Abdominal circumferences (in cm)						
	28.0	29.0	30.0	31.0	32.0	33.0	34.0
6.5	1,368	1,462	1,562	1,669	1,784	1,906	2.037
6.6	1,397	1,492	1,594	1,702	1,817	1,941	2,073
6.7	1,427	1,523	1,626	1,735	1,852	1,976	2,109
6.8	1,458	1,555	1,658	1,769	1,887	2,012	2,147
6.9	1,489	1,587	1,692	1,803	1,922	2,049	2.184
7.0	1,521	1,620	1,726	1,839	1,959	2,087	2,223
7.1	1,553	1,654	1,761	1,875	1,996	2,125	2,262
7.2	1,586	1,688	1,796	1,911	2,044	2,164	2,302
7.3	1,620	1,723	1,832	1,948	2,072	2,203	2,343
7.4	1,655	1,759	1,869	1,987	2,111	2,244	2,384
7.5	1,690	1,795	1,907	2,025	2,151	2,265	2,426
7.6	1,727	1,833	1,945	2,065	2,192	2,326	2,469
7.7	1,764	1,871	1,985	2,105	2,233	2,369	2,513
7.8	1,801	1,910	2,025	2,146	2,275	2,412	2,557
7.9	1,840	1,949	2,065	2,188	2,318	2,456	2,603
8.0	1,879	1,990	2,107	2,231	2,362	2,501	2,649
8.1	1,919	2,031	2,149	2,275	2,407	2,547	2,695
8.2	1,960	2,073	2,193	2,319	2,462	2,594	2,743
8.3	2,002	2,116	2,237	2,364	2,499	2,641	2,791
8.4	2,045	2,160	2,282	2,410	2,546	2,689	2,841
8.5	2,089	2,205	2,328	2,457	2,594	2,739	2,891
8.6	2,134	2,251	2,375	2,505	2,643	2,789	2,942
8.7	2,179	2,298	2,423	2,554	2,693	2,840	2,994
8.8	2,226	2,346	2,472	2,604	2,744	2,892	3,047
8.9	2,274	2,394	2,521	2,655	2,796	2,944	3,101
9.0	2,322	2,444	2,572	2,707	2,849	2,998	3,155
9.1	2,372	2,495	2,624	2,760	2,903	3,053	3,211
9.2	2,423	2,547	2,677	2,814	2,958	3,109	3,268
9.3	2,475	2,599	2,731	2,869	3,014	3,166	3,326
9.4	2,527	2,653	2,786	2,925	3,070	3,224	3,384
9.5	2,582	2,709	2,842	2,982	3,129	3,283	3,444

more difficult (e.g., low-weight and large-weight babies), cannot be overestimated. Critical decisions directing methods of delivery as well as directing whether to inhibit premature labor or allow labor, are more easily accomplished when accurate fetal weight is known.

b) *Total intrauterine volume (TIUV)* can be calculated from measurements made by the use of static scanner. In employing static scanning of the uterus in the anteroposterior, transverse, and sagittal planes, the following measurements should be obtained: L (longitudinal), T (transverse), and AP (anteroposterior). By using a simplified formula for the volume of an ellipse ($V = 0.5233 \times L \times T \times AP$), the intrauterine volume may be approximated. Plotting this value on a nomogram (Fig. 9–4), the *diagnosis of intrauterine growth retardation (IUGR) can be suspected if the TIUV for a pregnancy is 1.5 standard deviations below the predicted TIUV for the given gestational age.* Often this is the only accurate test that can alert the obstetrician to this high-risk problem, especially early in the pregnancy, since babies with IUGR show first a loss of amniotic fluid volume, followed by a decrease in body mass, and finally a slowing of head growth. IUGR may also be suspected with inappropriate head-to-abdominal circumference ratios, as noted in the previous section.

c) Routine use of the ultrasound in all pregnancies requiring *anniocentesis* allows this procedure to be safer, avoiding placental trauma and helping to localize pockets of fluid. Guessing to avoid the fetal injury and trying to locate fluid has no place in modern obstetrics.

d) More recently, *the maturation process of the placenta* has been examined, and findings in this area are most helpful in term pregnancies. Placental morphology on ultrasound showing evidence of maturity gives the

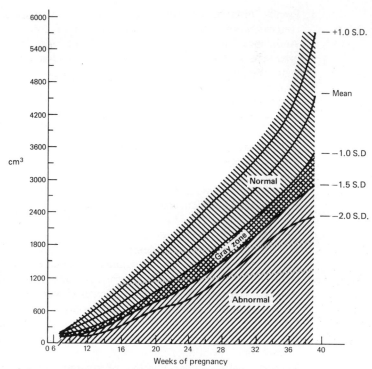

Figure 9–4. Determination of total intrauterine volume. (Adapted from Gohari P, Berkowitz, RL, Hobbin, DC: Am J Obstet Gynecol 127:255, 1977.)

physician another gauge of the estimated date of confinement when menstrual dates are inaccurate.

e) The use of ultrasound in the patient with *vaginal bleeding* of unknown etiology is paramount in differentiating placenta previa from abruption. If neither is present, the patient may then be examined to rule out the other etiologies of vaginal bleeding during gestation.

f) Finally, ultrasound's use in the *diagnosis of various congenital anomalies* is beginning to be explored. Anomalies involving the neural tube, craniofacial area, gastrointestinal tract, kidneys, heart, abdominal wall, and other organs have been reported.

3. *Clinical conditions in which most useful*

a) *IUGR.* Ultrasonography is perhaps the best laboratory method available for diagnosis of both symmetrical and asymmetrical growth retardation.

b) *Multiple gestation.* Presently the best measurement of assessing healthy fetuses. Biochemical tests often misleading.

c) *Rh isoimmunization.* Excellent method to demonstrate ascites; useful in transfusions by avoiding excessive radiation in fetus by standard x-ray techniques.

d) *Genetic diagnosis.* Paramount importance in evaluation of many congenital defects, inborn errors of metabolism, neural tube defects, and other genetically transferable diseases.

e) *Abortion.* Useful in evaluation of abortion, aiding in early clinical decision to perform dilatation and curettage.

f) *Ectopic pregnancy.* Can confirm intrauterine-extrauterine gestation.

g) *Tumors.* Allows determination of ovarian masses often difficult to diagnose during pregnancy, as well as helping to diagnose gestational trophoblastic disease with or without concomitant intrauterine gestation.

h) *Vaginal bleeding during pregnancy.* Allows determination of placenta as origin of bleeding versus other etiologies.

4. *Safety.* Many studies are now in progress to determine long-term infant-mother effects. To date, no long-term harmful effects have been established in human tissue studies.

5. *Use when combined with other tests.* Several investigators have generated data supporting the concept that during

routine ultrasonographic examination fetal tone and fetal breathing and gross body movement monitoring, and gross estimate of amniotic fluid volume should be performed, as well as routine determinations of BPD, fetal and placental position, etc. Fetal movements and breathing are discussed independently in later sections of this chapter. Some authors have devised scoring systems that help to identify pregnancies at higher risk for fetal distress, thus dictating the need for more extensive and intensive examination of the gestation to prevent death. Preliminary results utilizing such systems seem clinically promising.

D. *Amnioscopy/fetoscopy*. *Amnioscopy* is the examination of the color of the amniotic fluid through intact membranes at the cervix to evaluate the fetus for signs of distress in the last trimester of pregnancy. *Transabdominal amnioscopy* or *fetoscopy* is direct examination of the fetus and amniotic fluid through the abdomen during the second trimester for the diagnosis of congenital defects or inheritable diseases.

1. *Amnioscopy*

a) Amnioscopy was first introduced by Saling in 1962 as a diagnostic tool that was noninvasive yet allowed the practicing physician in his/her office to avoid fetal death by predicting which fetuses are at risk. This came in an era when only clinical parameters were followed (e.g., measurement of fundal height, clinical estimation of fetal weight). Ultrasound was in its infancy and amniocentesis had drawbacks since it was an "invasive" procedure. Saling felt that by examining the amniotic fluid for meconium staining, the physician could identify the fetus in jeopardy from hypoxia. He routinely recommended that amniotomy be performed on such patients and delivery effected.

b) *Meconium* colors the amniotic fluid in various shades of *yellow to green*. Also, if abruption or fetal demise occurs, a *port-wine color* can be seen. The instruments for amnioscopy are simple, involving amnioscopes of various sizes and a fiberoptic light source. Indications for the procedure originally included postmaturity, hypertensive disorders of pregnancy, isoimmunization pregnancies, and suspected fetal demise. More recently, wide screening of all "high-risk" pregnancies has been performed.

c) *Complications* from the procedure include premature rupture of the membranes (PROM), premature labor, bleeding, and infection. *The most frequent complication is PROM,* which occurs in 2 to 5 percent of the pregnancies examined. The major problem with amnioscopy is that although Saling was able to decrease perinatal mortality significantly, more recent studies have been unable to confirm this. This finding may be due to the fact that perinatal mortality rates are now much lower because of recent technical advances. Also, when groups are carefully randomized, antepartum meconium staining does not appear to have the same morbid significance as intrapartum staining. Finally, false-positives do occur with amnioscopy that are not confirmed by subsequent amniocentesis.

d) With the other more exact methods of evaluating high-risk pregnancies available, amnioscopy is practiced less frequently. It is a test that certainly can add knowledge in complicated pregnancies; however, its sole use seems unwarranted in determining obstetrical intervention. Knowledge gained from the method can alert the physician that further antepartum testing may be warranted.

2. *Fetoscopy*

a) Fetoscopy is an invasive procedure, not yet widely practiced, requiring extensive specialized training. It is best performed between the 17th and 20th week of gestation. The technology is still in its early stages of development, and complete visualization of the fetus and placenta is not yet possible. Only a 2 to 4 cm^2 area of visualization is presently possible with a depth of focus of about 2 cm. The instrument is introduced into the abdomen under strictly sterile technique through a 2.7-mm diameter canulla through which the lens is placed. Samples of fetal blood and small tissue samples can be obtained through an obturator contiguous with the larger cannula.

b) The major *complication* of fetoscopy is premature delivery. This occurs in 9 to 10 percent of pregnancies examined. The spontaneous abortion rate is only 3 to 6 percent. Other complications include mild abdominal pain, infection, and intermittent leakage of amniotic fluid.

E. *Fetal breathing.* Fetal chest wall movements have been documented for over 10 years in animals, but more recently, they have been studied in human gestations in the hope of identifying fetuses at risk. Although total comprehension of the mechanisms governing and surrounding fetal breathing motions (FBM) is less than completely understood, enough technology and understanding of the events is present for this parameter to be evaluated in the high-risk patient. Observation for FBM should be incorporated into every ultrasonographic examination of the high-risk pregnancy as the fetus reaches viability.

1. *Instrumentation.* The most readily available method for examining FBM by the practicing physician is by real-time B-mode sonography. This method has now proven consistently reliable in evaluating FBM. Quantification of this motion is now being extensively studied by various centers utilizing techniques to pick up the depth and frequency of the motions.

2. *Influencing factors*

a) FBM has not been reported in the first trimester or early second trimester. It has been reported to occur at 31 to 34 weeks, and there is a suggestion that intermittent diaphragmatic motion may occur even earlier. Whether breathing motions will eventually become an accurate predictor of gestational age remains to be elucidated.

b) Patterns
  (1) A *diurnal pattern* has been recorded, with the largest proportion of FBM occurring in the early morning hours and lowest activity recorded in late evening. A suggestion that this activity corresponds to the period of increased glucocorticoid levels remains to be documented.
  (2) FBM patterns have been correlated with *CNS activity*. During REM (rapid eye movement) sleep, an increase in FBM has been noted. An overall picture in FBM is evolving that relates CNS maturity to the development of regular, periodic FBM. The more mature the fetus, the more regular the cycles in utero, culminating with delivery of a term infant with normal neonatal respiratory patterns. The more immature the fetus, the more prolonged the apneic periods and the more irregular the cycles.
  (3) During *labor* FBMs have been shown to markedly decrease. More recent studies indicate that fetuses about to undergo labor show a decrease in FBM cycles.
  (4) Increased fetal breathing is seen with maternal ingestion of *glucose* loads. Peaks in FBM are seen after maternal meals.
  (5) In animal models, when PCO_2 is kept constant and hypoxemia induced, fetal gasping and a slow cessation of FBM are seen. Likewise, when PO_2 is maintained in the normal range and hypercarbia induced, FBM increases in both depth and rate. A correlation has been sought in human patterns.
  (6) Four distinct patterns have been demonstrated in term fetuses:
      (a) Regular crescendo-decrescendo
      (b) Irregular slow
      (c) Periodic accelerated
      (d) Hiccups

It has been difficult to correlate these patterns in the normal fetus with fetuses at high-risk either in the antepartum or intrapartum state. The main correlation of low-Apgar-score, poor-outcome babies has been with the *absence* of FBM, defined as the absence of FBM or the absence of an episode of FBM of at least 60-second duration during a 30-minute observation period. The presence of FBM defined as a minimum of one episode of fetal breathing of at least 60-second duration within a 30-minute observation period correlates better with good fetal-neonatal outcome.

F. *Fetal movements.* Mothers frequently report fetal movements during pregnancy. However, the technology has only recently become available to examine what women have related historically for centuries. *Quickening* is noted from the 16th to 20th week of gestation, with multiparous women discerning motion at an earlier time than nulliparous women. Detailed examination of various motions by the fetus can now be made over lengthy periods of time.

1. *Measurement*

   a) *Perception of motion by mothers* is helpful and records of motion can be kept easily at home. If examination takes place for a limited period several times during each day, a range of "normal" activity may be calculated and compared to "normal" standards. When mothers report no perceptible movement, the normal examination period (e.g., 15–30 minutes) should be extended. Usually, if the mother lies quietly and concentrates on perceiving motion, she will register motion. However, maternal obesity, placental location, and amount of amniotic fluid can inhibit perception.

   b) Many types of *instruments* have been devised to examine motion, including special tocodynamometers, various strain gauges, and more recently, real-time ultrasound scanners. While some authors report many more movements are recorded by instruments than mothers, other authors find that good correlation exist, with women reporting 80 percent of motions noted by electronic equipment.

2. *Patterns.* Four types of fetal movements (FM) have been recorded:
    a) *Rolling* movements last longer than 3 seconds and are easily perceived by the mother. On ultrasound these motions are complex limb and body movements causing distortion of the abdominal wall.
    b) *Simple* movements last 1 to 3 seconds and on real-time scanning are shown to be simple movements of the trunk and/or limb.
    c) *High-frequency* (isolated and repetitive) movements last less than 1 second and are observed when abrupt chest and abdominal wall movements occur resembling neonatal startle movements or hiccups.
    d) *Respiratory movements* have been discussed previously.

3. *Normal movements*
    a) An extensive study not only of "quantitative" but of "qualitative" motion by fetuses at various stages of development has been published. *A continuum of movements* is described as the fetus develops, with no abrupt changes seen after birth. What an observer sees in the new born is also consistent with movement patterns observed of the term infant in utero before delivery.
    b) *Mothers with normal pregnancies perceive motion* early in the second trimester, with rolling movements increasing from 22 to 23 weeks until 36 to 37 weeks, when FMs decrease slightly to term. Simple movements are perceived as the first movements by the mother and thereafter slowly decrease until 36 to 37 weeks, at which time they increase slightly until term.
    c) A *daily average of FM* has been quantitated: 200 FM

at about 20 weeks; 575 FM at 32 weeks; and a slow decrease after 32 weeks to 282 FM at term.

(1) There has been *a diurnal FM pattern* reported, with more activity documented to occur in the evening hours and during maternal REM sleep. However, this pattern has not been found consistently in all groups studied.

(2) More recent studies utilizing *electromyographic fetal recordings* have shown that fetuses exhibit rest-activity cycles, but preliminary data suggest this is unrelated to maternal sleep-waking patterns.

(3) Prior to labor, no change in FM is seen, although fetal breathing movements have been shown to decrease. Furthermore, FM increases during the active phase of *labor.*

(4) Following meals or an *increase in maternal glucose levels,* FM increases. However, more recent strictly controlled studies reveal no increase in FM but a distinct increase in fetal breathing after a glucose load.

(5) There is no difference in activity between male or female fetuses, age of mother, parity, or ethnic origin. The fetuses of smokers, as well as users of various sedatives and hypnotic drugs, show decreased activity.

4. *Responses to stimuli.* Numerous stimuli have been used to elicit fetal activity in the hopes of adding another noninvasive technique that will allow easy evaluation of the fetus in the antepartum period. Fetuses do respond to sounds, external light, touch, and motion associated with ultrasound scanning; however, the tests are presently insufficiently discriminatory to help in making accurate predictions of fetuses at risk on a large-scale screening basis.

5. *Decreased fetal motion. The obstetrician should be alarmed if a mother reports decreased FM at any point past*

fetal viability. Sandonsky has referred to this state as a "movement alarm signal." He has documented that FM decreases dramatically before fetal death in utero and that this finding occurs hours before any abnormal fetal heart rate abnormality. Other investigators have supported the findings that FMs are a better predictor of impending death in utero than are estriol levels. Certainly, these findings suggest that *if mothers report declining FM in their pregnancy, further immediate examination of the pregnancy using other antenatal screening tests is warranted.* During routine sonographic examination of pregnancies, fetal position, flexion or extension of extremities, and activity should also be recorded.

G. *pH monitoring*. Because of concerns about the cost-effectiveness of fetal monitoring and the rising cesarean section rates, as well as questions about evaluating fetal distress clinically versus electronically, obstetricians have been seeking a more reliable method to determine the need for operative intervention in pregnancies in which there is electronic evidence of fetal distress. Death or injury to an infant during the intrapartum course remains deeply unsatisfying and is tragic for physician and mother alike. Yet the accurate diagnosis of fetal distress during this critical period of time remains difficult.

Since the initial development of fetal scalp blood sampling, the technology involved in this monitoring technique has advanced to the point that a pH electrode can be attached to the fetus at all times during labor. *Results of more recent studies indicate that the diagnosis of fetal distress can be more accurately made if this parameter is known in addition to the other data provided by routine fetal monitoring.*

1. *Indications* for measurement of scalp pH include:
   a) Pesistent abnormal FHR tracings
   b) Meconium staining of the amniotic fluid
   c) Severe variable decelerations
   d) Any other high-risk condition that requires clarification

2. *Contraindications are few and include:*
   a) Fetuses known to have coagulation defects
   b) Maternal bleeding disorders
   c) Documented active genital infections such as herpes
3. *Techniques*
   a) Both the intermittent and continuous techniques require that the fetus be vertex, the cervix dilated 3 cm or more, the membranes be ruptured, and the station of the fetus be at least -1.
   b) *Intermittent scalp sampling.* Various kits are available, and most include a conical endoscope that attaches to an available light source, sponges for cleansing the fetal scalp, a guarded scalpel, heparinized glass capillary tubes, and a magnet. The patient may be placed in the lithotomy or Sims position and the endoscope introduced. Visualization and cleansing of the fetal scalp over an area not directly over a fontanelle or suture line are followed by controlled puncture of the scalp. As the blood forms a droplet, the heparinized tube is used to collect the specimen. Less than 100 μl of blood is needed for accurate determination of pH. More is necessary if P_{CO_2}, base deficit, and bicarbonate levels are also to be determined. The capillary tube is sealed at one end, the steel mixer rod introduced into the tube, and a magnet used to mix the heparin with the blood. The specimen is then rapidly sent for acid-base determination. *It is very important to apply pressure to the puncture site on the fetal scalp and observe it after obtaining the specimen, since rare fetal deaths from hemorrhage have resulted.* Factors known *not* to influence values obtained by this method include whether the sample was collected during the presence or absence of a uterine contraction, the use of agents on the fetal scalp in an effort to produce hyperemia, whether or not the fetus has a large caput, and the effect of multiple incisions to collect the sample.
   c) *Continuous tissue measurement.* The same positioning

and method is used for permanent attachment of an electrode to the fetal scalp. Presently, electrodes may be screwed or glued into place depending on the system used. The technique associated with placement is slightly more difficult but is easily learned. After attachment, the pH determination is made automatically every 15 seconds and is recorded synchronously on the same paper trace as FHR and uterine contractions. The electrode can be displaced during pelvic examination but can easily be replaced. This problem has been reported to occur as frequently as 85 percent of the time.

4. *Discussion*

A major factor in perinatal mortality and eventual poor neonatal outcome is fetal asphyxia. Some studies have related cerebral palsy to intrapartum hypoxic episodes. Hypoxic-anoxic episodes in the fetus result in a change of metabolism to an anaerobic cycle producing increasing quantities of lactic acid and subsequent metabolic acidosis as the interval of the insult lengthens. While FHR monitoring is 95 percent accurate in predicting neonates with good Apgar scores, its accuracy in predicting poor outcomes is notoriously low, 20 to 40 percent.

Saling has reported that a fetal pH of 7.20 to 7.25 is an indication for intervention. While isolated intermittent scalp pH measurements have been shown to be helpful in evaluating FHR patterns and in avoiding unnecessary intervention based on FHR patterns classically thought of as fetal distress, there is still a substantial percentage of labors in which the diagnosis is erroneous, e.g., fetuses with pH of 7.20 and good Apgar scores. Various authors have reported false-positive rates of 10 to 50 percent. A basic rule that has evolved is: *Never act on a single pH determination.* Factors that can affect scalp pH measurement include maternal acidosis or hyperventilation and failures inherent to the technique, such as obtaining the specimen too slowly.

5. *Tissue pH*. More recently, examination of FHR tracings in conjunction with continuous tissue pH has greatly improved the definition of fetal distress and aided in the study of the underlying pathophysiology of distress states. Tissue pH (tpH) has been found to average 0.04 pH units lower than simultaneously obtained blood pH. Also, a relative fall of tpH is seen as labor progresses, at a rate of approximately 0.01 pH units per hour. Uterine contractions that are associated with "good" FHR tracings show no change or a slight rise in tpH. Fetal accelerations and early decelerations have not been found to be associated with abnormal tpH values. However, greater deviations from normal (tpH 7.25) are seen in tpH values progressing from patterns of reduced variability to patterns showing late decelerations and, finally, to states of tachycardia. Patterns showing moderate bradycardia, defined as FHR of 100 to 119 bpm for any length of time, are innocuous and have been shown repeatedly to coexist with normal tpH. Likewise, sinusoidal patterns of FHR tracings occurring in the absence of fetal acidosis are not ominous predictions of near fetal demise and the need for intervention. Variable decelerations are the most common deceleration pattern seen in FHR tracings. Fetal outcome has always been difficult to predict with these patterns. However, Young has devised a nomenclature where reclassification of variable deceleration into subpopulations allows better prediction of fetal outcome associated with tpH. Variable decelerations are divided into three patterns:

a) Those with no consistent configuration in relation to uterine contractions.

b) Those with a "late component" with FHRs that do not return to the base line at the end of a contraction.

c) Those with late onset but recovery at the time of the end of the contraction. Young found significantly decreased tpH in the patterns that have a "late component" associated with the variable pattern.

Although further work must be done, a better understanding of FHR patterns is evolving. The relationship to the development of fetal acidosis and the patterns in which the acidosis becomes progressive and irreversible and require obstetrical intervention are becoming more clearly defined.

H. *Amniocentesis.* Amniocentesis is one of the most commonly practiced procedures in obstetrics. Previously, amniocentesis was limited to third-trimester examinations of the amniotic fluid for evaluation of fetal maturity and/or fetal distress. Now, second-trimester amniocentesis for prenatal diagnosis has become common with the advent of technology capable of determining new hormones, errors in metabolism, and chromosomal abnormalities.

1. *Genetic amniocentesis*

   a) *Second-trimester* amniocentesis is performed between 14 and 18 weeks. Amniotic fluid volume is too small before this period to allow technical success; additionally, the uterus is relatively inaccessible under the pelvic brim. At 12 weeks, only 50 ml of fluid is present. This increases to 100 ml at 14 weeks, 175 ml at 18 weeks, and 325 ml at 20 weeks. If termination of the pregnancy is desired based on laboratory results, this can be accomplished before the point of legal fetal viability. Placental size in second-trimester taps is also a problem. Ultrasonography should be used to avoid needle punctures of placental vessels and to locate an optimal site or "window" for the tap.

   b) *Indications* for second-trimester amniocentesis include pregnancy in older women (35 years or older), family history of chromosomal abnormality or documented chromosomal abnormality in one parent, family history of errors of metabolism, and previous children born with chromosomal anomalies, neural tube defects, or inborn errors in metabolism. When amniocentesis is combined with tissue sampling via fetoscopy, the diagnosis of many other fetal diseases and genetically transferrable disorders is possible.

c) *Technique*
  (1) Before amniocentesis the patient is asked to empty her bladder, and the physician should examine the pregnancy ultrasonographically. Intrauterine gestation should be confirmed as well as fetal viability and age. The placental site must be found and a suitable "window" as free as possible from placental tissue isolated.
  (2) Measurement by sonogram of the depth of the amniotic sac from maternal skin surface is taken.
  (3) Under sterile conditions, a local anesthetic is applied and a 20- or 22-gauge needle of at least 3½ inches in length is introduced into the preselected site.
  (4) Approximately 20 ml of fluid is withdrawn and placed in sterile containers for study, since bacteria can greatly inhibit growth of the cells. Amniotic fluid is rapidly replaced. Monitoring of the pregnancy immediately after amniocentesis is unwarranted, since intervention at this time would be nonproductive. For this reason, genetic amniocentesis can be an office procedure, provided ultrasound equipment is available.
  (5) Controversy exists as to whether all Rh-negative mothers should receive a prophylactic minidose of Rho Gam to prevent sensitization secondary to leakage of fetal erythrocytes into the maternal bloodstream.
d) *Counseling.* Although over 95 percent of genetic amniocentesis reveal "normal" fetuses, some fetuses are found to be abnormal or are found to have defects not thought to be present. Counseling services must be an integral part of the perinatal team since "abnormal" findings dictate that a decision must be made to terminate the pregnancy or "ready" the home environment for delivery of the abnormal child.
2. *Third-trimester amniocentesis*
  a) *Indications.* Amniocentesis done in the third trimester

is usually performed to evaluate fetal maturity and fetal distress, e.g., Rh isoimmunization problems. The fluid obtained must be kept refrigerated to avoid breakdown of the phospholipids, which causes falsely low lecithin: sphingomyelin (L/S) ratios. If Δ OD 450 is being measured in evaluating bilirubin levels, the tube should not be exposed to sunlight since this will decrease the amplitude of the bilirubin curve and give a false reading. Contamination of the specimen with blood can also confuse results; however, L/S values greater than 2 usually represent evidence of pulmonary maturation. Meconium contamination also produces variable L/S results.

b) *Technique*

   (1) This procedure should be performed in a setting where immediate surgical intervention is possible should complications from the procedure arise.

   (2) The patient is asked to empty her bladder.

   (3) The physician should examine the gestation by sonography for fetal age, viability, congenital anomalies, and adequacy of the amount of amniotic fluid present. He or she should localize the placenta and note the position of the fetus. The area of the fetal neck and, more commonly, the area of the fetal extremities are two locations most frequently used for selection of fluid.

   (4) An optimum "window" with a pocket of fluid and minimal overlying placental tissue is selected and a measurement made sonographically from maternal skin surface to fluid. If placental tissue must be traversed, an area away from the area of insertion of the umbilical cord is sought. The procedure is then identical to the technique described with genetic amniocentesis.

   (5) At the termination of the procedure, fetal heart tones are periodically monitored to ascertain that the fetus is not in jeopardy secondary to one of the rare complications of the procedure. Interven-

tion would be dictated at this stage for fetal survival should fetal distress be detected.

3. *Risks.* The risks of amniocentesis include cord accidents, hemorrhage, permanent needle marks on the baby, premature labor, Rh sensitization of the mother, infection, amniotic fluid embolism, leaking membranes, and fetal lacerations and/or demise. *Major catastrophies from this procedure are rare, occurring in less than 1 percent of procedures.* Long-term risks in the United States — including perinatal problems, congenital defects, fetal loss and neonatal complications — have not been found to be increased over controlled populations not undergoing amniocentesis.

I. *Amniography.* Amniography is an invasive technique involving the injection of a radiopaque substance into the amniotic cavity for visualization of the fetus and placenta. The technique, which began in the 1930s has now largely been replaced by sonographic examination of the same structures. Its main uses at present are involved with identifying fetal congenital defects that cannot be defined clearly by ultrasound.

BIBLIOGRAPHY

Estriol

Gabbe SG, Hogerman DD: Clinical application of estriol analysis. Clin Obstet Gynecol 21:353, 1978

Goebelsmann U: The uses of oestriol as a monitoring tool. Clin Obstet Gynecol 6:22, 1979

Greene JW, Touchstone JC: Urinary estriol as an index of placental function. Am J Obstet Gynecol 85:1, 1963

Tulchinsky D: Use of biochemical indices in the management of high-risk obstetric patients. Clin Perinatol 7:413, 1980

Human Chorionic Gonadotropin

Okagaki T: Pregnancy tests. In Scirra JJ (ed): Gynecology and Obstetrics, Vol 3. Philadelphia, Harper & Row, 1979

Osathanondh R: Endocrine tests in obstetrics and gynecology, Part 1. Curr Probl Obstet Gynecol 3(6):5, 1980

Osathanondh R, Tulchinsky D: Placental polypeptide hormones. In Tulchinsky D, Ryan KJ (eds): Maternal-Fetal Endocrinology. Philadelphia, Harper & Row, 1980

Human Placental Lactogen

Frieson HG, Singer W: Human placental lactogen and chorionic thyrotropin. In Goodwin JW, Godden JO, Chance GW (eds): Perinatal Medicine, the Basic Science Underlying Clinical Practice. Baltimore, Williams and Wilkins, 1976

Hobbins JC, Berkowitz RL: Current status of human placental lactogen. Clin Obstet Gynecol 21:363, 1978

Tyson JE: Changing role of placental lactogen and prolactin in human gestation. Clin Obstet Gynecol 23:737, 1980

Varner MW, Hauser KS: Current status of human placental lactogen. Semin Perinatol 5:123, 1981

α-Fetoprotein

Crandall BF, Lebherz TB, Freihube R: Neural tube defects: maternal serum screening and prenatal diagnosis. Pediatr Clin North Am 25:619, 1978

Lau HL: Fetal surveillance. In Aladjem S, Hoed EV (eds): Obstetrical Practice. St. Louis, Mosby, 1980

Lau HL, Linkins SE: Alpha-protein. Am J Obstet Gynecol 124:533, 1976

Nadler HL, Simpson JL: Maternal serum AFP screening: promise not yet fulfilled. Obstet Gynecol 54:333, 1978

β₁-Glycoprotein

Horne CH, Towler CM: Pregnancy-specific β_1-glycoprotein: a review. Obstet Gynecol Surv 33:761, 1978

Sorensen S: An electroimmuno-assay of the pregnancy-specific β_1-glycoprotein (SP_1) in normal and pathological pregnancies, and its clinical value compared to HCS. Acta Obstet Gynecol Scand 57:193, 1978

Creatinine Phosphokinase
Kerenyi T, Sarkozi L: Diagnosis of fetal death in utero by elevated amniotic fluid CPK levels. Obstet Gynecol 44:215, 1974

Diamine Oxidase
Carrington ER, Frishmuth GJ, Oesterling MJ, et al.: Gestational and postpartum plasma diamine oxidase values. Obstet Gynecol 39:426, 1972

Weingold AB, Southern AL: Diamine oxidase as an index of the fetoplacental unit. Obstet Gynecol 32:593, 1968

Oxytocinase
Carter ER, Goodman LV, Dehaan RM, Sobota JT: Serum oxytocinase levels: a clinical laboratory and clinical appraisal. Am J Obstet Gynecol 119:76, 1974

Henseleigh PA, Cheatum SG, Spellacy WN: Oxytocinase and human placental lactogen for prediction of intrauterine growth retardation. Am J Obstet Gynecol 129:675, 1977

Fetal Monitoring
Banta HD, Thacker SB: Costs and benefits of electronic fetal monitoring: a review of the literature. DHEW Pub. No. 79–3245. US Dept HEW, April 1979.

Caldeyro-Barcia R, Pose SV, Alvarez H: Am J Obstet Gynecol 73:1238, 1957

El-Sahwi S, Gaafar AA, Topozada HK: A new unit for evaluation of uterine activity. Am J Obstet Gynecol 98:900, 1967

Gratacos JA, Paul RH: Antepartum fetal heart rate monitoring, nonstress test versus contraction stress test. Clin Perinatol 7:387, 1980

Hobbins JC, Freeman R, Queenan JT: The fetal monitoring debate. Obstet Gynecol 54:103, 1979

Jarrell SE, Sokol RJ: Clinical use of stressed and nonstressed monitoring techniques. Clin Obstet Gynecol 22:617, 1979

Miller FC, Paul RH: Intrapartum fetal heart rate monitoring. Clin Obstet Gynecol 22:561, 1979

Ultrasound

Hertz RH, Zador IE: Ultrasound cephalometry: a clinical discussion. Clin Obstet Gynecol 22:561, 1979

Hobbins JC: Diagnostic Ultrasound in Obstetrics, Vol 3, Clinics in Diagnostic Ultrasound. Baltimore, Williams and Wilkins, 1979, pp 1–192

Hobbins JC: Use of ultrasound in complicated pregnancies. Clin Perinatol 7:397, 1980

Sabbagha RE: Ultrasonography in obstetrical practice. In Aladjem S, Hoed EV (eds): Obstetrical Practice. St. Louis, Mosby, 1980

Amnioscopy

Salana LR, Schulman H, Lin C: Routine amnioscopy at term. Obstet Gynecol 47:521, 1976

Saling E: Amnioscopy. Clin Obstet Gynecol 9:472, 1966

Fetoscopy

Elias S: Fetoscopy in prenatal diagnosis. Semin Perinatol 4:199, 1980

US Dept HEW: Antenatal Diagnosis. NIH Pub. No. 79–1973, April 1979

Fetal Breathing Monitoring

Dierker LJ Jr , Hertz RH, Timor-Tritsch I, Rosen MC: Fetal respiration: a review of two techniques for observation. Clin Obstet Gynecol 22:593, 1979

Manning FA, Platt LD: Human fetal breathing monitoring—clinical considerations. Semin Perinatol 4:311, 1980

Rosen MG, Hertz RH, Dierker LJ Jr, et al.: Monitoring fetal movement. Clin Obstet Gynecol 6:335, 1979

Fetal Movements

Ianniruberto A, Tajani E: Ultrasonographic study of fetal movements. Semin Perinatol 5:175, 1981

Patrick J: Fetal activity and fetal breathing movements as methods for monitoring the fetus using ultrasound. Oral presentation at a mini-symposium on fetal monitoring at SGI Meeting, St. Louis, March 1981

Sadovsky E: Fetal movements and fetal health. Semin Perinatol 5:131, 1981

Timor-Tirtsch I, Dierker LJ, Hertz RH, Rosen MG: Fetal movement: a brief review. Clin Obstet Gynecol 22:583, 1979

pH

Quilligan EJ: Monitoring the fetus using acid base status. Clin Obstet Gynecol 6:309, 1979

US Dept HEW: Antenatal Diagnosis: Intrapartum Fetal Distress. NIH Pub. No. 79–1973, April 1979

Young BK: The relationship of fetal pH and heart rate: new. In Lauerson NH, Hochberg HM (eds): Clinical Perinatal Biochemical Monitoring. Baltimore, Williams and Wilkins, 1981

Young BK, Katz M, Wilson SJ, Klein SA: Continuous fetal tissue pH monitoring in labor. In Young BK (ed): Perinatal Medicine Today. New York, AR Liss, Inc., 1980

Amniocentesis

Fuchs F: Volume of amniotic fluid at various stages of pregnancy. Clin Obstet Gynecol 9:449, 1966

Queenan JT: When and how to do amniocentesis. Contemp Obstet Gynecol 15(2):61, 1980

Turnbull AC, Fairweather DV, Hibbard BM et al.: An assessment of the hazards of amniocentesis. Br J Obstet Gynecol (Suppl 2) 85:1, 1978

US Dept HEW: Anetenatal Diagnosis: Report of a Consensus. NIH Pub. No. 79–1973, April 1979

Amniography

Caterini H, Sama J, Iffy L, et al.: A reevaluation of amniography. Obstet Gynecol 49:373, 1976

Rubino SM: Diagnosis of an intact hydatidiform mole with coexistent fetus by amniography. Obstet Gynecol 46:364, 1975

10

The Powers, Passenger and Passage

Jeffrey W. Ellis, M.D.

PRACTICE PRINCIPLES

The *three critical factors* affecting labor are the strength and coordination of the uterine contractions (*powers*), the size and position of the fetus (*passenger*), and the size and configuration of the bony pelvis and soft tissues (*passage*). The treatment of dysfunctional labor will involve individual assessment of each of these factors.

POWERS: THE EXPULSIVE FORCES

A. The forces involved in the expulsion of the fetus and placenta are both involuntary and voluntary:
 1. The involuntary contractions of the uterus.
 2. The voluntary contractions of the abdominal and diaphragmatic muscles.
B. Uterine contractions
 1. *Physiology.* Uterine contractions are initiated by pacemakers located in the cornual areas of the uterine fundus. Individual contractions are initiated by a single

pacemaker. The contraction spreads downward from the pacemaker at a rate of 2 cm/second, thus involving the entire myometrium in approximately 15 seconds. Normal uterine contractions are characterized by fundal dominence. There is a decreasing gradient of intensity and duration of the myometrial contraction from the fundus to the lower uterine segment. Therefore, the contractions in the area of the fundus are the longest and the most intense. During normal labor, intrauterine pressures range between 35 and 55 mm Hg, with a resting tonus between contractions of 8 to 12 mm Hg. Contractions creating intrauterine pressures of 100 mm Hg may occur.

2. *Anatomic changes.* After a contraction occurs in the upper uterine segment, the myometrial fibers do not completely relax, but rather remain relatively fixed at a shorter length. As labor progresses, the uterine cavity becomes progressively smaller. The presenting part is forced downward into the cervix. As retraction of the upper uterine segment progresses, the lower uterine segment develops and with the cervix is pulled upward over the presenting part.

3. *Frequency and duration of contractions.* During the early phases of labor, contractions occur irregularly every 15 to 20 minutes. As labor progresses, the interval between contractions decreases to every 2 to 3 minutes. The average contraction has a duration between 30 and 90 seconds. The duration of the contractions tend to decrease as they increase in frequency.

C. *Voluntary contractions.* Intrauterine pressure is increased considerably after forceful contractions of the abdominal muscles are combined with a fixed diaphragm following forced inspiration. This increase in intrauterine pressure aids in expulsion of the fetus after complete cervical dilatation. As the presenting part distends the perineum, the patient will maintain an almost involuntary urge to push. Voluntary contractions will have no effect on cervical dilatation and effacement.

PASSENGER

Structurally, the fetus is composed of two oval parts, the head and the body. During labor, the head is the most critical, since it must adapt to the various diameters of the maternal pelvis.

A. *Sutures.* The sutures (Fig. 10–1) of the fetal skull are membranous spaces between the cranial bones. Palpation of the sutures aids in identification of the fetal position.
  1. The sagittal suture lies between the parietal bones and extends from the anterior to the posterior fontanelle.
  2. The frontal suture lies between the frontal bones.
  3. The coronal sutures lie between the frontal and parietal bones.
  4. The lambdoidal sutures lie between the parietal bones and the occipital bone.
B. *Fontanelles.* The fontanelles (Fig. 10–1) are irregular membrane-filled spaces at the intersection of sutures.
  1. The *anterior fontanelle* is shaped like an irregular diamond and lies at the junction of the sagittal, frontal, and coronal sutures. It is the largest fontanelle, measuring 2 × 3 cm in the term infant.
  2. The *posterior fontanelle* is shaped like a triangle and lies at the junction of the sagittal and lambdoidal sutures.
  3. The *temporal fontanelles* lie at the junction of the lambdoidal and temporal sutures.
C. *Diameters of the fetal skull* (Fig. 10–2)
  1. *Biparietal diameter.* The greatest transverse diameter of the skull, extending between the parietal bosses.
  2. *Bitemporal diameter.* The shortest transverse diameter of the skull, extending between the two temporal sutures.
  3. *Suboccipitobregmatic diameter.* The shortest anterioposterior diameter of the skull, extending from the middle of the anterior fontanelle to the under surface of the occipital bone at the junction with the neck.
  4. *Occipitomental diameter.* The longest anteroposterior diameter of the skull, extending from the chin to the most distant point on the vertex.

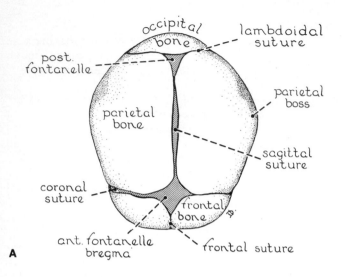

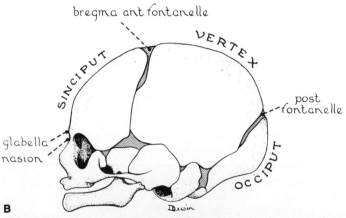

Figure 10-1. Superior (**A**) and lateral (**B**) views of the fetal skull showing sutures and fontanelles. (From Oxorn H, Foote WR: Human Labor and Birth, 4th ed. New York, Appleton-Century-Crofts, 1980, pp 39, 43.)

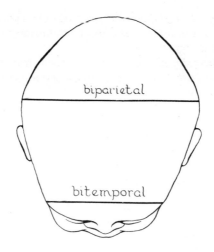

A

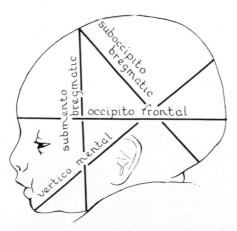

B

Figure 10-2. Landmarks and diameters of the fetal skull. **A.** Transverse diameters. **B.** Anteroposterior diameters. (From Oxorn H, Foote WR: Human Labor and Birth, 4th ed. New York, Appleton-Century-Crofts, 1980, pp 39, 43.)

5. *Occipitofrontal diameter.* Extends from a point above the root of the nose to the most prominent portion of the occipital bone.
6. *Submentobregmatic diameter.* Extends from the center of the anterior fontanelle to the junction of the neck and lower jaw.

PASSAGE: THE NORMAL PELVIS

A. *Gross anatomy*
   1. The pelvis is composed of four bones:
      a) *Sacrum*
      b) *Coccyx*
      c) *Two innominate bones* each formed by the fusion of the *ilium, ischium,* and *pubis*
   2. Articulation is through four joints:
      a) *Symphysis pubis*
      b) *Sacrococcygeal joint*
      c) *Two sacroiliac joints*
   3. The pelvis is divided by the *linea terminalis* into the *false pelvis* (above) and the *true pelvis* (below). The false pelvis has no obstetric significance.
   4. The true pelvis is divided into three *planes:*
      a) Plane of the pelvic inlet
      b) Plane of the midpelvis
      c) Plane of the pelvic outlet
B. *Pelvic inlet* (Fig. 10–3)
   1. *Boundaries*
      a) The upper border of the pelvis anteriorally
      b) The linea terminalis laterally
      c) The sacral promontory posteriorly
   2. *Anterior-posterior diameters*
      a) *True conjugate*
         (1) Extends from the middle of the sacral promontory to the superior margin of the pubis.
         (2) It is the true anatomical anterior-posterior diame-

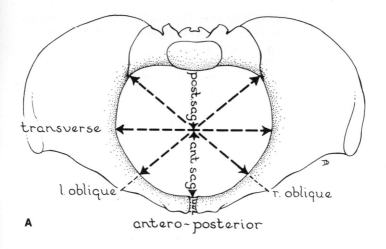

A

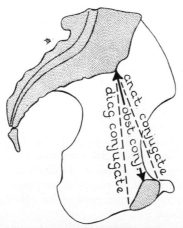

B

Figure 10-3. Pelvic inlet. **A.** Anteroposterior view. **B.** Sagittal section. (From Oxorn H, Foote WR: Human Labor and Birth, 4th ed. New York, Appleton-Century-Crofts, 1980, p 27.)

ter of the inlet but is not the shortest distance between the sacral promontory and the pelvis.
b) *Obstetric conjugate*
   (1) Extends from the middle of the sacral promontory to the innermost point of the pubis.
   (2) It is the *shortest distance* between the sacral promontory and the pubis.
   (3) In most cases, it represents the smallest diameter of the inlet through which the presenting part must pass.
c) *Diagonal conjugate*
   (1) Extends from the middle of the sacral promontory to the lowest margin of the pubis.
   (2) This is the only diameter of the inlet that can be measured manually.
   (3) Subtracting 1.5 cm from the diagonal conjugate will approximate the length of the obstetric conjugate.
3. *Transverse diameter*
   a) Formed as a right angle to the true conjugate representing the greatest distance between each linea terminalis.
   b) This diameter can only be determined by radiographic evaluation.
C. *Pelvic midplane* (Fig. 10–4)
   1. *Boundaries*
      a) apex of the pubic arch
      b) ischial spines
      c) lower portion of the sacrum near the junction of the fourth and fifth sacral vertebrae
   2. *Anterior-posterior diameter.* Extends from the inferior margin of the pubic symphysis to a point on the lower portion of the sacrum, passing through the level of the ischial spines.
   3. *Transverse diameter* (bispinous diameter). The distance between the tips of the ischial spines.
   4. *Posterior sagittal diameter.* Extends from the bispinous

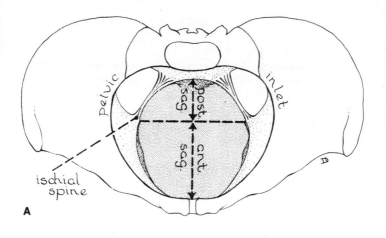

A

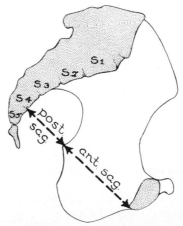

B

Figure 10-4. Pelvic midplane. **A.** Anteroposterior view showing the anteroposterior and transverse diameters. **B.** Sagittal section showing the anteroposterior diameter. (From Oxorn H, Foote WR: Human Labor and Birth, 4th ed. New York, Appleton-Century-Crofts, 1980, p 29.)

diameter to the junction of the fourth and fifth sacral
vertebrae.

D. *Pelvic outlet* (Fig. 10–5)
   1. *Boundaries.* The outlet is composed of two triangles.
      a) *Anterior triangle.* The area under the pubic arch
         bounded by the inferior margin of the symphysis pubis
         and the two ischial tuberosities.
      b) *Posterior triangle.* Bounded by the tip of the sacrum,
         sacrospinous ligaments, and the ischial tuberosities.
   2. *Anterior-posterior diameter*
      a) Extends from the inferior margin of the symphysis
         pubis to the sacrococcygeal joint.
      b) Due to the mobility of the sacrococcygeal joint, the
         anterior-posterior diameter will increase by up to 2 cm
         as the presenting part moves through the outlet.
   3. *Transverse diameter.* The distance between the inner
      surfaces of the ischial tuberosities.
   4. *Posterior sagittal diameter.* Extends from the middle of
      the transverse diameter to the sacrococcygeal joint.

E. *Average pelvic diameters* (Fig. 10–6)
   1. *Inlet*
      a) True conjugate, 11.0–11.5 cm
      b) Obstetric conjugate, 10.5–11.0 cm
      c) Diagonal conjugate, 12.0–13.5 cm
      d) Transverse, 13.0–13.5 cm
   2. *Midplane*
      a) Anterior-posterior, 12.0 cm
      b) Transverse, 10.5 cm
      c) Posterior sagittal, 4.5–5.0 cm
   3. *Outlet*
      a) Anterior-posterior, 9.5–11.5 cm
      b) Transverse, 10.5–11.0 cm
      c) Posterior sagittal, 9.0 cm

F. *Classification of the pelvis.* The pelvis is classified according
   to four basic shapes (Figs. 10–7 to 10–9). The Caldwell-
   Maloy classification is most commonly used and is based on
   the shape of the inlet. The transverse diameter of the inlet
   divides the inlet into anterior and posterior segments.

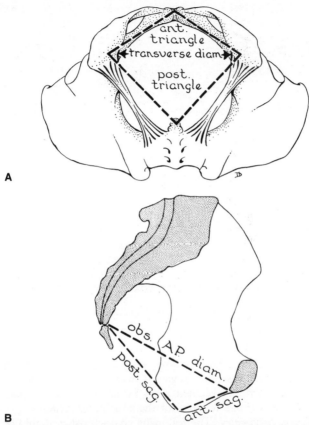

Figure 10-5. Pelvic outlet. **A.** Inferior view. **B.** Sagittal section. (From Oxorn H, Foote WR: Human Labor and Birth, 4th ed. New York, Appleton-Century-Crofts, 1980, p 31.)

1. The shape of the posterior segment determines the pelvic type: *gynecoid, android, anthropoid, platypelloid.*
2. The shape of the anterior segment determines the *tendency.*
3. Most patients will have a mixed type of pelvis, for

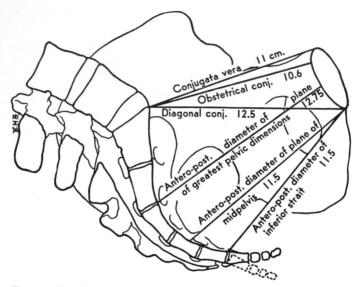

Figure 10-6. Diagram showing various pelvic planes and diameters.
Conjugata vera, true conjugate. (From Hellman LM, Pritchard JA:
Williams Obstetrics, 14th ed. New York, Appleton-Century-Crofts, 1971,
p 293.)

example, a gynecoid type with an android tendency
(rounded posterior segment with a narrow, wedge-
shaped anterior segment). See Table 10–1 for a comparison of various features of the four pelvic types.

G. *Clinical pelvimetry.* The following characteristics should be
   evaluated during manual assessment of the pelvis:

1. *Diagonal conjugate*	Subtract 1.5 cm to determine anteroposterior diameter of the inlet
2. *Transverse of the mid-pelvis*	Normally 10 cm or greater
3. *Pelvic side walls*	Straight, divergent, convergent

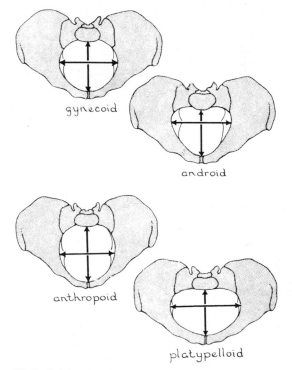

gynecoid

android

anthropoid

platypelloid

Figure 10–7. Pelvic inlet (Caldwell-Moloy classification). (From Oxorn, H, Foote WR: Human Labor and Birth, 4th ed. New York, Appleton-Century-Crofts, 1980, p 33.)

4. *Sacrum*	Concave, straight, forward, or backward inclination
5. *Sacrosciatic notch*	Wide, narrow
6. *Subpubic angle*	Wide, narrow
7. *Transverse of outlet*	Normally 10.5 cm or greater
8. *Mobility of coccyx*	Mobile, rigid

H. *X-Ray pelvimetry.* Radiographic examination of the pelvis will enable relatively accurate measurement of the pelvic

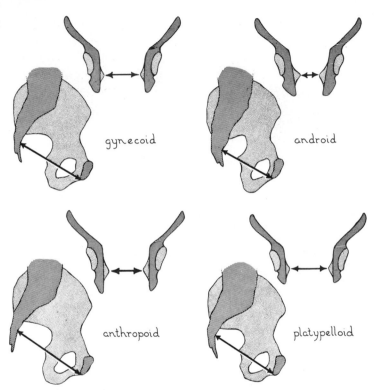

Figure 10-8. Midpelvis (Caldwell-Moloy classification). (From Oxorn H, Foote WR: Human Labor and Birth, 4th ed. New York, Appleton-Century-Crofts, 1980, p 35.)

diameters, including several that cannot be determined manually. There is considerable disagreement regarding the value of x-ray pelvimetry in the management of labor. The long-term effects of maternal and fetal irradiation are unknown, though some reports suggest an increase in the rate of malignancy in children radiated in utero. Single anteroposterior and lateral views of the pelvis will deliver approximately 1 roentgen to the fetal gonads and maternal

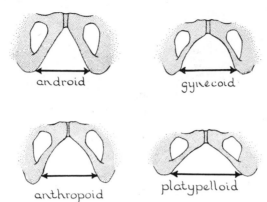

Figure 10-9. Pelvic outlet (Caldwell-Moloy classification). (From Oxorn H, Foote WR: Human Labor and Birth, 4th ed. New York, Appleton-Century-Crofts, 1980, p 37.)

ovaries. For details regarding the techniques and interpretation of x-ray pelvimetry, the reader is referred to *Williams Obstetrics*, 16th edition, p 285–86.

FETOPELVIC RELATIONSHIPS

Practice Principles

During the course of pregnancy, the fetus will assume a variety of postures in relation the the uterus and pelvis. The terms lie, presentation, presenting part, attitude, and position are used to describe these relationships, and the course of labor and delivery will depend on them.

A. *Lie*
    1. *Definition.* The relationship of the long axis of the fetus to the long axis of the mother.
    2. *Types of lie*
       a) *Longitudinal.* The long axis of the fetus is parallel to the long axis of the mother.

TABLE 10–1. PELVIC TYPES

	Gynecoid	Android	Anthropoid	Platypelloid
Incidence	50%	20%	25%	5%
Inlet shape	Round, transverse, oval	Rounded triangle, short posterior segment	Long oval	Transverse oval, short posterior segment
Inlet				
Anteroposterior	Adequate	Adequate	Long	Shortened
Transverse	Adequate	Adequate	Adequate	Long
Midpelvis				
Anteroposterior	Adequate	Shortened	Long	Shortened
Transverse	Adequate	Shortened	Adequate	Long
Sacrum	Curved, average length	Straight, forward inclination	Curved, long	Curved
Sidewalls	Usually straight	Usually convergent	Straight	Straight
Sacrosciatic notch	Usually wide	Narrow	Wide	Narrow
Ischial spines	Not prominent	Prominent	Variable	Variable
Outlet				
Anteroposterior	Long	Short	Long	Short
Transverse	Adequate	Narrow	Adequate	Adequate
Subpubic angle	Wide	Narrow	Narrow	Wide

   b) *Transverse.* The long axis of the fetus is perpendicular to the long axis of the mother.
   c) *Oblique.* The long axis of the fetus forms an oblique angle with the long axis of the mother. This is an unstable lie that will convert to either longitudinal or transverse during labor.
B. *Presentation/presenting part*
   1. *Definition.* The presenting part is the most dependent part of the fetus in the birth canal. The presenting part determines presentation.
   2. *Types of presentation*
      a) Cephalic (longitudinal lie)
      b) Breech (longitudinal lie)
      c) Shoulder (transverse lie)
C. *Attitude*
   1. *Definition.* The relationship of fetal parts to each other, specifically the relationship between the head and the trunk. The fetal head may assume an attitude of complete flexion, complete extension, or points in between.
   2. *Types*
      a) *Complete flexion.* The fetal chin approaches the chest. The occiput becomes the reference point for determining position in the pelvis.

      b) *Complete extension.* The occiput approaches the back. The chin becomes the reference point. Complete extension with a cephalic presentation is termed *face presentation.*
      c) *Incomplete extension.* When the most dependent part of the fetus is the anterior fontanelle, this is termed *sinciput presentation.* When the most dependent part is the brow, this is *brow presentation.*
D. *Position/variety* (Fig. 10–10)
   1. *Definition. Position* is the relationship of an arbitrary reference point on the fetus to the right or left side of the maternal pelvis. *Variety* is the relationship of the reference point to the anterior, transverse, or posterior portions of the maternal pelvis.

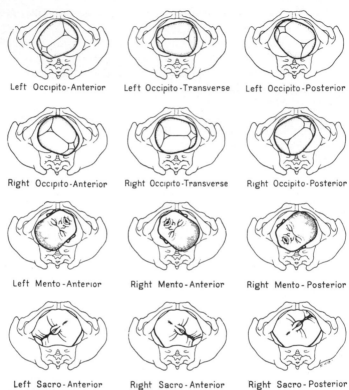

Left Occipito-Anterior   Left Occipito-Transverse   Left Occipito-Posterior

Right Occipito-Anterior   Right Occipito-Transverse   Right Occipito-Posterior

Left Mento-Anterior   Right Mento-Anterior   Right Mento-Posterior

Left Sacro-Anterior   Right Sacro-Anterior   Right Sacro-Posterior

Figure 10-10. A. Left positions in occiput presentations, with fetal head viewed from below. **B.** Right positions in occiput presentations **C.** Left and right position in face presentations. **D.** Left and right positions in breech presentations. (From Pritchard JA, MacDonald PC: Williams Obstetrics, 16th ed. New York, Appleton-Century-Crofts, 1980, p 297.)

2. *Types.* For each reference point, there are eight possible locations. In a cephalic presentation with complete flexion of the head, the reference point is the occiput. The occiput may be straight anterior (OA), left occiput anterior (LOA), left occiput transverse (LOT), left

occiput posterior (LOP), straight posterior (OP), right occiput posterior (ROP), right occiput transverse (ROT), or right occiput anterior (ROA). Reference points for other presentations are the chin (mentum) in face presentation, the brow in brow presentation, the sacrum in breech presentation.

BIBLIOGRAPHY

Caldeyro-Barcia R, et al.: A better understanding of uterine contractility through simultaneous recording with an internal and a seven channel external method. Surg Gynecol Obstet 91:641, 1950

Caldwell WE, Moloy HC: Anatomical variations in the female pelvis and their effect in labor with a suggested classification. Am J Obstet Gynecol 26:479, 1933

Cibils LA, Zuspan FP: Pharmacology of the uterus. Clin Obstet Gynecol 11:34, 1968

Mengert WF: Estimation of pelvic capacity. JAMA 138:169, 1948

Reynolds SRM: Physiology of the Uterus. New York, Hafner, 1965

Thoms H: The uses and limits of roentgen pelvimetry. Am J Obstet Gynecol 34:150, 1937

11

Labor and Delivery

Jeffrey W. Ellis, M.D.

PRACTICE PRINCIPLES

Labor, and delivery of the newborn, is a normal physiologic process requiring little intervention in most cases. A thorough knowledge of the processes involved is mandatory so that the obstetrician may *assist* in normal labor and delivery and *intervene* appropriately when abnormalities develop.

PRODROMES OF LABOR

The following signs and symptoms often occur as preliminary events before the onset of labor.

A. *Lightening* is the settling of the presenting part into the true pelvis. As the uterus descends slightly, pressure on the diaphragm is relieved and breathing becomes easier. Pressure from the presenting part may lead to urinary frequency and pelvic pain.
   1. In *primigravidas,* lightening begins approximately two to three weeks before the onset of labor. Failure of lightening to occur in a primigravida is suggestive of a fetopelvic disproportion.

   2. In *multiparas,* lightening generally does not occur until the onset of labor.

B. *Passage of the mucus plug.* As the cervix becomes partially effaced and dilated, the plug of mucus that filled the endocervical canal is expelled. Occasionally, the mucus plug is blood-tinged ("bloody show").

C. *Cervical effacement and dilatation.* Progressive cervical effacement and dilatation often occur beginning three to four weeks before the onset of labor. Primigravidas may become completely effaced prior to the onset of labor.

D. *Vaginal secretions* increase several days before the onset of labor.

E. *False labor.* Uterine contractions of variable frequency and intensity are common during the final month of pregnancy (Braxton-Hicks contraction).

LABOR

A. Labor is the physiologic process by which the uterus expels, or attempts to expel, the products of conception. During the initial evaluation of a patient with uterine contractions, it is necessary to differentiate *true labor* from *false labor.* The following criteria are used to establish the diagnosis:

	True Labor	**False Labor**
Contractions		
Interval	Regular with a gradually shortening interval	Irregular with no interval shortening
Duration	Gradual increase	No change
Intensity	Gradual increase	No change
Cervical changes	Progressive dilatation and effacement	No change
Presenting Part		
Descent	Progressive descent	No change

	True Labor	**False Labor**
Fixation	Presenting part remains fixed between contractions	Presenting part may recede between contractions
Location of pain	Back and abdomen	Abdomen only
Effects of sedation	Contractions do not stop	Contractions stop

B. If doubt exists regarding the diagnosis of labor, the patient may be observed for a one to two-hour period and then reexamined. True labor will lead to demonstrable cervical changes.

Admission Evaluation

Upon admission to the hospital a brief history and physical examination are performed. The patient's prenatal record should be reviewed. If no previous records are available, a standard prenatal history should be obtained.

A. *History*. The following information should be obtained from all patients:
   1. Time of onset of contractions.
   2. Frequency of contractions.
   3. Symptoms of membrane rupture.
   4. Presence of bleeding. If present, determine the time of onset, duration, quality, and amount.
   5. Time of the last intake of solid food or liquids.
   6. The patient should also be specifically questioned regarding the presence of headache, visual disturbances, and abdominal pain unrelated to contractions.
   7. Inquire about the character and frequency of recent fetal movements.
B. *Physical examination*. A complete physical examination should be performed to detect intercurrent disease or factors that may complicate labor and delivery. The following

evaluation of the pregnancy should be performed:

1. *Abdominal examination.* Fetal lie and presentation, fetal heart rate, and fundal height. Note any abdominal tenderness that occurs between contractions.

2. *Pelvic examination.* A pelvic examination *should not* be performed in the presence of any vaginal bleeding until appropriate evaluation of the bleeding has been done. In the absence of vaginal bleeding, the following examinations should be performed:

   a) *Speculum examination.* Note evidence of ruptured membranes, uterine bleeding, and lesions that may indicate an active herpes genitalis infection.

   b) *Digital examination.* Perform a digital examination using aseptic technique to determine cervical dilatation and effacement, station, and fetal position and attitude.

      (1) *Dilatation.* The determination of cervical dilatation involves digital measurement of the diameter of the cervical os. The distance is expressed in centimeters, with 10 cm considered "complete" dilatation. Care should be taken not to stretch the cervix during examination, as this may give a falsely high measurement.

      (2) *Effacement.* The process of cervical thinning before or during labor is termed effacement. The degree of effacement is expressed as a percentage of the length of the uneffaced cervix. The normal uneffaced cervix averages approximately 2 cm in length. A cervix that is 1 cm in length is termed 50 percent effaced. When the cervix becomes as thin as the lower uterine segment, it is termed 100 percent effaced.

      (3) *Station.* Station describes the location of the lowest point of the presenting part in the pelvis. The reference point is the level of the maternal ischial spines, designated *zero station.* Points above and below the level of the ischial spines are measured in centimeters from the reference point.

If the lowest point of the presenting part is 2 cm above the level of the ischial spines, this is designated −2 station. If the lowest point of the presenting part is 2 cm below the level of the ischial spines, this is designated as +2 station. Some authors use an alternate system of designating station in which the long axis of the birth canal is arbitrarily divided into thirds. For example, if the lowest point of the presenting part is one-third of the distance from the ischial spines to the perineum, it is designated as +1 station. If more than one physician is evaluating a patient in labor, it is mandatory that the same system of station designation is used.

3. *Clinical pelvimetry.* The bony pelvis and soft tissues are manually examined. The characteristics of the pelvis are noted.

LABOR ROOM ORDERS

Basic orders for patients in labor may differ among hospitals according to physician preference and institutional tradition or protocol. Orders will be modified according to specific complications. Orders should be specified for the following:

- Diet
- Activity-position
- Vital signs
- Patient preparation
- Labor monitoring
- Intravenous fluids
- Intake and output
- Laboratory studies
- Analgesia-sedation

A. *Diet.* Because gastric emptying essentially ceases with the onset of labor, the patient should receive nothing by mouth (NPO) to prevent possible regurgitation and aspiration. Ice chips and small amounts of water may be given for patient comfort.

B. *Activity-position.* In early labor, the patient may ambulate or sit in a chair as long as membranes are intact and analgesics have not been given. The patient should remain in bed during active labor, after rupture of membranes, or if analgesics have been administered. The left lateral decubitus position will displace the uterus from the inferior vena cava and increase renal and uterine perfusion.

C. *Vital signs.* Blood pressure, pulse, and respiratory rate should be determined every hour with oral temperature determinations every three to four hours. More frequent determinations may be necessary according to the clinical circumstances.

D. *Patient preparation*
   1. *Perineal shave.* If an episiotomy is anticipated, the hair on the perineum may be shaved. Complete shaving of the vulva is uncomfortable and unnecessary.
   2. *Enema.* Evacuation of the rectum and sigmoid colon may prevent fecal soilage at the time of delivery. A Fleets enema or 500 ml tap water enema may be given. *Contraindications* to the use of enemas are:
      a) Ruptured membranes with an unengaged presenting part (possible cord prolapse)
      b) Undiagnosed vaginal bleeding
      c) Imminent delivery

E. *Labor monitoring.* Continuous electronic monitoring of fetal heart rate and uterine contractions has become routine in many institutions. If electronic monitoring is not used or is unavailable, the fetal heart rate should be determined by auscultation every 15 minutes during the first stage of labor and after every contraction during the second stage. Auscultation should begin with the onset of a uterine contraction and continue for 30 seconds after the contraction has stopped.

F. *Intake and output.* Accurate hourly determinations should be made. Urine should be checked for specific gravity and for the presence of glucose, protein, and ketones.

G. *Intravenous fluids.* A solution of 5 percent dextrose in Ringer's lactate or saline should be administered through a secure 16-or-18-gauge indwelling catheter. Fluid should be administered at a rate of 100 to 125 ml/hour in most cases. Intravenous fluids will prevent dehydration during labor and will provide a route for administration of analgesic and other medications.

H. *Laboratory studies*
   1. Hemoglobin and hematocrit determination and urinalysis should be done on all patients at admission. Blood type and Rh factor, RPR, and rubella should be known, and if not documented, obtained. Other studies (PT/PTT, electrolytes, BUN, Cr, CXR, EKG, etc.) should be performed as clinically indicated.
   2. A blood specimen should be sent to the blood bank so that blood may be typed immediately and crossmatched if necessary.

I. *Analgesia-sedation.* Standing orders for analgesia and sedation should not be written. The physician should evaluate the status of the patient and fetus before administering any medication.

MECHANISM OF LABOR IN VERTEX PRESENTATIONS

The mechanism of labor involves a series of changes in the position and attitude of the fetus that allow it to adapt or accommodate to various segments of the pelvis during labor and delivery. The *cardinal movements of labor* are engagement, descent, flexion, internal rotation, extension, external rotation, and expulsion (Fig. 11–1). These movements do not occur separately and independently, but rather in combination during the course of descent.

A. *Engagement.* This is the mechanism by which the biparietal diameter of the head passes through the pelvic inlet. Clinically, the fetus is engaged when the lowest point of the presenting part is at or below the level of the maternal ischial

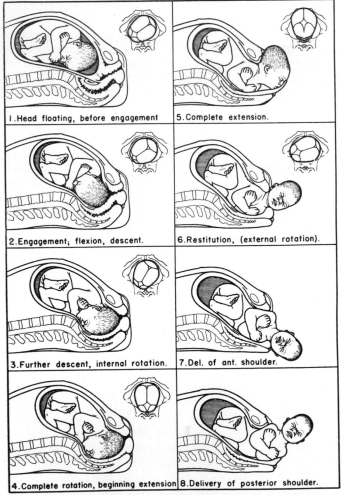

Figure 11–1. Principal movements in the mechanism of labor and delivery; LOA position. (From Pritchard JA, MacDonald PC: Williams Obstetrics, 16th ed. Appleton-Century-Crofts, 1980, p 397.)

spines. In primigravidas, engagement generally occurs approximately two weeks before term. In multiparas, engagement generally does not occur until early labor. The anteroposterior diameter of the head enters the pelvis in either the transverse or oblique diameter of the pelvic inlet (the longest diameter of the head enters the longest diameter of the inlet). The head is considered *synclitic* if the sagittal suture is equidistant from the symphysis and the sacral promontory. The head is *asynclitic* if the sagittal suture is deflected either anteriorly or posteriorly. In *anterior asynclitism,* also called anterior parietal bone presentation, the sagittal suture lies closer to the sacral promontory than to the symphysis. In *posterior asynclitism,* also called posterior parietal bone presentation, the sagittal suture lies closer to the symphysis. Engagement in asynclitism presents the smallest transverse diameter of the head, thus aiding in passage through the inlet.

B. *Descent.* The presenting part is progressively pushed into the pelvis by the force of the uterine contractions, and in the second stage, by voluntary contractions of the abdominal muscles. The degree of descent is measured by change in station. As the head descends through the pelvis, various degrees of *molding* of the head may occur. In order to accommodate to the different diameters of the pelvis, the head may change shape, thus reducing certain cephalic diameters. Movement of the cranial bones occurs at suture lines, and actual overlapping of the bones may occur.

C. *Flexion.* As the descending head meets resistance, flexion occurs. Resistance may occur at the cervix and pelvic side walls or floor. As flexion occurs, the suboccipitobregmatic diameter of about 9.5 cm replaces the larger occipitomental (12.0 cm) and occipitofrontal (10.5 cm) diameters. The presenting anteroposterior diameter of the head is then reduced by approximately 3.0 cm.

D. *Internal rotation.* As the head descends into the midpelvis, rotation occurs so that the sagittal suture occupies the anteroposterior diameter of the pelvis. This occurs because the anteroposterior diameter of the midpelvis is larger than the transverse diameter. Internal rotation normally begins when the presenting part has reached the level of the ischial spines and is completed as the head transverses the midpelvis. Several factors are responsible for rotation. The levator ani, coccygeous, and ileococcygeous muscles form a V-shaped sling that tends to diverge anteriorly and superiorly. In addition to muscular anatomy, the largest diameter of the midpelvis is the anteroposterior.

E. *Extension.* As descent progresses, the occiput contracts the inferior margin of the symphysis pubis. The symphysis acts as a fulcrum, and as further force is applied to the head, extension occurs. The head is born by extension with the occiput, forehead, face, and chin successively passing over the perineum.

F. *External rotation.* The head turns to an oblique position to resume its normal relationship to the shoulders. Further external rotation of the head occurs as the shoulders rotate to an anteroposterior position within the midpelvis.

G. *Expulsion.* After external rotation is completed, the anterior shoulder appears beneath the symphysis pubis and the posterior shoulder distends the perineum. After delivery of the shoulders, the body of the infant is extruded by no specific mechanism.

CLINICAL COURSE OF LABOR

A. *Three stages of labor*
   1. *First stage.* Begins with the onset of labor and ends at the point of complete cervical dilatation.
   2. *Second stage.* Begins with complete cervical dilatation and ends with delivery of the infant.
   3. *Third stage.* Begins with delivery of the infant and ends with delivery of the placenta.
B. *First stage*
   1. *Uterine contractions.* At the beginning of labor, uterine contractions are mild, occurring at regular intervals of 15

to 20 minutes. As labor progresses, the uterine contractions gradually increase in frequency, intensity, and duration. Frequency ranges from every 2 to 5 minutes; intensity ranges from 50 to 75 mm Hg; duration ranges from 45 to 90 seconds.

2. *Pattern of cervical dilatation* (Figs. 11–2, 11–3). Cervical dilatation proceeds with a characteristic pattern that may be demonstrated by graphic analysis. When cervical dilatation is plotted against time, a broad S-shaped curve results. The curve is divided into two well-defined phases, the latent and the active.

a) *Latent phase.* This phase is characterized by slow effacement and dilatation of the cervix to approxi-

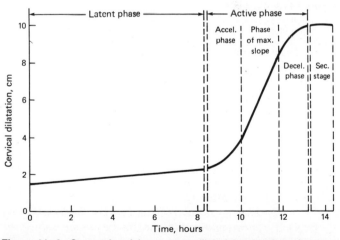

Figure 11–2. Composite of the average dilatation curve for nulliparous labor based on analysis of the data derived from the patterns traced by a large, nearly consecutive series of gravidas. The first stage is divided into a relatively flat latent phase and a rapidly progressive active phase. The active phase has three identifiable component parts—an acceleration phase, a linear phase of maximum slope, and a deceleration phase. (From Friedman EA: Labor: Clinical Evaluation and Management, 2nd ed. New York, Appleton-Century-Crofts, 1978, p 33.)

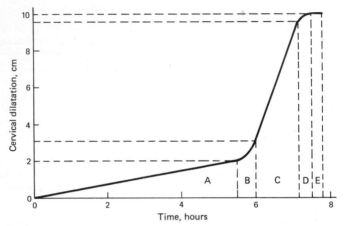

Figure 11–3. Composite of the average dilatation curve for multiparous labor: (A) latent phase, (B) acceleration phase, (C) phase of maximum slope, (D) deceleration phase, (B) through (D) active phase, and (E) second stage. (After Friedman EA:Labor:Clinical Evaluation and Management, 2nd ed. New York, Appleton-Century-Crofts, 1978.)

mately 3 to 4 cm. It begins with the onset of labor and ends with the beginning of the active phase of dilatation.

    (1) *In primigravidas,* effacement is generally complete before significant dilatation occurs. In *multiparas,* effacement and dilatation usually occur concomitantly.

    (2) *There is no correlation between the length of the latent phase and the course of the subsequent labor.*

b) *Active phase.* The active phase is characterized by a more rapid dilatation of the cervix. It begins at the point of an acute change in the rate of cervical dilatation and ends at complete cervical dilatation. The active phase is further divided into phases:

    (1) *Phase of acceleration.* At this time, there is a

transition between the slow dilatation of the latent phase and the rapid linear dilatation of the active phase.

(2) *Phase of maximum slope.* In normal labors, this phase is characterized by a linear progression of dilatation.

(3) *Phase of deceleration.* During this phase, there is an apparent slowing of the rate of cervical dilatation. The cervix retracts over the presenting part allowing descent to progress.

C. *Second stage.* During the second stage of labor, descent and expulsion of the fetus occur:

1. *Uterine contractions.* Uterine activity is usually at a maximum in this stage. Frequency ranges from 1½ to 3 minutes; intensity may exceed 75 mm Hg with voluntary contractions of the abdominal muscles; duration ranges from 60 to 90 seconds.

2. *Pattern of descent.* Descent of the presenting part usually begins during the phase of maximum slope of cervical dilatation. The maximum rate of descent corresponds to the deceleration phase of dilatation. During the second stage, normal descent occurs at a rate of greater than 1 cm/hour in primigravidas and greater than 2 cm/hour in multiparas.

D. *Duration of labor.* The duration of labor in any patient is determined by multiple factors: parity; pelvic size and architecture; fetal size, position, and attitude; consistency of the cervix; and frequency, intensity, and duration of uterine contractions. Table 11–1 presents mean values of various components of labor. A phase or stage of labor with a duration longer than the statistical limit is considered *prolonged.*

E. *Third stage*

1. *Placental separation.* After delivery of the infant and escape of the amniotic fluid, there is a sudden reduction in uterine size. As the area of the placental site decreases, the placenta thickens and begins to buckle. The developing tension leads to cleavage at the decidua spongiosa

**TABLE 11–1. MEAN VALUES OF VARIOUS COMPO-
NENTS OF LABOR**

	Mean	Statistical Limit (95%)
NULLIPAROUS LABOR		
Latent phase	8.6 hr	20.6 hr
Active phase	4.9 hr	11.7 hr
Deceleration	54 min	3.3 hr
Maximum slope	3.0 cm/hr	1.2 cm/hr
Second stage	57 min.	2.5 hr
MULTIPAROUS LABOR		
Latent phase	5.3 hr	13.6 hr
Active phase	2.2 hr	5.2 hr
Deceleration	14 min	53 min
Maximum slope	5.7 cm/hr	1.5 cm/hr
Second stage	14 min	50 min

(Modified from Friedman EA: Labor: Clinical Evaluation and
Management, 2nd ed. New York, Appleton-Century-Crofts, 1978,
p 49.)

layer. A hematoma then forms between the separating
placenta and the uterine wall.

2. *Placental expulsion*
   a) After separation, the placenta is forced into the lower
      uterine segment or upper portion of the vagina by the
      pressure of the developing hematoma and by the force
      of uterine contractions. Some form of manual inter-
      vention is often necessary to completely deliver the
      placenta, since maternal bearing down efforts are
      often insufficient. In the *Schultze mechanism* of
      placenta extrusion, the retroplacental hematoma pro-
      duces progressive inversion of the membranes. The
      glistening fetal surface of the placenta presents at the
      vulva, and blood does not escape externally until after
      delivery of the placenta. In the *Duncan mechanism* of
      placental extrusion, the initial area of placental sep-
      aration probably occurs at the periphery. Blood

dissects between membranes and uterine wall and is eventually visible at the vulva. The placenta enters the vagina in a sideways fashion and the rough maternal surface presents first at the vulva.

b) *Duration.* The average length of the third stage is 5 minutes. It is considered prolonged after 30 minutes.

MANAGEMENT OF LABOR AND DELIVERY

A. *First stage.* Management of the first stage of labor involves continuous evaluation of the fetus, the mother, and the progress of labor

1. *Evaluation of the fetus.* The *routine* assessment of the condition of the fetus is confined to evaluation of the fetal heart rate. Decelerations of the heart rate, loss of beat-to-beat variability, and changes in base-line heart rate mandate further evaluation. The presence of meconium-stained amniotic fluid is suggestive of fetal distress.

2. *Evaluation of the mother.* Vital signs and intake and output are evaluated hourly. The patient is instructed to report severe headache, visual disturbances, and any abdominal pain that is unrelated to contractions. The degree of labor pain should be assessed and the appropriate anesthesia or analgesia administered.

3. *Evaluation of the progress of labor.* The frequency, intensity, and duration of uterine contractions are noted. Vaginal examinations are performed to determine cervical effacement and dilatation, station and position, and attitude of the presenting part. Sterile gloves should be used, and the vulva should be cleansed with an antiseptic solution prior to the examination. *Vaginal examinations* are performed under the following conditions:

a) In normal labors, the vaginal examination should be performed every one to two hours. More frequent examinations will be indicated according to clinical conditions.

b) Before administration of anesthesia or analgesia.

      c) Immediately after spontaneous rupture of the membranes to detect possible cord prolapse.

      d) Upon detection of any abnormality of the fetal heart rate.

      e) When the patient experiences signs that the second stage of labor has started.

B. *Second stage*

  1. Clinical signs

      a) Slight vaginal bleeding may be noted.

      b) The patient has the urge to bear down with contractions.

      c) The patient may indicate the urge to defecate as the presenting part exerts pressure on the rectum.

  2. *Transfer to the delivery room. Sufficient time should be allowed before delivery to properly situate the patient in the delivery room.* Primigravidas should be moved to the delivery room when the presenting part begins to distend the vulva and perineum (crowning). Multiparas are moved to the delivery room when the cervix is about 8 to 9 cm dilated, since the second stage of labor may last only several minutes.

C. *Management of spontaneous delivery.* Preparation of the patient is as follows:

  1. *Positioning for delivery.* The patient is placed on the delivery table in the dorsal lithotomy position. The legs are secured in either stirrups or leg platforms. The buttocks should extend several inches over the edge of the delivery table.

  2. *Preparation of the delivery field.* The vulva, proximal thighs, perineum, and anal area are cleansed with an antiseptic solution. Sterile drapes are placed over the abdomen and legs and under the buttocks.

  3. *Anesthesia.* Several types of anesthesia may be used for delivery, with the choice determined by patient preference and the clinical situation.

D. *Episiotomy.* An episiotomy is an incision into the perineum and vagina that widens the vaginal opening.

1. *Advantages*
   a) It helps prevent or reduce the severity of perineal and vaginal lacerations. An episiotomy is easier to repair than a laceration, and healing is generally more satisfactory.
   b) Compression of the fetal head is reduced.
   c) The second stage of labor is shortened.
2. *Indications*
   a) When a vaginal or perineal tear is anticipated.
   b) In cases of breech or forceps delivery when the largest possible outlet is necessary.
   c) In cases of delivery of a premature infant when it is necessary to reduce head compression.
3. *Types of episiotomy*
   a) *Midline* (median). The perineum is divided in the midline down to a level immediately above the anal sphincter.
      (1) *Advantages* (vs mediolateral episiotomy)
         (a) Repair is easier.
         (b) Blood loss is reduced.
         (c) Healing is generally complete with an excellent anatomic result.
         (d) There is less pain during the puerperium.
         (e) Dyspareunia rarely occurs after healing.
      (2) *Disavantage.* Extension of the episiotomy through the anal sphincter and rectum may occur.
   b) *Mediolateral.* The perineum is divided by an incision directed approximately 45 degrees from the midline to a point just superior to the lateral margin of the anal sphincter.
      (1) *Advantages.* Extension of the episiotomy into the anal sphincter and rectum is less common than with the midline episiotomy.
      (2) *Disadvantages* (vs midline episiotomy)
         (a) Repair is more difficult.
         (b) Blood loss is greater.
         (c) Healing may be incomplete, with resultant

anatomic distortion of the vulva and perineum.

(d) Pain is greater during the puerperium.

(e) Dyspareunia may result due to faulty healing.

c) *Lateral.* A lateral episiotomy is often associated with excessive bleeding and poor healing. There are no advantages to this technique, which is obsolete.

4. *Choice of episiotomy.* The choice of episiotomy in a given clinical situation is somewhat controversial, since both the midline and mediolateral techniques have advantages and disadvantages. In cases of extension of the episiotomy into the anal sphincter or rectum, healing is complete after proper repair in 98 to 99 percent of cases. Rectovaginal fistula may result in less than 2 percent of cases, with spontaneous healing of the fistula often occurring. Extension of a midline episiotomy into the anal sphincter and rectum is associated with a short perineal body, a large infant, forceps delivery, breech delivery, and delivery in the occiput posterior position. The ultimate choice of episiotomy technique often depends upon institutional tradition and personal experience with complications.

5. *Timing of episiotomy*
   a) *Vertex presentations:* as the head begins to distend the perineum
   b) *Breech presentation:* prior to delivery of the head
   c) *Forceps delivery:* after application of the forceps. If a rigid perineum compromises application, an episiotomy should be performed prior to insertion of the blades.

6. *Timing of repair.* The episiotomy is usually repaired after delivery of the placenta and inspection of the vagina and cervix. If bleeding from the episiotomy is excessive before delivery of the placenta, bleeding vessels should be individually ligated. Tamponade with a gauze pad is also effective.

E. *Technique of delivery (occiput anterior position)*
  1. *Birth of the head.* The objectives of a slow, controlled
    delivery of the head are to prevent injury to the infant
    and to prevent or minimize lacerations of the maternal
    tissues.
    a) As the head begins to distend the vulva and perineum,
       the patient is instructed to begin slow, controlled
       bearing-down efforts with contractions. Erratic, force-
       ful bearing down may lead to a rapid uncontrolled
       delivery of the head. An episiotomy may be per-
       formed at this time.
    b) To aid in a slow, controlled delivery, the *Ritgen
       maneuver* may be used. After the occiput has de-
       scended below the symphysis, a hand is placed over
       the vertex, and slight pressure is exerted to prevent
       rapid expulsion of the head. Excessive pressure
       should never be applied. The other hand is covered
       with a towel and the fingers are placed behind the
       maternal anus. Forward pressure is then exerted on
       the infant's chin, and the head is delivered by slow
       extension. The head is generally delivered between
       contractions to enable slow delivery and maximum
       control. If the chin is held up behind the perineum, a
       finger is inserted into the vagina below the chin and
       slight forward pressure is exerted to complete de-
       livery.
    c) The nose, mouth, and oral pharynx are gently suc-
       tioned with a bulb syringe. Prolonged and vigorous
       aspiration should be avoided, since this may lead to
       vagal stimulation and bradycardia.
    d) The neck is then palpated for the presence of coils of
       unbilical cord. A loose cord may be easily slipped over
       the head. If the cord is tight or if several loops are
       present, it should be doubly clamped, cut and un-
       wound.
    e) The head should be supported as external rotation
       occurs.

2. *Birth of the shoulders*
   a) After external rotation is completed, the shoulders have rotated to an anteroposterior position. Spontaneous delivery will then often occur.
   b) If spontaneous delivery does not occur, the patient is instructed to bear down slowly. The head is then grasped in both hands either over the parietal bones or over the face and occiput.
   c) Gentle downward traction is applied until the anterior shoulder is delivered beneath the symphysis.
   d) Gentle upward traction is then applied until the posterior shoulder is delivered over the perineum.
   e) *Excessive traction and bending of the neck must be avoided since brachial plexus injuries may result.*
3. *Birth of the trunk and lower extremities*
   a) After delivery of the shoulders, the remainder of the body usually delivers spontaneously.
   b) If spontaneous delivery does not occur, gentle traction may be applied to the head in the direction of the long axis of the body. The shoulders may be grasped if additional traction is necessary to effect delivery. Bearing-down efforts by the mother may aid in completing delivery.
   c) *Traction should not be applied at the axilla since brachial plexus injuries may result.*
4. Immediate care of the infant
   a) After delivery, the infant is cradled on the physician's arm with the head held down to promote drainage of tracheobronchial secretions. Care should be taken to avoid hyperextension of the infant's head.
   b) Secretions from the nose, mouth, and oral phyarynx are aspirated with a bulb syringe.
5. *Clamping of the umbilical cord*
   a) The umbilical cord should be doubly clamped and cut as soon as is convenient. Normally, the cord is clamped 3 to 4 cm from the skin surface of the infant. The cord should be left longer if an umbilical hernia or

omphalocele is present. If the infant is premature or severely depressed, a long cord segment should be left to allow for insertion of umbilical catheters or injection of medications.

b) If the infant is held below the level of the vulva after delivery, up to 80 to 100 ml of placental blood will enter the infant's circulation. The benefits and disadvantages of the procedure are disputed. In cases of infants affected by maternal-fetal blood group incompatability, the cord should be clamped immediately to prevent the entry of additional red blood cells that may contribute to subsequent hyperbilirubinemia.

c) Samples of blood are then obtained from the portion of the cord still attached to the placenta. The samples are evaluated for fetal blood type and the presence of antibody (direct Coombs test).

d) The cut end of the cord is then inspected for the presence of two arteries and one vein.

F. *Management of the third stage*

1. The uterine fundus is palpated for evidence of placental separation, *signs of which include:*
   a) The uterus changes from a flattened and discoid shape to a globular shape.
   b) The uterine fundus rises.
   c) There is a sudden gush of blood from the vagina.
   d) The portion of the umbilical cord outside of the vulva lengthens. The umbilical cord does not recede when the uterus is elevated.

2. Uterine massage and other manipulation should be avoided until evidence of placental separation is present. Premature attempts at delivery may lead to uterine inversion or partial placental separation and hemorrhage.

3. After the placenta has separated, the patient should bear down while gentle traction is applied to the cord.

4. If these efforts fail or if the patient is under anesthesia, *manual expression* may be necessary. Gentle traction is applied to the cord. The fingers of the other hand are

placed over the lower uterine segment immediately above the symphysis. The uterus is then simultaneously pushed cephalad and down towards the maternal spine. If tension is then felt in the cord, complete separation has not occurred and further attempts at expulsion should be postponed for several minutes. If no tension is felt in the cord, continued cephalad and downward pressure should be applied until the placenta becomes visible at the introitus.

5. The placenta is then slowly delivered to prevent tearing of the membranes. Torn membranes should be grasped with ring forceps and removed by gentle traction.

6. The maternal surface of the placenta should be examined for the presence of missing fragments, and the membranes should be examined for the presence of torn vessels. Manual exploration of the uterus is necessary if retained placental fragments or accessory lobes are suspected.

7. Drugs are commonly administered to decrease subsequent bleeding by promoting myometrial contraction. Though probably not necessary in most patients, the following drugs may be administered: *oxytocin* (Pitocin, Syntocinon), *ergonovine maleate* (Ergotrate), *methylergonovine* (Methergine), and prostaglandin E_2. The choice of drug and route of administration have been shown to make little difference in the degree of postpartum bleeding.

   a) *Oxytocin* (possible routes and dosages)

      (1) 10 units IM after delivery of the infant (or with delivery of the anterior shoulder).

      (2) 10 units IM after delivery of the placenta.

      (3) 10 or 20 units in 1 liter of intravenous fluid. A 200- to 300-ml bolus of fluid is given either after delivery of the infant or after delivery of the placenta. The rate of infusion is then decreased to 100 to 125 ml/hour.

    (4) Bolus intravenous administration of undiluted oxytocin is considered to be contraindicated by many authorities because of a potent vasodilating effect that may lead to an acute drop in blood pressure.

  b) *Ergot derivatives: ergonovine maleate, methylergonovine* (possible routes and dosages)

    (1) 0.25 to 0.5 mg IM after delivery of the placenta.

    (2) The intravenous administration of these drugs should be avoided. Severe hypertension, depression of the sinoatrial node, cardiac arrhythmias and cardiac arrests have been reported.

  c) Because of the high incidence of pospartum hemorrhage associated with the following clinical conditions, these patients should receive either oxytocin or ergot derivatives after delivery; overdistended uterus (multiple gestation, large infant, hydramnios), history of previous postpartum hemorrhage, high parity, prolonged labor, rapid labor, oxytocin-induced or stimulated labor, and general anesthesia with the use of agents causing myometrial relaxation.

8. *Manual removal of the placenta.* Active intervention to remove the placenta will be necessary in the following circumstances:

  a) If there is excessive vaginal bleeding due to incomplete separation.

  b) If there is suspicion of retained placental fragments or membranes.

  c) If separation and expulsion have not occurred after 30 minutes from the time of delivery of the infant.

  d) *Technique*

    (1) General anesthesia should be administered.

    (2) The fundus of the uterus is pushed downward towards the pelvis using the abdominal hand.

    (3) The other hand is inserted through the vagina into the uterine cavity.

(4) The margin of the placenta is identified and a cleavage plane is established by gentle finger dissection.

(5) The fingers are gently swept between the placenta and uterine wall until the entire placenta is separated.

(6) The placenta is grasped and withdrawn slowly.

(7) If there is unusual difficulty in separating the placenta, further efforts should cease and placenta accreta should be suspected.

9. *Inspection of the maternal soft tissues.* After delivery of the placenta, the cervix, vagina, vulva, perineum, and rectum should be inspected for injury.

a) *Cervix.* The posterior portion of the vagina is exposed using either retractors or by depressing the vaginal floor with the fingers. The anterior lip of the cervix is grasped with ring forceps and pulled towards the introitus. Deep lacerations or areas or bleeding should be repaired using either interrupted or continuous sutures. After repair, the patency of the endocervical canal should be evaluated by digital examination.

b) *Vagina.* The outer portion of the vagina may be exposed by depressing the vaginal floor with the fingers or with a retractor. Examination of the upper vagina may require retractors. If lacerations are present, bleeding vessels should be individually ligated and the vaginal mucosa closed with a continuous suture. Small hematomas generally do not require repair. If the hematoma appears to enlarge, the vaginal mucosa over the hematoma should be incised and the bleeding vessels ligated.

c) *Vulva.* Small lacerations of the vulva are common, especially after uncontrolled deliveries. Most small lacerations do not require repair. If there is active bleeding or if a large defect is present, repair is necessary. Bleeding vessels should be individually ligated and the skin reapproximated using interrupted sutures. Bleeding in the periurethral area can usually be stopped by applying pressure with a gauze pad. If repair is necessary, fine grade sutures are used. The urethra should be avoided, since urethral strictures may result. If significant periurethral urethral edema is anticipated, resultant urethral obstruction may be avoided by placement of a Foley catheter for 24 to 48 hours.

d) *Perineum.* Four degrees of perineal laceration are described:

(1) *First-degree laceration.* The laceration involves the forchette, perineal skin, or vaginal mucosa with no involvement of underlying muscle. Repair with interrupted sutures is necessary only if bleeding is present or the defect is large.

(2) *Second-degree laceration.* The laceration involves the forchette, perineal skin or vaginal mucosa, and underlying muscles. Repair is required to restore the normal anatomy of the perineum. The muscles are reapproximated using interrupted sutures.

(3) *Third-degree laceration.* The laceration has extended to involve the anal sphincter. The perimuscular fascia overlying the severed ends of the sphincter is reapproximated using interrupted sutures. Sutures placed only through the sphincter muscle will usually tear through.

(4) *Fourth-degree laceration.* The laceration has further extended to involve the rectum. Repair is mandatory to prevent the development of a rectovaginal fistula. The *technique of repair* is as follows:

(a) A finger is inserted into the rectum to evaluate the extent of the laceration.

(b) The rectal wall is closed using interrupted fine suture placed through the muscularis layer of the rectal wall. The sutures are

placed 0.5 cm apart and should not protrude
into the rectal lumen.

(c) The fascia overlying the rectum is reapproximated using interrupted sutures.

(d) A rectal exam is again performed to ensure
that there are no defects in the rectal
closure.

(e) The anal sphincter is reapproximated.

(f) The remainder of the repair is described
under *Episiotomy repair* below.

10. *Manual exploration of the uterus.* In the following situations, manual exploration of the uterus is required before
repair of the episiotomy or lacerations. General anesthesia may be required:

a) If retention of placental fragments or membranes is
suspected.

b) After forceps delivery if uterine injury is suspected.

c) After vaginal delivery of a patient who has undergone
a previous cesarean section.

d) If an acquired or congenital uterine anomaly is
suspected.

11. *Episiotomy repair.* There are numerous techniques of
episiotomy repair. All are designed to obtain exact
anatomic reapproximation of severed tissues:

a) All bleeding vessels should be individually ligated.

b) The vaginal mucosa is reapproximated using a continuous suture. The initial suture is placed approximately 1 to 2 cm above the apex of the vaginal incision
to ensure inclusion of retracted vessels or extension of
the incision. The continuous suture is carried to the
hymenal ring.

c) The severed edges of the fascia and muscles are
reapproximated using either interrupted or continuous sutures. Two layers of closure may be necessary.

d) The skin of the perineum is reapproximated using
either interrupted sutures or a continuous subcuticular
suture.

12. *Postpartum note.* The following format may be used to summarize the delivery in the medical record:

	Example
1. Procedure	Spontaneous vaginal delivery
2. Obstetrician	Dr. _____
3. Assistants	Dr. _____
4. Anesthesia	Pudendal block
5. Placental delivery	Spontaneous
6. Episiotomy	Midline
7. Lacerations	First-degree laceration of the perineum
8. Blood loss	495 ml
9. Condition of infant	Male; Apgar score: 8 (one minute)/9 (five minute)
10. Complications	None

INDUCTION OF LABOR

A. *Indications.* Induction of labor is indicated when prolongation of the pregnancy would place the mother or fetus in jeopardy *and* when vaginal delivery is not contraindicated by maternal or fetal factors.

B. *Contraindications*
   1. The following contraindications to induction of labor are similar to the contraindications to vaginal delivery:
      a) Known or suspected fetopelvic disproportion
      b) Placenta previa
      c) Uterine scar (previous cesarean section, myomectomy, or unification procedure)
      d) Transverse lie
   2. Many authorities also consider the following to be contraindications to induction of labor but not necessarily contraindications to vaginal delivery:
      a) Breech presentation

b) Uterine overdistention (hydramnios, multiple gestation)

c) Grand multiparity (very controversial, especially when intrauterine pressure monitoring is available)

C. *Physical factors.* Successful induction of labor is more likely to occur in near-term or term pregnancies when the cervix is soft, partially dilated, and partially effaced. A convenient system for predicting the success of induction is the *Bishop scoring system* (Table 11–2). Five factors are evaluated: cervical consistency, cervical effacement, cervical position, cervical dilatation, and station of the presenting part. Values are assigned to each factor, with a total score ranging from zero to 13 points. The likelihood of successful induction of labor increases as the point total becomes higher.

D. *Methods of inducing labor*

1. *Amniotomy.* Spontaneous labor follows artificial rupture of the membranes in approximately 90 percent of patients who are near term with high Bishop scores. In preterm pregnancies, the incidence of spontaneous labor decreases with decreasing gestational age. The principal risks of amniotomy are cord prolapse and amnionitis if labor is prolonged. Amniotomy should be performed only if the fetus is definitely to be delivered within 24 hours.

a) *Technique*

(1) In general, amniotomy should be performed only when the presenting part is firmly applied to the cervix, and preferably when the presenting part is engaged. If amniotomy is performed with an unengaged or floating presenting part, there is increased risk of cord prolapse.

(2) Two fingers are inserted into the vagina using aseptic technique. The membranes are palpated and the station of the presenting part noted. If the umbilical cord is palpated through the membranes, amniotomy is not performed.

TABLE 11–2. Bishop Scoring Factors

Scoring criteria	0	1	2	3	Total Possible Score: 13
Cervical consistency	Firm	Medium	Soft	—	2
Cervical position	Posterior	Midposition	Anterior	—	2
Cervical effacement	0–30%	40–50%	60–70%	< 80%	3
Cervical dilation	Closed cervix	1–2 cm dilation	3–4 cm dilation	5–6 cm dilation	3
Station of fetal head	–3	–2	–1/0	+1/+2	3

    (3) The membranes are ruptured using a suitable hook device (Amnihook), making certain not to injure the presenting part.

    (4) The vaginal fluid is allowed to escape slowly with the vaginal fingers remaining in place to detect cord prolapse.

    (5) No attempt should be made to displace the presenting part upward, since cord prolapse may result.

    (6) Stripping of the membranes from the cervix should be avoided, as this might lead to separation of a low-lying placenta.

2. *Oxytocin*

   a) *Physiology*. The following properties of exogenous oxytocin must be considered during its clinical use in induction or augmentation of labor:

    (1) The response of the uterus is a dose-dependent increase in contractility.

    (2) The dosage needed to initiate contractions depends on the reactivity of the myometrium.

    (3) Dosages above the level needed to initiate contractions will increase both the amplitude and frequency of contractions.

    (4) After a certain contraction frequency is exceeded, uterine tonus will increase. Further dosages of oxytocin may increase uterine tonus to high levels.

    (5) The sensitivity of the myometrium to exogenous oxytocin gradually increases until term.

    (6) The half life of exogenous oxytocin is between three and six minutes.

    (7) Oxytocin has an antidiuretic effect somewhat less than vasopressin. A clinically significant antidiuretic effect is seen only when prolonged high doses are used.

   b) *Administration*. Because of the potentially serious consequences of uterine overstimulation, oxytocin must be administered in a dilute concentration through a continuous infusion pump. Close supervision of administration is mandatory:

(1) Before administration of oxytocin, continuous electronic monitoring of fetal heart rate and uterine contractions is instituted.

(2) A convenient oxytocin solution is prepared by adding 10 units of oxytocin (Pitocin, Syntocinon) to 1000 ml of 5 percent dextrose in water or a balanced saline solution, the final oxytocin concentration of which will be 10 milliunits (mU) per milliliter (1 mU/0.1 ml).

(3) A two-bottle technique of infusion should be used. In the primary intravenous line, the patient should recieve fluid that contains no oxytocin. The fluid containing oxytocin is connected to the main intravenous fluid line through a Y-connector. This technique will ensure that the patient does not receive large quantities of oxytocin if the intravenous line is inadvertently allowed to run at a high rate.

(4) The oxytocin solution should be administered using a continuous infusion pump mechanism (Harvard pump, I-vac pump).

(5) The infusion is started at a rate of 2 mU (0.2 ml/minute). The infusion rate may be increased by 2 mU/minute at 15-to 20-minute intervals until the optimum pattern of contractions is achieved. Increasing the rate at more frequent intervals is inappropriate, since maximal uterine response to oxytocin is not realized for 15 to 20 minutes.

(6) Optimally, the uterine contractions should be moderate to strong in intensity, occurring every three minutes and lasting 45 to 60 seconds. Complete relaxation of the uterus should occur between contractions.

(7) An infusion of 2 mU/minute will be sufficient to

initiate contractions in most term pregnancies. A dosage up to 16 mU/minute may be necessary, and even higher dosages may be necessary in preterm pregnancies.

(8) Successful induction of labor is unlikely if adequate contractions cannot be obtained with an infusion of 30 to 40 mU/minute.

(9) Close monitoring during oxytocin administration is mandatory. Because of the risks inherent with oxytocin administration, many centers require that an attendant be present continuously. Prolonged contractions or elevated uterine tonus may adversely effect placental circulation and lead to fetal hypoxia.

(10) Oxytocin administration should be stopped immediately if the following signs of overstimulation develop:

(a) The duration of the uterine contractions exceeds 90 seconds.

(b) Late deceleration of the fetal heart rate develop.

(c) The uterus does not relax between contractions.

(d) More than four contractions occur in a 10-minute period.

(e) After the signs of overstimulation resolve, the infusion may be restarted with a lower maintenance dosage.

3. *Prostaglandins*. Prostaglandins have been used widely to initiate uterine contractions for midtrimester pregnancy terminations. Their clinical use for induction of labor is currently under investigation. The major disadvantage of prostaglandins is hypercontractility.

GENERAL TEXTS

Friedman EA: Labor: Clinical Management and Evaluation, 2nd ed. New York, Appleton-Century-Crofts, 1978

Oxorn H: Human Labor and Birth, 4th ed. New York, Appleton-Century-Crofts, 1980

Pritchard JA, McDonald PC: Williams Obstetrics, 16th ed. New York, Appleton-Century-Crofts, 1980

BIBLIOGRAPHY

Brandt ML: Mechanisms and management of the third stage of labor. Am J Obstet Gynecol 25:662, 1933

Friedman EA: Cervimetry: an objective method for the study of cervical dilation in labor. Am J. Obstet Gynecol 71:1189, 1956

Friedman EA: The functional division of labor. Am J Obstet Gynecol 109:274, 1971

Friedman EA: Labor in multiparas. Obstet Gynecol 8:691, 1956

Friedman EA: Primigravid labor. Obstet Gynecol 8:691, 1955

12

Obstetric Analgesia and Anesthesia

William Gottschalk, M.D.

PRACTICE PRINCIPLES

All anesthetic-analgesic procedures involve risks to the mother and to the fetus.

All anesthetic-analgesic agents cross the blood-brain barrier.

All anesthetic-analgesic agents cross the placenta.

Definition

- *Analgesia:* Abolition of painful sensations.
- *Anesthesia:* Abolition of all sensations.

CAUSES OF MATERNAL MORTALITY

Anesthesia, since its inception, has been a significant cause of maternal mortality (it is usually ranked first to fourth).

A. *Complications with general anesthesia*
  1. *Aspiration* of gastric contents
     a) Particulate matter (food)
     b) Gastric juices (pH 2.5)
  2. *Complications with hypoxia,* hypercarbia, acidosis, sec-

ondary to complications resulting from the use of potent anesthetic agents, and/or muscle relaxants.

3. *Airway management problems* (for example, endotracheal intubation misadventures).

B. *Regional blocks*

1. Local anesthetic intoxication

   a) *Overdosage.* Over 95 percent of the complications resulting from the administration of local anesthetics are caused by abnormally high levels of circulating local anesthetics.

   b) *Allergic reactions.* Allergic reactions are limited to ester-linked local anesthetics (e.g., procaine, 2-chloroprocaine, tetracaine).

   c) *Hypotension.* Secondary to the administration of a regional block such as epidural, caudal, and subarachnoid block, hypotension occurs more frequently during pregnancy than in the nonpregnant state, because hypotension is secondary to the blocking of spinal segments containing sympathetic nerves and to the compression of the inferior vena cava by the gravid uterus.

   However, hypotensive episodes related only to sympathetic blockade are easily reversed.

   d) *High doses.* Administration of imprudently high doses of local anesthetic in the course of a subarachnoid block. The pregnant patient needs a third to a half the quantity of local anesthetic she would need in the nonpregnant state for a similar level of block.

GENERAL MANAGEMENT PRINCIPLES

A. No anesthesia that causes or has the potential to cause a loss capable of depriving the patient of consciousness should ever be administered without the presence of:

1. Personnel trained in anesthesia and its complications.

2. Modern anesthesia equipment equal in quality to that used in the operating room.

3. Resuscitation equipment and drugs as normally expected in other situations in which patients' lives may be at risk because of anesthesia.

B. The administration of a regional block in a labor room makes it advisable to have *within easy reach* the drugs and equipment necessary to manage complications resulting from the injection of a local anesthetic as well as complications resulting from the blocks themselves.

MATERNAL CHANGES AFFECTING ANESTHESIA

A. While anesthesia effectuates changes in maternal physiology and fetal physiology, changes in normal physiology due to pregnancy alter the usual management of the patient and the expected effects of anesthesia.

B. *Diminished functional residual capacity* and the *increased effective alveolar ventilation* tend to speed up the rate of induction of inhalation anesthesia. With highly potent vapors such as halothane, enflurane, and methoxyflurane unwanted depths of anesthesia are reached significantly faster. Although the increased cardiac output of pregnancy slows the rate of induction of anesthesia, this effect is masked by the more significant respiratory changes.

C. Great care should be employed in the administration of subarachnoid blocks in pregnancy because of the *diminished volume of the subarachnoid space.* This is possibly due to the engorgement of the internal venous plexus that occupies space in the epidural space, thereby compressing and diminishing the subarachnoid space. The amount of local anesthetics necessary to achieve an epidural block is possibly diminished in pregnancy. However, this point is controversial.

D. The diminished concentrations of circulating plasma cholinesterases during pregnancy do not appear to be of clinical significance. These enzymes are necessary for the metabolism of substances used in anesthesia such as succinylcholine (a depolarizing muscle relaxant) and local anesthetics of the ester-linked type (procaine, 2-chloroprocaine, tetracaine).

TRANSPLACENTAL PASSAGE OF ANALGESICS AND ANESTHETICS

A. All anesthetic and analgesic agents used in anesthesia cross the placental barrier. However, muscle relaxants, whether depolarizing or nondepolarizing, do not cross the placenta in clinically significant amounts.
B. All analgesic and anesthetic agents pass through biologic membranes such as the blood-brain barrier or the placenta by simple diffusion. Factors influencing transplacental passage of anesthetic and analgesic agents are (in order of importance):
   1. Lipid solubility.
   2. Degree of ionization (the less ionized the more readily the drug passes the placenta).
   3. Molecular weight (drugs having molecular weights over 1000 do not cross the placenta in significant amounts). The molecular weight of protein-bound fractions of administered drugs should be considered as the sum of the drug plus the protein.
   4. Of lesser importance are the maternal-fetal concentration gradient and exchange membrane surfaces and thicknesses. Changes in maternal or fetal cardiovascular physiology may also play a role in the transplacental passage of analgesic-anesthetic drugs.

ALTERATIONS OF LABOR ATTRIBUTABLE TO ANESTHESIA

A. Alterations of normal labor attributable to analgesic or anesthetic agents, administered in usually accepted concentrations, are difficult to evalute. Alterations of labor patterns attributed to anesthesia without prior careful evaluation of possible obstetrical causes can be misleading and result in delaying diagnosis of more probable causes.

B. Potent anesthetic vapors are effective myometrial depressants: they can arrest uterine contractions, and in the third stage of labor they may lead to postpartum hemorrhage as a result of a lack of myometrial tone. Regional anesthetic methods can alter the normal progression of labor in a variety of ways and through various mechanisms:

1. In-vitro local anesthetics can alter myometrial contractions. However, the usual amounts of local anesthetics administered in the course of a subarachnoid, epidural, paracervical, or pudendal block are insufficient to alter normal spontaneous or oxytocin-induced uterine contractile patterns.

2. All blocks that relax the pelvic musculature may interfere with internal rotation and flexion, and may therefore prolong the second stage of labor.

3. All blocks that anesthetize the perineum deprive the parturient of the urge to bear down, also thereby potentially prolonging the second stage of labor.

C. *Sensory deprivation does not necessarily imply that the patient has been deprived of the motor ability to bear down.* Specifically, this is true of pudendal blocks and all other blocks that involve only sacral segments. However, in the case of lumbar-epidural blocks, low concentrations of local anesthetics will not block motor fibers to the extent that there will be interference with normal efforts at bearing down. As to subarachnoid blocks the concentrations of local anesthetics necessary to block motor nerves are higher than those necessary to block sensory nerves. Therefore, if a sensory block is administered to level T_{10}, the motor blockade, because of the dilutional factor, will not affect motor nerves above T_{12}, allowing the patient to bear down voluntarily.

D. Epinephrine, occasionally used as an adjuvant to local anesthetics in order to prolong regional blocks and diminish the uptake of local anesthetic agents, may diminish uterine tone and the intensity and frequency of uterine contractions by stimulating β-adrenergic receptors.

E. Perhaps the single most important fact to be remembered about alteration of labor secondary to the administration of regional blocks and systemic analgesics is that their *injudicious use during the latent phase of labor may delay the onset of the acceleration phase of spontaneous labor*. However, any effect caused by these agents and techniques can be reversed by the administration of oxytocin.

LOCAL ANESTHETICS

A. *Physiology.* Local anesthetics are weak bases usually prepared for clinical use as hydrochloride salts. Depending on the pK_a (the pH at which half of the substance is ionized and half un-ionized), different concentrations of the drug will be in the cationic (ionized form) or base form (un-ionized). Today's concept of the way local anesthetics block impulse transmission attributes to the base the role of passing through biologic membranes (nerve membranes, placenta); however, it is the cationic form that blocks the nerve impulse propagation. Hence, local anesthetics with high pK_a's such as bupivacaine will have more of the drug in the ionized form at physiologic pH (7.4) than local anesthetics such as mepivacaine with lower pK_a's. It follows that local anesthetics with high pK_a's will not cross the placental barrier as readily as local anesthetics with lower pK_a's.

B. *Chemical structure.* Local anesthetics can be divided into two groups on the basis of chemical structure. (Fig. 12–1). All local anesthetics bear a striking resemblance to each other; however, the linkage between the aromatic and the aliphatic moiety is what differentiates them into amide-linked local anesthetics and ester-linked local anesthetics.

   1. *Amide-linked.* All of the most recently synthesized local anesthetics—bupivacaine, etidocaine, mepivacaine,

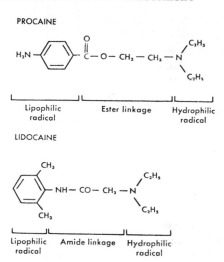

Figure 12–1. Chemical structure of procaine and lidocaine.

lidocaine — are amide-linked local anesthetics. These drugs are metabolized by hepatic microsomal enzymes both by the mother and fetus or neonate.

2. *Ester-linked.* Ester-linked local anesthetics such as procaine, 2-chloroprocaine, and tetracaine are metabolized by plasma cholinesterases. In the case of 2-chloroprocaine, the elimination half-life is only 21 seconds in the mother and 43 seconds in the neonate (Table 12–1).

C. *Neonatal effects*

1. Molecular weight, pK_a, route, and rate of metabolism play a major role in the effect of these drugs on the neonate. While it is true that depression secondary to the effect of local anesthetics on the fetus is rare except after paracervical blocks, studies of more discrete changes — neurobehavioral effects — are probably much more common and may interfere with early adaptation to

TABLE 12–1. LOCAL ANESTHETICS COMMONLY USED IN OBSTETRICS

Local Anesthetic	Molecular Weight	Protein Binding	pK_a	Maternal: Fetal Ratio at Birth	Neonatal Elimination Half-Life (hr)	Anesthesia Potency	Latency	Duration
Procaine (Novocaine)	236	66	8.9	—	—	1	Moderate	Short
2-Chloroprocaine (Nesacaine)	307	—	8.7	—	43 (sec)	2	Fast	Very short
Tetracaine (Pontocaine)	264	75	8.2	—	—	15	Very slow	Long
Lidocaine (Xylocaine)	271	50	7.9	2:1	3	3	Fast	Moderate
Mepivacaine (Carbocaine)	285	65	7.7	3:2	9	3	Fast	Moderate
Bupivacaine (Marcaine)	325	95	8.1	4:1	2	15	Moderate	Long

extrauterine life. It now appears that local anesthetics that cross the placenta readily or are eliminated slowly (lidocaine, mepivacaine) cause more problems than local anesthetics that cross the placenta with difficulty or are rapidly eliminated (bupivacaine and 2-chloroprocaine).

2. Hepatic microsomal enzymes are not as fully developed in the newborn as in the adult; renal excretion may be impaired; the blood-brain barrier may be more permeable in the newborn than in the adult.

D. *Clinical characteristics.* While it is possible to predict the clinical characteristics of local anesthetics by examination of their chemical structure, this is beyond the scope of this book. However, some of the more important clinical characteristics are listed below (Table 12–2).

Paracervical Block

A. *Technique and physiology.* A paracervical block consists of the injection of a local anesthetic into the nerve-rich zones at the base of the broad ligament. This space also contains the uterine arteries and veins, as well as the ureters. Paracervical blocks interrupt the sensory pathways that emanate from the uterus and cervix, and hence they are useful only in management of the pain of the first stage of labor. The technique involves the transvaginal administration of a local anesthetic, in the fornices, on either side of the cervix (3 to 4 or 8 to 9 o'clock).

B. *Advantages*
   1. Simplicity of instrumentation and ease of administration.
   2. It is readily accepted by the patient in labor and when successful gives excellent analgesia during the first stage of labor.

C. *Disadvantages and complications*
   1. Postparacervical block fetal bradycardia. The administration of a local anesthetic in the paracervical areas can result in a 20 to 70 percent incidence of postparacervical

TABLE 12-2. CONCENTRATIONS AND DOSAGES USUALLY RECOMMENDED FOR VARIOUS BLOCKS*

Local Anesthetic	Available Concentration %	Local Infiltration %	Subarachnoid (mg.) VAGINAL	Subarachnoid (mg.) CESAREAN	Epidural (%)† VAGINAL DELIVERY SEGMENTAL	Epidural (%)† VAGINAL DELIVERY STANDARD	Epidural (%)† CESAREAN	Pudendal Blocks %	Paracervical %	Maximum Amounts (mg/kg)
Procaine (Novocaine)	1, 2, 10	0.5	—	—	—	—	—	1–2	1	12
2-Chloroprocaine (Nesacaine)	2–3	0.5–1	—	—	—	—	—	2–3	2	15
Tetracaine (Pontocaine)	1 (powder)	0.05	3	6–8	—	—	—	—	—	2
Lidocaine (Xylocaine)	1–1.5 2–5	1–1.5 5–	25–30	50–70	1–2 (4–6)	1–2 (6–10)	1.5–2 (16–20)	1	1	6
Mepivacaine (Carbocaine)	1–2	1–2	—	—	1–2 (4–6)	1–2 (6–10)	1.5–2 (16–20)	1	1	6
Bupivacaine (Marcaine)	0.25, 0.5, 0.75	0.06–0.125	—	—	0.125–0.5 (4–6)	0.125–0.5 (6–10)	0.375–0.75 (16–20)	0.25–0.5	0.125 0.5	2

*Higher concentrations for epidural blocks are only recommended when muscle relaxation is necessary.

†Recommended dosage of percent concentration indicated is given in parentheses (in ml).

block fetal bradycardia. This is a true bradycardia unrelated to uterine contractions and has been attributed to:
   a) Large quantities of local anesthetics passing the placental barrier.
   b) Increase in uterine tone.
   c) Decrease in intervillous space perfusion due to increased uterine artery vasoconstriction.
2. Failure to produce analgesia in 10 to 20 percent of parturients.
3. Retroperitoneal infections.
4. Hematomas.
5. Maternal local anesthetic intoxication.

Pudendal Block

A. *Technique and physiology.* A pudendal block involves the administration of a local anesthetic into Alcock's canal as it courses under the ischial spine. This technique blocks the pudendal nerve, which is made up of the anterior primary division of S_2, S_3, and S_4. The pudendal nerve divides into three major branches: the inferior hemorrhoidal nerve, the perineal nerve, and the dorsal nerve of the clitoris. The pudendal block may be administered through the perineum or transvaginally. The latter is the most frequent route of administration.
B. *Advantages*
   1. Instrumentation is simple.
   2. Good pain relief is achieved during the second stage of labor.
   3. Progress of labor is usually not altered; however, a pudendal block eliminates the afferent limb of the reflex that urges the parturient to bear down.
   4. Landmarks necessary for performing the block are easily identifiable.
   5. No special postanesthetic surveillance is necessary.
   6. It is readily accepted by patients.
   7. It results in enough analgesia to allow the physician to

perform low forceps and low midforceps deliveries. However, the addition of inhalation analgesia is recommended. The combination of pudendal block and inhalation analgesia gives considerably more comfort to the parturient than either of these techniques alone.

8. Pudendal blocks allow the obstetrician to work safely without the assistance of an anesthesiologist or nurse anesthetist.

C. *Disadvantages*

1. It does not give as predictable an area of anesthesia as do low spinals, caudals, and epidural blocks, nor is the area of anesthesia as wide.

2. It is often difficult to gauge the optimal time of administration.

3. The pudendal artery and veins are in close proximity to the pudendal nerve.

4. Failure to obtain good analgesia may lead to repeated injections, which can result in local anesthetic overdosage.

5. It does not relieve the pain sensations emanating from the uterus and cervix (T_{10}–T_{11}–T_{12}).

D. *Indications*

1. Absence of an anesthesiologist; at the time of delivery, a pudendal block is the safest form of regional anesthesia an obstetrician can administer.

2. Spontaneous vaginal deliveries, including assisted breech deliveries.

3. Low forceps deliveries (vertex on the perineum in direct occipitoanterior position).

4. Simple midforceps deliveries.

5. Repair of low vaginal or perineal lacerations.

6. Minor surgical procedures involving the perineum and/or lower vagina.

7. Procedures that may require a weighted vaginal speculum and will be performed under local infiltration or paracervical block.

E. *Contraindications*
1. The obstetrician's lack of thorough knowledge of the pertinent anatomy and technique and of knowledge of the pharmacology of local anesthetics.
2. Lack of knowledge and skill in preventing, promptly diagnosing, and effectively treating systemic toxic reactions and other complications.
3. Intrauterine manipulations (the cervix and uterus are innervated by lower thoracic segments).
4. Difficult midforceps rotations.
5. Infection of the perineum, perianal, labial, or ischiorectal space.

F. *Complications*
1. Vaginal and ischiorectal hematomas.
2. Retroperitoneal infections.
3. Infections of the acetabulum or femoral head.
4. Toxic reactions to local anesthetics.
5. Abolition of the desire of the parturient to bear down.

REGIONAL ANESTHESIA

General Principles

Regional anesthetic blocks have become the preferred way of handling analgesia-anesthesia during labor, vaginal delivery, and cesarean section, in part because they alter maternal physiology in more predictable ways than general anesthetics. They also affect the baby, in the usual controlled clinical situations, less perceptibly than other techniques. They have in common the fact that they allow mothers to remain conscious at the birth of their child and leave them able to participate. These techniques also make participation by the husband more feasible. Pain relief can be extended over prolonged periods of time without significantly altering fetal or neonatal well-being. Selective use of one regional technique over another allows for significant flexibility over the course of labor, vaginal delivery, or cesarean section. Local anesthetics used to perform these blocks present a variety of physical and chemical characteristics and physiological and pharmacologic effects that make some local anesthetics preferable to others, depending on the clinical situation (Table 12–1).

A. *Physiology*
  1. Fundamental to understanding the uses of regional techniques in obstetrics is the knowledge of pain perception and nerve distribution.
  2. During the *first stage of labor,* pain is due to myometrial contractions and stretching of the uterine cervix. Nerve endings in these structures are stimulated and transmit impulses via A-delta fibers and c fibers that traverse the uterine plexus, the middle hypogastric plexus, the superior hypogastric plexus, and the upper lumbar and lower thoracic sympathetic chains; they enter the white rami communicantes to reach the posterior roots at T_{10}, T_{11}, and T_{12}. Pain sensations at the end of the first stage of labor may become sufficiently severe as to cause pain spread to the first and second lumbar segments. Pain sensations travel along single nerve fibers from the uterus to the spinal cord, the nerve cells themselves being in the dorsal ganglia. It is believed that, thereafter, synapses in the dorsal horn of the thoracic spinal cord transmit the pain sensations to other nerve fibers by way of the contralateral and ipsilateral spinothalamic tracts.
  3. Pain and pressure sensations during the *second stage of labor* are mediated by fibers originating in the lower vagina, vulva, and perineum that reach the spinal cord via the anterior primary divisions of the second, third, and fourth posterior sacral roots.
B. *Regional blocks*
  1. *Subarachnoid block*
    a) *Technique and physiology.* Subarachnoid block consists in the injection of a local anesthetic into the

subarachnoid space. Once injected, the local anesthetic mixes with the cerebrospinal fluid. Hence the specific gravity of the injected local anesthetic is of considerable importance considering its spread. In obstetrics, only hyperbaric solutions of local anesthetics are used. (Hyperbaric: solutions of specific gravity greater than that of CSF.) Hyperbaric solutions are usually made by mixing the local anesthetic with 5 to 7.5 percent dextrose in water.

The technique of a subarachnoid block for obstetrical purposes consists of the introduction of an appropriate needle between lumbar vertebral spinous processes (usually L_2–L_3, L_3–L_4, or L_4–L_5). The needle is advanced until puncture of the dura occurs; the local anesthetic solution is then injected.

b) *Advantages*
   (1) Simple to perform with available drugs and equipment
   (2) Clear end point (CSF)
   (3) Predictable side effects (hypotension)
   (4) Effects on the fetus are usually avoidable and treatable, and are secondary to changes in maternal physiology
   (5) Allows the patient to remain awake at delivery
   (6) Good muscle relaxation
   (7) Serious complications are very rare
   (8) Local anesthetic intoxication virtually impossible because of the small amounts injected

c) *Disadvantages*
   (1) Frequent hypotension (20 to 90 percent depending on the level of sensory blockade, e.g., T_{10}–T_5)
   (2) Postpuncture headache (due to traction on pain-sensitive structures in the skull due to the drop in CSF pressure resulting from CSF leakage)
   (3) Neurologic damage (very rare)
   (4) Poorly accepted by some

    (5) "Segmental" blocks not practicable

    (6) In the usual setting cannot be continued for prolonged periods of time

d) *Indications*

    (1) When general anesthesia is contraindicated or undesirable

    (2) When pain relief is necessary but wakefulness is desirable

    (3) When a major regional block is necessary for a relatively short period of time

    (4) When loss of consciousness is to be avoided but good muscle relaxation is required

    (5) When the fetus is to be spared the potential systemic effects of local anesthetics (small quantities of local anesthetics are used)

e) *Contraindications for subarachnoid, lumbar-epidural, and caudal blocks*

    (1) Hypotension present or expected

    (2) Hypovolemia, whether from dehydration, blood loss, or expected blood loss (a major contraindication to any block involving the thoracolumbar nervous system)

    (3) Infections at the site of the contemplated puncture

    (4) Anticoagulation therapy

    (5) Active central nervous system disease

    (6) Patient refusal (perhaps even patient ambivalence)

    (7) Untrained personnel

    (8) Unavailability of medications and equipment necessary for the management of complications arising from these blocks, or unavailability of equipment and medications necessary for life-support measures

    (9) Absence of monitoring equipment

    (10) Absence of a guaranteed intravenous access to the systemic circulation

f) *Hypotension*

(1) Of all side effects or complications secondary to subarachnoid blocks administered during gestation, hypotension is the most common. It occurs in 20 percent of subarachnoid blocks administered for vaginal delivery with sensory levels up to T_{10}, and in over 85 percent of subarachnoid blocks administered for cesarean section with levels up to T_5. Hypotension is caused by the combination of sympathetic blockade and inferior vena cava compression.

(2) *Management.* It is advisable to attempt to prevent hypotension secondary to subarachnoid or epidural blocks. The patient should be "preloaded" with 500 to 1000 ml of a lactated Ringer's solution, to increase the circulatory volume acutely, and the uterus should be displaced to the left to relieve inferior vena cava compression. Following the administration of a major block, blood pressures and other vital signs should be monitored with great frequency. Should the systolic blood pressure drop below 100 mm Hg, intravenous fluid should be rapidly infused. If the blood pressure does not quickly return to acceptable levels, a vasopressor should be administered.

The choice of a vasopressor in obstetrics demands that it not reduce intervillous space perfusion. Therefore, all vasoactive substances causing significant vasoconstriction (α-adrenergic-receptor stimulants) are not recommended. Ephedrine which has principally β- but some α-adrenergic properties is the vasopressor of choice. It can be administered intravenously in doses of 10 to 25 mg. It has been recommended by some that 50 mg ephedrine be administered intramuscularly at the time of the institution of the subarachnoid block. However, the use of vasopressors

precludes the administration of ergot derivatives.
The sequential or simultaneous use of ergotrate
derivates and/or vasopressors has been responsible for reported maternal deaths secondary to
sudden hypertensive crisis with resulting heart
failure and cerebrovascular accidents.

2. *Lumbar-epidural blocks*
   a) *Technique and physiology*
      (1) A lumbar-epidural block involves the injection of
          a local anesthetic solution into the lumbar-
          epidural space.
      (2) The epidural space extends from the base of the
          skull to the tip of the caudal canal. For all
          practical purposes, the epidural space is limited
          ventrally by the dura and dorsally by the ligamen-
          tum flavum. The single most important difference
          between a subarachnoid and an epidural block is
          that injections into the epidural space are made in
          a virtual space filled with nerve roots, blood
          vessels, fat, and areolar tissue. While dilution of
          the local anesthetic by cerebrospinal fluid is of
          major consideration in subarachnoid blocks, it
          does not occur in the epidural space. Hence, the
          extent of the block is dependent on the mass of
          local anesthetic injected (volume × concentra-
          tion).
      (3) An epidural block gives the anesthesiologist
          greater flexibility both in choosing the extent of
          the block and the quality of the block (sensory,
          sympathetic, motor). By injecting small volumes
          of local anesthetics it is possible to block only
          certain specific nerve roots as they pass through
          the epidural space. It is also possible to avoid
          motor blockade by utilizing low concentrations of
          local anesthetics. For example, bupivacaine,
          0.125 to 0.25 percent, does not interfere with
          motor function; however, bupivacaine, 0.75 per-

cent, while affording good pain relief, will also give a significant measure of muscle relaxation.

(4) By carefully limiting the volume of local anesthetics administered during the first stage of labor (4 to 5 ml) one can achieve a "segmental epidural block" involving nothing but segments T_{10}–L_2. This will spare the sacral segments and therefore not interfere with the parturient's reflex bearing-down efforts; neither will it block painful sensations during the second half of labor. By maintaining low concentrations of local anesthetics it is also possible to avoid motor weakness of the abdominal muscles, thereby allowing the parturient to effectively push during the second stage of labor.

(5) In the course of a "standard epidural block" all segments from T_{10} to S_5 are blocked. This is accomplished by the administration of 6 to 10 ml of local anesthetics injected during the course of labor and will block all segments involved in pain perception during the first and second stages of labor; however, it will interfere with reflex bearing-down efforts.

b) *"Single-shot" vs. "continuous" epidural block.* While there is some risk in the placement of a catheter in the subarachnoid space, because the nerve roots are devoid of any covering except pia mater, the placement of a catheter in the epidural space presents few risks and allows for the repeated injection of local anesthetic (continuous block) and maintenance of anesthesia for several hours. However, with the advent of long-acting local anesthetics for epidural use, such as bupivacaine and etidocaine, single-shot epidural blocks can also be varied in length of action (35 to 40 minutes in the case of 2 percent 2-chloroprocaine or 3 to 4 hours with 0.75 percent bupivacaine).

c) *Epidural for cesarean section.* Epidural for cesarean sections can be performed either as a "single-shot" or as a "continuous" epidural block depending on the local anesthetic administered and the expected duration of the procedure (Table 12–2).

d) *Advantages*
(1) Segmental blockade of T_{10}–L_2 is feasible.
(2) Repeated injections can be performed through a catheter placed in the epidural space. This requires only one needle puncture.
(3) Muscular blockade can be avoided or produced, depending on the concentration of the local anesthetic.
(4) Duration of the block can be controlled by appropriate choice of the local anesthetic and avoidance or addition of a vasoconstrictor, which slows down local anesthetic reabsorption (epinephrine, phenylephrine) and prolongs the block.

e) *Disadvantages*
(1) Sympathetic blockade increases the incidence of hypotension.
(2) Large quantities of local anesthetics can cause systemic intoxication if injected in a vessel or in a highly vascular area.
(3) Inadvertent subarachnoid injection can cause a "total spinal" block.
(4) Large quantities of local anesthetic can cause neurobehavioral changes in the newborn.
(5) Inadvertent dural puncture with a large-bore epidural needle can cause a high incidence of postpuncture headache (the larger the bore, the higher the incidence).

3. *Caudal Blocks*
a) *Techniques and physiology*
(1) The caudal canal is contained between the anterior and posterior tables of the sacrum; it is

filled with the same tissues as the epidural space and is continuous with it.

(2) Like lumbar-epidural blocks, caudal blocks can be administered to maintain analgesia during the first and second stages of labor. However, it is not possible to block only thoracic or lumbar segments without also blocking sacral segments. It is possible to extend the block to the levels necessary to perform a cesarean section; however, very large quantities of local anesthetics would be necessary. This problem is related to the fact that injections of local anesthetics into the caudal canal results in the escape of large volumes of the injected substance from the canal through the anterior sacral foramina to the perirectal space, where they serve no useful purpose.

(3) Caudal blocks can be administered either as a single-shot or as continuous blocks.

(4) A single-shot technique consists of the introduction of a needle between the cornua of the sacrum through the sacro-coccyxgeal membrane and into the caudal canal. Local anesthetics are then injected. A continuous-block technique consists of the introduction of a needle in a similar manner as in the single-shot technique; however, a catheter is then threaded 5 cm cephalad and left in place for later reinjections.

b) *Advantages*. These are the same as epidural block; however, it is possible to block only the sacral segments and thereby avoid sympathetic blockade. This is only of use during the second stage of labor.

c) *Disadvantages*

(1) Disadvantages are the same as those of a lumbar-epidural block, however, special precautions must be taken not to let the needle slip lateral to the sacral cornua and puncture the rectum, vagina, and even the fetal presenting part.

(2) Inadvertant subarachnoid or intravascular injections are potentially more dangerous in view of the larger quantities of local anesthetics that usually need to be injected.

(3) The area where the caudal blocks are administered is frequently contaminated. The presence of a high incidence of sacral and anatomic variations may make the performance of a caudal block difficult.

d) *Contraindications*. These are the same as for a lumbar-epidural block. However, the presence of a pilonidal cyst contraindicates the administration of a caudal block.

GENERAL ANESTHESIA

A. *Complications*
   1. Changes in respiratory and cardiovascular physiology.
   2. The fact that no mother in labor can be considered to have an empty stomach, regardless of when her last meal was ingested; gastric juices of a pH of less than 2.5 can, if aspirated, produce severe respiratory and cardiovascular changes that may lead to death or to permanent respiratory damage. (Aspiration of gastric contents is the most prevalent cause of maternal mortality attributable to anesthesia.)
   3. Anesthetic vapors such as ether, chloroform, enflurane, isoflurane, and halothane, are potent myometrial depressants.
   4. Rapid transplacental passage of volatile anesthetic vapors may anesthetize and depress the fetus.
B. *Indications*
   1. *General considerations*. The administration of general anesthesia implies the need for a technique that either requires unconsciousness or makes unconsciousness unavoidable in the face of other anesthetic requirements.

General anesthesia is *never* to be administered when it is not absolutely medically indicated.

2. Refusal of a regional technique.
3. When hypovolemia is present and anesthesia is necessary, and local infiltration or other minor blocks are insufficient.
4. Bleeding.
5. Unmanageable patients.
6. Intrauterine manipulations, when no regional technique can be utilized.
7. Any surgical situation when time is of the essence (e.g., fetal distress).

C. *Contraindications*
   1. Lack of trained personnel
   2. Lack of adequate equipment
   3. Refusal by patient

D. *Relative contraindications*
   1. Full stomach
   2. Asthma
   3. Anatomic distortion of face and neck

E. *Techniques*
   1. All techniques of general anesthesia that result in loss of laryngeal reflex integrity must involve *airway protection* such as is afforded by an endotracheal tube. In view of the potentially lethal effects of aspiration of acid gastric juices, at pH lower than 2.5, *the administration of antacids 30 minutes before induction of anesthesia is highly recommended* (e.g., Riopan, 30 ml; Maalox, 30 ml; Gelusil, 30 ml). The administration of antacids does not replace the well-ordered precautions rcommended to prevent aspiration of gastric contents.
   2. Techniques of general anesthesia must take into consideration the *myometrial-depressant effect* of anesthetic gases such as halothane, enflurane, isoflurane, ether, and chloroform; however, nitrous oxide, cyclopropane, ketamine, barbiturates, narcotics, and muscle relaxants, do not depress the myometrium. Myometrial relaxation

may at times be desirable in the management of special situations, such as trapped second twin, uterine inversion, and retained placenta.

3. The most common technique of general anesthesia used in obstetrics, whether for vaginal delivery or cesarean section, combines a "rapid induction" that minimizes the risks of maternal aspiration, as well as fetal depression, with a "balanced anesthesia" technique that causes light anesthesia and good muscle relaxation. This technique also generally avoids myometrial and fetal depression, without increasing maternal risks.

F. *Sequence of necessary steps*
   1. Preoxygenation — 5 minutes
   2. *d*-Tubocurarine, 3 mg IV (to prevent fasciculations caused by succinylcholine)
   3. Thiopental (4 mg/kg or less), IV bolus
   4. Succinylcholine (0.5–1.0 mg/kg), IV bolus
   5. Digital pressure on the cricoid cartilage to prevent passive regurgitation
   6. Rapid, unhesitating, oral endotracheal intubation
   7. Nitrous oxide is added to the oxygen (4 liters nitrous oxide/2 liters oxygen)
   8. Succinylcholine drip to maintain muscle relaxation (or other muscle relaxant)
   9. This is continued until after the birth of the baby, when the administration of narcotics, benzodiazepines, or low concentrations of volatile anesthetic agents may be administered to supplement nitrous oxide. Multiple variations on this theme exist. For example, ketamine, 0.3 to 0.5 mg/kg, may be substituted for thiopental (step 3) in cases where hypovolemia is suspected and hypotension is feared.

      Ketamine is a dissociative agent that stimulates the sympathetic nervous system. It can be a potent respiratory depressant for the fetus if used in inappropriate doses. However, it has the advantage over rapid-acting barbiturates of altering neurobehavior in the newborn to a lesser extent than thiopental.

G. *Inhalation analgesia*

1. With few exceptions *anesthetic gases are potent analgesics.* Inhalation analgesia implies the administration of inhalation anesthetic agents in subanesthetic concentrations; it allows the patient to remain conscious although experiencing analgesia.

2. *Recommended concentration* of common anesthetic agents: nitrous oxide, 30 to 40 percent; diethyl ether, 2 percent; chloroform, 0.1 to 0.5 percent; cyclopropane, 3 to 5 percent; methoxyflurane, 0.2 to 0.8 percent.

3. In systemic sedation and analgesia, care must be taken to differentiate between the need for sedation and the need for analgesia. All sedatives, tranquilizers, narcotics, and hypnotics cross the placental barrier. They may therefore affect the fetus and newborn. The unnecessary administration of sedatives and narcotics must be avoided during the latent phase of labor, since it may prolong it.

4. Tranquilization may be achieved by means of the administration of:
   a) Hydroxizine, 50 to 100 mg IM.
   b) Promethazine.

5. Diazepam is contraindicated, as are the other benzodiazapines. They can cause flaccidity in the newborn and derange its temperature-regulating mechanisms. What is more, diazepam has a prolonged elimination half-life and may compete for bilirubin binding sites (probably due to preservatives).

H. *Narcotics*

1. *All narcotics cross the placental barrier rapidly.* At equipotent doses no major differences exist between narcotics with regard to respiratory depression. However, major differences in elimination time and peak concentration do exist for various narcotics and various routes of administration. For example, the effect of an IM injection of morphine sulfate occurs in the second hour; analgesia lasts four to six hours. The peak effect of meperidine occurs in 40 to 50 minutes, while analgesia may last three hours. Intravenous administration of

narcotics reach their peak in minutes, but their effectiveness diminishes rapidly thereafter.

2. Rapid intravenous administration of a bolus of narcotics
will result in the almost immediate appearance of the
drug in the fetal circulation. Moreover, concentrations in
the fetus may be higher than the concentration in the
mother. This problem may last for as long as 30 minutes.
Therefore, it is advised that if narcotics are to be
administered intravenously, they should be administered
slowly over several circulation times. The advantage of
intravenous administration of narcotics is that it allows
the physcian to "titrate" the doses administered

3. Narcotic analgesia can be potentiated by the administration of low concentrations of nitrous oxide (30 to 40
percent). This can also be achieved by low concentrations
of methoxyflurane (0.5 percent).

4. Narcotics can be reversed by the administration of
narcotic antagonists such as *N*-allyl noroxymorphone,
naloxone (Narcan). This modern narcotic antagonist,
although a narcotic derivative, has no agonistic properties
and therefore will not cause respiratory depression.
Narcotic antagonists belong to the family of opiods and
hence cross the placenta rapidly.

PSYCHOLOGIC ANALGESIA
Psychologic support for the woman in labor has been part of her
management throughout the ages, in all civilizations. More or
less scientific approaches to the problem however, are relatively
new.

A. *Natural childbirth.*This method, introduced by Grantly
Dick-Read in 1933, is dedicated to breaking the vicious cycle
of fear-tension-pain through a series of prenatal lectures and
exercises.

B. *Psychoprophylactic method.* In 1947, Velvovski, a Russian
physician, introduced the concept of the "psychoprophylactic method." The method is based on the Pavlovian

conditioned-reflex theory. Lamaze introduced the method in France, and it was popularized in the United States by Karmel.

At present the psychoprophylactic method (Lamaze method) is the most popular in the United States.

C. *Hypnosis.* Used throughout the ages, hypnosis can be used both for vaginal deliveries and cesarean sections; however, the method is time-consuming and unpredictable.

D. *Acupuncture.* Acupuncture is another method that approaches the problem of the pains of childbirth without the use of pharmacologically active agents; it appears to have limited success both here and in the Orient.

E. *Advantages.* Do not rely on drugs that may cross the placenta and affect the fetus.

F. *Disadvantages*
   1. May be inadvisedly proselytized and should not be used to the exclusion of other methods if these other methods are necessary.
   2. In the absence of medication, labor may lead to hyperventilation with a resulting drop in P_{CO_2}, maternal respiratory alkalosis, vasoconstriction of the uterine bed, diminished intervillous space perfusion, altered maternal-fetal gas exchanges, fetal hypoxia, and fetal metabolic acidosis.

BIBLIOGRAPHY

Bromage PR: Epidural Analgesia. Philadelphia, WB Saunders, 1978

Caton D: Ob anesthesia: the first 10 years. Anesthesiology 33:102, 1970

Clinik EW: Perineal nerve block; an anatomic and clinical study in the female. Obstet Gynecol 1:137, 1953

Cosmi EV: Obstetric Anesthesia and Perinatology. New York, Appleton-Century-Crofts, 1981

Covino BG, Vassallo HG: Local anesthetics. In Mechanisms of Action and Clinical Use. New York, Grune & Stratton, 1976

Lamaze F: Painless Childbirth: the Lamaze Method. New York, Pocket Books, 1972

Levinson G, Shnider SM: Anesthesia for Obstetrics. Baltimore, Williams & Wilkins, 1979

Marx GF, Cosmi EV, Wollman SB: Biochemical status and clinical condition of mother and infant at C/S. Anesth and Analg 48:986, 1969

Scanlon JW, Brown WV, Weiss JB, et al.: Neurobehavioral responses of newborn infants after maternal epidural anesthesia. Anesthesiology 40:121, 1974

Scanlon JW, Ostheimer GW, Lurie AO, et al.: Neurobehavioral responses and drug concentrations in newborns after maternal epidural anesthesia with bupivaccaine. Anesthesiology 45:400, 1976

13

Resuscitation of the Depressed Newborn

Diane R. Gomez, M.D.

PRACTICE PRINCIPLES

Profound neurologic sequelae or loss of life itself await the newborn who fails to make an uncomplicated transition from intrauterine to extrauterine life. Neonatal asphyxia—i.e., combined hypoxemia and hypercapnea—can result from maternal, placental, or fetal factors, and calls upon delivery room personnel to perform emergency procedures to maintain adequate ventilation and circulation in the depressed newborn.

ANTICIPATION

Numerous antenatal and perinatal conditions should alert medical personnel to the infant potentially at risk for birth asphyxia. Communication with the pediatrician provides him or her with an opportunity to anticipate and prepare for problems that may arise.

The following is a list of events that constitute risk factors that may threaten fetal well-being.

A. *Maternal factors*
   1. Toxemia
   2. Fever (maternal infection, chorioamnionitis)
   3. History of maternal infection (TORCH, etc.)

   4. Prolonged rupture of membranes (> 24 hours)
   5. Abruptio placentae or placenta previa
   6. Polyhydramnios or oligohydramnios
   7. Primigravida (> 35 years of age)
   8. Age greater than 40 or less than 16
   9. Drug addiction or ethanol abuse
  10. Hypotension
  11. Chronic disease
      a) Cardiovascular
      b) Pulmonary
      c) Diabetes mellitus (also gestational diabetes)
      d) Renal
      e) Hematologic
      f) Metabolic
  12. Malignancy
  13. Chronic medications
  14. Previous neonatal death
  15. Cephalopelvic disproportion
B. *Fetal factors*
   1. Prematurity (< 38 weeks)
   2. Postmaturity (> 42 weeks)
   3. Multiple gestation
   4. Intrauterine growth retardation
   5. Abnormal presentation
   6. Meconium staining
   7. Umbilical cord prolapse
   8. Persistent fetal tachycardia (> 160 beats/min)
   9. Loss of beat-to-beat variability
  10. Late or variable decelerations
  11. Decreased fetal scalp pH
  12. Immature lecithin-sphingomyelin ratio or lung profile
  13. Abnormal stress or nonstress testing
  14. Sudden decrease in estriols or HPL
  15. Erythroblastosis fetalis
C. *Labor and delivery factors*
   1. Prolonged labor
   2. Precipitous labor

3. Version
4. Forceps delivery or vacuum extraction
5. Cesarean section
6. Anesthesia-analgesia
7. Traumatic delivery

EQUIPMENT

It is essential that necessary equipment be available and inspected to ensure proper function. Every delivery room should contain the following:

- Overhead radiant warmer
- Towels
- Flow-through infant resuscitation bag with tailpiece, capable of administering 100 percent oxygen
- Face-masks of various sizes
- Oxygen source
- Suction source (bulb syringe, DeLee suction device, wall suction, etc.)
- Suction catheters (5 and 8 French)
- Stethoscope
- Laryngoscope with #0 and #1 straight (Miller) blades
- Endotracheal tubes (2.5-, 3.0-, and 3.5-mm internal diameter)
- Syringes
- Needles (including #23 and #25 Butterfly needles)
- Umbilical venous catheters (3.5 and 5 French)
- Three-way stopclock
- Scalpel blade
- Transport incubator with oxygen source
- Medications
  Sodium bicarbonate, 0.45 mEq/cc
  Epinephrine 1:10,000
  Dextrose, 10 percent solution
  Normal saline
  Calcium gluconate, 10 percent solution
  Naloxone

BIRTH ASPHYXIA: PRIMARY VS. SECONDARY APNEA

Dawes' animal studies (using the rhesus monkey) describe the natural history of birth asphyxia, demonstrate the changes in physiologic parameters during total asphyxia and resuscitation, and underscore the critical importance of time with regard to intervention, recovery, and permanent neurologic impairment or death (Fig. 13-1).

A. Within seconds of clamping the cord of a normal fetal monkey whose head has been covered by a warm saline bag, a short series of rapid gasps commence, along with thrashing muscular efforts. Moments later, these activities cease and heart rate falls precipitously. At this time, the animal experiences a brief period of *primary apnea,* during which cyanosis and then pallor ensue.

B. This is followed by a series of gasping efforts that gradually weaken and terminate in the last gasp, heralding the period of *secondary* or *terminal apnea.* During the animal's second rally, blood pressure has begun to drop; during the period of secondary apnea, both heart rate and blood pressure continue to fall.[1] From the onset of asphyxia, acid-base parameters undergo changes: pH and PO_2 drop; PCO_2 and blood lactate rise, reflecting inadequate compensatory anaerobic metabolic processes.

C. During the period of *primary apnea,* spontaneous respirations can be induced by various sensory stimuli; during *secondary apnea,* respirations cannot be elicited by stimulation alone. Instead, artificial ventilatory measures must be instituted, at which point heart rate and blood pressure will begin to rise. *Time is paramount:* the longer the delay in establishing resuscitative efforts, the longer the time to the first gasp and subsequent regular respirations, and the greater the potential for central nervous system damage or death.

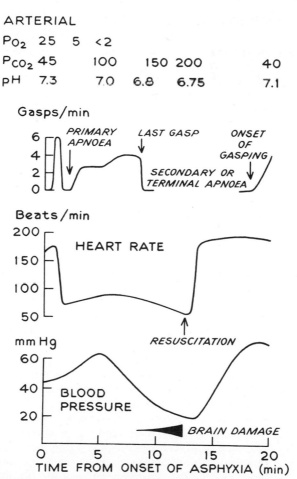

Figure 13–1. Asphyxia and resuscitation in the rhesus monkey. (Reproduced with permission from Dawes GS: Foetal and Neonatal Physiology. Copyright © 1968, by Year Book Medical Publishers, Inc., Chicago.)

ASSESSMENT

Appropriate assessment of the severity of birth depression is essential in determining the mode and dispatch of management.

A. *Apgar scoring system.* A useful guideline for immediate evaluation is the classic Apgar scoring system (Table 13–1). This consists of a rating of 0, 1, or 2 for each of five objective signs: *Heart rate, respiratory effort, muscle tone, reflex irritability,* and *color.* The *Apgar score* — the sum of the independent scores — is to be ascertained at one and five minutes of life, i.e., after both the head and feet of the infant are visible. A score of 7 to 10 indicates a normal infant; a score of 4 to 6, a moderately depressed infant; a score of 0 to 3 is indicative of a severely depressed newborn.[2]

B. *Interpretation of the Apgar scoring system.* The one-minute Apgar score identifies the infant in need of immediate assistance. The five-minute score not only reflects the effects of resuscitative efforts or the infant's own ability to rally, but is believed to correlate with neonatal morbidity and mortality.[3] Dr. Apgar herself has warned of the misconception of waiting until a full minute has passed before resuscitating a severely depressed baby. She also has recommended that the score be assigned by someone other than the individual who is delivering the baby, since he or she tends to be involved emotionally with the outcome of the delivery and may unconsciously fail to make an accurate assignment, thereby delaying active intervention.

   1. *Heart rate.* The normal heart rate is between 120 and 160 beats/minute. Low rates tend to be associated with moderate to severe asphyxia and signify decreased cardiac output. One notable exception is congenital heart block, where the normal heart rate for the infant is approximately 60 beats/minute.

   2. *Respiratory rate.* Respiratory activity should commence by 30 seconds of life and then improve and stabilize progressively. Respiratory rate may vary between 30 and 60/minute. Low respiratory rates reflect asphyxia, respi-

TABLE 13–1. APGAR SCORING SYSTEM

Sign	0	1	2
Heart rate	Absent	< 100/min	> 100/min
Respiratory effort	Absent	Slow or irregular	Good; crying
Muscle tone	Flaccid	Some flexion of extremities	Good flexion, active motion
Reflex irritability	Absent	Grimace	Cough, sneeze, cry
Color	Blue or pale	Body pink extremities blue	Completely pink

ratory acidosis, maternal sedation, sepsis, or central nervous system insult. Rapid respirations suggest hypoxia, hypovolemia, metabolic acidosis, pneumothorax or pneumomediastinum, or the respiratory distress syndrome.

3. *Muscle tone.* All infants should be active and demonstrate recoil when a limb is hyperextended and then released. Poor muscle tone or flaccidity may mean severe asphyxia, maternal sedation, or congenital central nervous system disease. Tone is acquired in a cephalad direction; therefore, very young prematures normally may demonstrate less flexion in the upper — and even the lower — extremities.

4. *Reflex irritability.* Squeezing or flicking of the feet, and suctioning or insertion of a nasal cathether should elicit movement.

5. *Color.* All infants are cyanotic at delivery. Color improves once ventilation is established. *Acrocyanosis* (blue feet, hands, and lips) is acceptable initially, but the trunk and mucous membranes should become pink. *Persistent cyanosis,* i.e., perfusion of unoxygenated blood, may mean compromised cardiac output, congenital heart disease, polycythemia, or pulmonary anomaly or disease. *Pallor* indicates peripheral vasoconstriction resulting from profound acidosis, hypovolemia, or anemia.

C. *Rapid assessment.* A practical shortcut rating utilizes two of the above parameters: heart rate and muscle tone. *A baby with a heart rate above 100 beats/minute, and good flexion or activity tends to require little or no assistance. On the other hand, an infant who is bradycardic and flaccid almost invariably will have a poor or absent respiratory effort, cyanosis, or pallor, and will not be responsive to stimulation alone. Such infants require immediate assistance.*

RESUSCITATION

Resuscitation of the depressed newborn should follow a systematic and orderly sequence (Fig. 13–2). Ongoing assessment of the infant's condition will determine the indication for and mode of intervention. It must be remembered that unnecessary procedures may result in iatrogenic complications, while delay in instituting appropriate measures may further the degree of birth depression.

A. *Obstetrician clears airway.* When the infant's head appears, and before the shoulders are delivered, the obstetrician should suction the mouth, then nares, with a bulb syringe. If the nares are suctioned first, the infant may gasp and aspirate the oral contents. After delivery, the cord is clamped and cut.

B. *Infant placed under radiant warmer.* The baby should be placed under a radiant warmer. Do not cover the infant with a towel, for the baby's skin must be exposed to the source of radiant heat for it to be effective. The head should be lower than the feet in order to promote bronchial drainage and prevent aspiration. The head and neck should be maintained in neutral or "sniffing" position. Molding and edema of the occiput may result in increased flexion of the neck and airway compromise. This can be remedied by placing a folded towel or blanket under the infant's shoulders.

C. *Dry face and body.* Quickly, the infant's face and body should be dried to prevent heat loss through evaporation. Hypothermia will increase the infant's oxygen consumption and, if prolonged, can produce metabolic acidosis and hypoglycemia.

D. *Clear airway.* The oropharynx should be suctioned gently with a bulb syringe. Vigorous suctioning with a catheter, or immediate passage of a nasogastric tube, should be avoided as either may produce bradycardia or apnea of vagal etiology.[4]

E. *One-minute Apgar: 7–10.* An active, pink infant should be observed until after the five-minute Apgar to ensure continued well-being. This is a suitable time for appropriate identification, vitamin K administration to prevent hemorrhagic disease of the newborn, and either silver nitrate 1 percent ophthalmic preparation or intramuscular penicillin

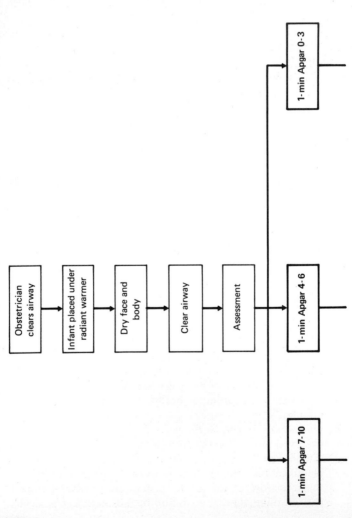

Obstetrician clears airway → Infant placed under radiant warmer → Dry face and body → Clear airway → Assessment

1-min Apgar 0-3

1-min Apgar 4-6

1-min Apgar 7-10

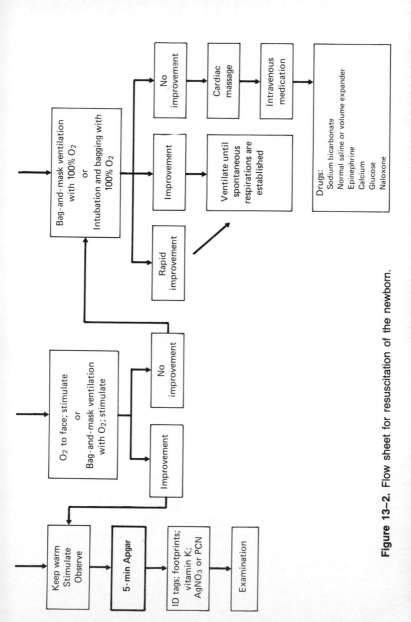

Figure 13–2. Flow sheet for resuscitation of the newborn.

for protection against gonococcal ophthalmia neonatorum. Brief examination will preclude overlooking even subtle problems or anomalies.

F. *One-minute Apgar: 4–6.* The newborn who is *mildly to moderately depressed* demands accurate assessment to administer proper assistance and to avoid unnecessary intervention. This is the infant most likely in *primary apnea,* or approaching the last gasp prior to secondary apnea.

1. If the baby has spontaneous respirations, oxygen can be waved over the baby's face during gentle stimulation, e.g., flicking the feet or further drying of the skin with a soft cotton towel. Jack-knifing, slapping, hot-and-cold water pouring, and dilatation of the anal sphincter are melodramatic and to be disapprobated. Furthermore, a high flow of cold, unhumidified oxygen directly stimulating the posterior pharynx may produce vagal stimulation and result in reflex apnea and/or bradycardia.

2. The precordium should be auscultated or the base of the umbilical cord palpated for pulsations.

3. The first breath of an infant may necessitate exertion of negative pressures from 40 to 80 cm of water.[5] If the anesthesia bag is to provide the infant's first breath, a pressure up to 60 cm of water may be necessary to expand the lungs. Thereafter, pressures of 20 to 25 cm of water should be adequate, although infants with severe hyaline membrane disease may continue to require higher pressures.

4. Proper technique is a prerequisite to successful positive pressure ventilation with bag-and-mask. (Remember that most Ambu-type ventilators deliver oxygen to the mask only when squeezed.) An appropriate-size mask should cover the infant's mouth and nose with no air leak. Oxygen-rich gas at approximately 5 liters/minute should be delivered at a rate of 30 to 40 inflations/minute. Expiration should be slightly longer than inspiration to preclude carbon dioxide retention. Adequacy of ventilation can be assessed by observation of chest motion,

auscultation of breath sounds, or prompt improvement of heart rate and color. Since the opening pressure of the stomach is less than the opening pressure of the lung, sustained bag-and-mask ventilation may produce gastric distention and limit tidal volume secondary to decreased diaphragmatic excursions. Placement of a nasogastric tube will then relieve overinflation of the stomach.

5. Within 30 to 60 seconds of positive pressure breathing, a mildly to moderately depressed infant should recover and begin to establish spontaneous respirations. Iatrogenic pneumothorax is always a risk, and overaggressive bagging should therefore be avoided.

6. An infant who responds quickly will not need exogenous buffers to remedy a probable acidosis, but will self-correct over time. Follow-up of these infants should include monitoring of pH and blood gases, along with periodic glucose determinations, especially if the infant will not be fed immediately. Asphyxiated infants, especially small ones, can deplete their cardiac and hepatic glycogen stores, placing them at risk for hypoglycemia.

G. *One-minute Apgar: 0–3.* The severely depressed, brady-cardic, flaccid infant constitutes a *medical emergency*. The onset of *secondary apnea* heralds brain damage, which can be halted only when adequate resuscitative measures are instituted.

1. Some neonatologists feel that even a severely asphyxiated infant first should be given a trial of bag-and-mask ventilation, resorting to endotracheal intubation only if the infant fails to respond to the former. Others maintain that an Apgar score of less than 3 is an immediate indication for intubation.[6] This is especially true when airway obstruction or meconium aspiration is suspected, and intubation will avoid the development of acute gastric distention.

2. *Intubation.* The laryngoscope should be held between the thumb and index finger of the left hand, while the baby's chin is grasped with the third and fourth fingers of the

same hand. This leaves the small finger available to apply pressure over the thyroid cartilage to move the larynx posteriorly, thereby facilitating visualization of the vocal cords. The laryngoscope is introduced to the right or left side of the mouth and moved to a midline position; while depressing the tongue, it is advanced until the blade tip lodges in the vallecula (i.e., the space between the base of the tongue and epiglottis). A lifting or rocking action of the blade will bring the vocal cords (which will appear as an inverted V) into view. An endotracheal tube of appropriate size should be inserted from the right side of the mouth and advanced between the vocal cords to approximately 2 cm below the glottis. While the endotracheal tube is being held in place, it can be attached to the resuscitation bag and the child ventilated with 100 percent oxygen at a rate of 50 breaths/minute. Careful auscultation of equal breath sounds over both lung fields will testify to proper placement.

H. *Cardiac massage.* If the heart rate fails to rise over 70 beats/minute following a series of lung inflations, cardiac massage should be instituted. Two techniques are practiced:

   1. Holding the chest in both hands, with the fingertips on the spine, the thumbs are placed on the body of the sternum at the junction of the middle and lower thirds. The sternum is then compressed approximately two-thirds of the distance to the vertebral column at a rate of 100 to 120 compressions per minute. Pressure over the inferior third of the sternum will be ineffective and may lacerate the underlying liver.

   2. With the infant on a firm surface or with one hand supporting the infant's back, the index and middle fingers of the free hand are placed over the middle third of the sternum and the chest is depressed as above.

The effectiveness of massage can be assessed by palpation of femoral or umbilical cord pulses. Cardiac resuscitation should be alternated with ventilatory resuscitation in a 3:1 ratio in order to provide optimal support.

I. *Intravenous therapy*. A severely asphyxiated baby may require volume and metabolic resuscitation as well. Inefficient anaerobic metabolism produces large amounts of lactic acid, which reduces the pH and thereby depresses the myocardium, the central nervous system, and the pulmonary and peripheral vasculature. If the Apgar score remains 3 or below after several minutes of assisted ventilation, or is 5 or less at five minutes, alkali therapy is indicated.

  1. *Cannulation*
     a) Peripheral vasoconstriction may preclude peripheral administration of medications through either a 25- or 23-gauge Butterfly. However, in a number of infants it is feasible, and the infant recovers dramatically as soon as alkali is infused.
     b) A more accessible, but more hazardous, route is provided by the umbilical vessels. The umbilical vein tends to be more expeditious than the umbilical arteries. The umbilical arteries may be in spasm and, via the umbilical vein, the drugs will be reaching their target organs (heart, lungs, brain) by the shortest possible route (i.e., umbilical vein to ductus venosus to inferior vena cava to atria).
     c) A 5 French umbilical venous catheter (or a feeding tube) can be joined to a three-way stopcock to which one syringe of normal saline (for volume) and one syringe of sodium bicarbonate (for buffer) can be attached. The line should be flushed with normal saline. This creates a closed system for medications and avoids the introduction of a potentially fatal air embolus.
     d) The umbilical cord should be held at the base, prepped with an antiseptic, and neatly severed with a scalpel blade approximately 1 to 1.5 cm from the abdominal wall. The fingers supporting the base can control bleeding while cannulation takes place. The vein can be identified as a single, thin-walled, oval vessel; the arteries, normally two in number, are

smaller, thick-walled, and round, usually with tightly constricted lumens. The catheter should be inserted into the vein along a superficial, cephalad plane. It is acceptable procedure to advance the catheter only until blood flow can be demonstrated by gentle suction on the syringe. Umbilical tape then can be secured around the base of the cord to stabilize the catheter while medications are infused. Ideally, the catheter should be advanced through the ductus venosus and into the inferior vena cava (approximately 8 to 10 cm). However, in attempting this the catheter may become lodged in an hepatic vessel.

e) Complications of umbilical venous catheterization include thrombosis, adventitial hemorrhage and hepatic necrosis. The frequency of these dangers appears to increase with the amount of time the catheter remains in place; an exception is hepatic necrosis, which is believed to be related to the hypertonicity of the solutions being administered.[7]

2. Medications (Table 13–2)

   a) *Sodium bicarbonate*

      (1) Sodium bicarbonate (0.45 mEq/ml) should be pushed *slowly* at a dosage of 2 mEq/kg. *Adequate ventilation must attend sodium bicarbonate administration to eliminate the carbon dioxide being produced.* As acidosis is corrected, peripheral perfusion should improve.

      (2) Adult and pediatric preparations of sodium bicarbonate are hypertonic solutions. (Isotonicity calls for 1 mEq/ml of sodium bicarbonate to 5 ml of water.) In addition to being suspect in cases of hepatic necrosis, administration of alkali or any hypertonic solution has been linked with intracranial hemorrhage, especially in premature infants. Judicious employment of metabolic resuscitation, avoidance of sodium bicarbonate administration greater than 8 mEq/kg, and slow infusion rate are imperative.

TABLE 13–2. DRUGS FOR RESUSCITATION

Drug	Dosage	Indication
Sodium bicarbonate, 0.45 mEq/ml	2 mEq/kg	Metabolic acidosis
Epinephrine, 1:10,000 solution	0.1 ml/kg or 0.5–1.0 ml total dose	Asystole or bradycardia
Dextrose, 10% solution	2 ml/kg	Hypoglycemia
Calcium gluconate, 10% solution	100 mg/kg *slowly*	Decreased cardiac output
Crystalloid or Plasma	10–20 ml/kg	Hypotension or hypovolemia
Albumin, 5% solution	1 gm/kg	Hypotension or hypovolemia
Naloxone	0.01 mg/kg	Previous maternal sedation with narcotics or maternal narcotic abuse

b) *Normal saline.* Blood pressure may drop when acidosis is relieved, necessitating volume expansion with normal saline or colloid. Either 10 to 20 ml/kg of normal saline or plasma, or 1 gm/kg of 5 percent albumin should correct hypotension.

c) *Epinephrine*
  (1) Lack of improvement or slow or decelerating heart rate should be followed by epinephrine 1:10,000 at a dosage of 0.1 ml/kg or 0.5 to 1 ml, given by umbilical catheter. Prior treatment with alkali will render adrenergic receptors responsive to pressor agents.
  (2) Intracardiac administration of medications should be reserved for the infant in asystole with no other immediate approach available, as this may cause injury to tiny coronary arteries.

d) *Calcium.* Ten percent calcium gluconate, 100 mg/kg, given over five minutes, may be utilized to support cardiac function. Rapid infusion can produce bradycardia or cardiac arrest.

e) *Glucose.* Most term infants have sufficient glycogen stores to meet their requirements for labor and delivery. Prolonged asphyxia and resuscitative efforts speed the infant, especially the small or premature infant, toward hypoglycemia by exhausting endogenous supplies. Ten percent dextrose in water, 2 ml/kg by IV push, followed by a continuous infusion of $D_{10}W$ at a rate of 65 ml/kg/24 hours is recommended.

f) *Naloxone*
  (1) Infants depressed from maternal analgesia and anesthesia may require prolonged manual ventilation.
  (2) Meperidine administered to the mother, between one and three hours prior to delivery, can produce central respiratory depression in the infant. This can be reversed by a narcotic antagonist such as naloxone hydrochloride (Narcan neonatal prepa-

ration, 0.01 mg/kg), given via an intravenous, intramuscular, or subcutaneous route.

(3) It must be remembered that a narcotic antagonist administered to the infant of an addicted mother will precipitate acute narcotic withdrawal in the baby.

g) *Additional medications.* Isoproterenol, dopamine, atropine, and cardioversion rarely find a place in the resuscitation of the depressed newborn.

MANAGEMENT OF MECONIUM ASPIRATION

Asphyxiation in utero leads to reflex ischemia of the gastrointestinal tract. This is believed to presage relaxation of the anal sphincter and hyperperistalsis of the gut, leading to fetal passage of meconium. Meconium aspiration prior to or during birth can result in airway obstruction, ventilation-perfusion abnormalities, and subsequent respiratory distress. Gregory's study has demonstrated a 56 percent incidence of meconium in the trachea of infants with meconium-stained amniotic fluid. A number of these infants (approximately 17 percent) had meconium in the trachea but none in the mouth or larynx; therefore, lack of visualization of meconium above the vocal cords does not preclude an aspiration syndrome.[8] The *amount* and *consistency* of the meconium, along with the *degree of birth depression,* constitute determinants of medical management.

A. *Immediate suctioning* of the oropharynx and nares by the obstetrician, *as soon as the infant's head is delivered,* is crucial to successful treatment.

B. Thin, watery, yellow or green meconium-stained fluid should be suctioned further with a suction catheter or bulb syringe. Aggressive intubation and suctioning of a vigorous, crying infant covered with thin meconium is not advised. Following the five-minute Apgar, if stable, gastric lavage should be performed to prevent later aspiration of stomach contents should the baby gag and vomit.

C. Management of the infant smeared with pea-soup, particulate meconium is unequivocal. The pharynx should be suctioned while the vocal cords are being visualized. After an endotracheal tube has been introduced, suctioning may be accomplished either by suction catheter and saline lavage or by direct suctioning by mouth, i.e., sucking on the endotracheal tube (through a gauze pad or face mask) as the tube is being withdrawn from the trachea. With the latter method, repeated intubations may be necessary if copious amounts of meconium are present. If the infant remains depressed, resuscitation may proceed as with any other asphyxiated baby. *Remember: bag-and-mask ventilation in a depressed, meconium-stained infant will drive the meconium deep into the lungs and can generate meconium pneumonitis unless the airway is cleared initially.*

D. This immediate treatment should be followed by careful observation and postural drainage; a chest roentgenogram and arterial or capillary blood gases should be obtained when warranted by the infant's clinical condition. Sudden deterioration of such a newborn may mean *pneumothorax* or *pneumomediastinum.* Shift of the apical impulse, decreased breath sounds, descent of the liver edge, asymmetrical transillumination of the chest, or hypotension with weak pulses lend support to this diagnosis.

BIBLIOGRAPHY

Anderson JM, et al.: Hyaline membrane disease, alkaline buffer treatment and cerebral intraventricular hemorrhage. Lancet 1:117, 1976

Apgar VA: proposal for a new method of evaluation of the newborn infant. Anesth Analg 33:260, 1953

Behrman RE, et al.: Treatment of the asphyxiated newborn infant. J Pediatr 74:981, 1969

Cordero L, Hon EH: Neonatal bradycardia following nasopharyngeal stimulation. J Pediatr 78:441, 1971

Dawes GS: Foetal and Neonatal Physiology. Chicago, Year Book Medical, 1968

Gregory GA: Resuscitation of the newborn. Anesthesiology 43:225, 1975

Gregory GA, et al.: Meconium aspiration in infants—a prospective study. J Pediatr 85:848, 1974

Karlberg P: The adaptive changes in the immediate postnatal period, with particular reference to respiration. J Pediatr 56:585, 1960

Larroche J: Umbilical catheterization: its complications (Symposium on Artificial Ventilation, Paris, 1969). Biol Neonate 16:101, 1970

Osthaimer GW: Resuscitation of the depressed neonate. Contemp Obstet Gynecol 15:27, 1980

Simmons MA, et al.: Hypernatremia and intracranial hemorrhage in neonates. N Engl J Med 291:6, 1974

REFERENCES

1. Dawes GS: Foetal and Neonatal Physiology. Chicago, Year Book Medical, 1968
2. Apgar V: A proposal for a new method of evaluation of the newborn infant. Curr Res Anesth Analg 33:260, 1953
3. Drage JS, et al.: The Apgar score as an index of infant morbidity. Dev Med Child Neurol 8:141, 1966
4. Cordero L Jr, Hon EH: Neonatal bradycardia following nasopharyngeal stimulation. J Pediatr 78:441, 1971
5. Karlberg P: The adaptive changes in the immediate postnatal period, with particular reference to respiration. J Pediatr 56:585, 1960
6. Behrman RE, et al.: Treatment of the asphyxiated newborn infant. J Pediatr 74:981, 1969
7. Larroche J: Umbilical catheterization: its complications (Symposium on Artificial Ventilation, Paris, 1969). Biol Neonate 16:101–116, 1970
8. Gregory GA, et al.: Meconium aspiration in infants—a prospective study. J Pediatr 85:848, 1974

14

Postpartum Care
Jeffrey W. Ellis, M.D.

PRACTICE PRINCIPLES

The puerperium is a period of approximately six weeks beginning after the delivery of the placenta and ending when the reproductive organs have returned anatomically to the normal nonpregnant state. Care during the immediate postpartum period involves promoting patient comfort and recognizing and treating complications.

POSTPARTUM ORDERS

After delivery, the following orders should be specified:

- Diet
- Activity
- Vital signs
- Intake and output
- Intravenous fluids
- Perineal care
- Bowel care
- Bladder care

- Breast care
- Medications:
    Analgesia
    Hypnotics
    Lactation suppression
- Laboratory studies

A. *Diet.* The patient may be started on a regular diet when she has recovered from anesthesia and her vital signs are stable. If a third- or fourth-degree laceration of the perineum occurred during delivery, the patient should be placed on a low-residue diet for several days to avoid overdistention of the rectum and sphincter. Diets previously prescribed should be reinitiated.

B. *Activity.* The patient may be allowed normal ambulation and activity when she has recovered from anesthesia and vital signs are stable. Frequent ambulation should be encouraged to prevent lower-extremity thrombophlebitis.

C. *Vital signs.* Temperature, pulse, respirations, and blood pressure should be monitored four times a day throughout hospitalization. More frequent assessment will be necessary if, for example, blood loss was excessive at delivery or if the patient was hypertensive during pregnancy.

D. *Intake and output.* An accurate record of oral and intravenous intake and all fluid output should be maintained every two hours for at least the first 12 hours after delivery on all patients. If normal, it should then be recorded every eight hours.

E. *Intravenous fluids.* A solution of 1000 ml of 5 percent dextrose in Ringer's lactate plus 20 units of oxytocin should run at a maintenance rate of 125 cc/hour. This may be discontinued when the patient recovers from anesthesia, tolerates a diet, and maintains normal vital signs.

F. *Perineal care.* The perineal area may be painful and swollen for several days after delivery, especially if an episiotomy was performed or lacerations repaired. Routine care should involve cleansing and drying the area three times a day. Pain relief may be obtained with the following:

1. Ice packets to the perineum, p.r.n.
2. Warm sitz baths, t.i.d.
3. Dermoplast or Americaine Spray, p.r.n.
4. Proctofoam cream, p.r.n.
5. Heat lamp to perineum, p.r.n.
6. Witch hazel pads, p.r.n.

G. *Bowel care*
1. The following may be administered if a bowel movement has not occurred by the third postpartum day:
   a) Dulcolax suppository
   b) Fleets enema
   c) Milk of magnesia, 30 ml orally
2. Patients who have undergone repair of a third- or fourth-degree laceration should be placed on a stool softener, dioctyl sodium sulfosuccinate (Colace), one tablet twice a day, and should not receive enemas, rectal suppositories, or rectal temperature determinations.

H. *Bladder care.* Urinary retention may result from an atonic bladder or urethral edema. Catheterization may be performed every four to six hours if the patient is unable to void. If a third catheterization is required, an indwelling catheter should be inserted and left in place for 48 hours. Each micturition and defecation should be followed by a careful cleansing of the perineum and vulva from above downward.

I. *Breast care.* Breast engorgement will often occur on the second or third postpartum day. Symptomatic relief may be obtained on the non-breast-feeding patient with the following:

1. Breast binder, p.r.n.
2. Ice packs p.r.n.
3. Warm, moist heat, p.r.n.
4. Nipple fissures may be treated with an emollient cream (Masse Nipple Cream)

J. *Medications*
   1. *Analgesics*
      a) Codeine, 30 or 60 mg p.o. q4h p.r.n.
      b) Aspirin, 10 grains p.o. q4h p.r.n.
      c) Acetaminophen, 10 grains p.o. q4h p.r.n.
   2. *Hypnotics*
      a) Flurazepam (Dalmane), 30 mg p.o. h.s. p.r.n.
      b) Secobarbital (Seconal), 100 mg p.o. h.s. p.r.n.
   3. *Lactation suppression*
      a) Bromocryptine mesylate (Parlodel), 1 capsule p.o.
         b.i.d. for 14 days
K. *Laboratory studies.* The patients' hemoglobin and hematocrit should be obtained on the second postpartum day. Maternal blood type and Rh, if not known, should be obtained as soon as possible. Other laboratory studies may be ordered to assess specific symptoms.

POSTPARTUM EVALUATION
During daily patient rounds, the following areas should be evaluated:

- Vital signs
- Character and amount of lochia
- Bowel function
- Urinary function
- Breasts
- Uterus
- Perineum
- Extremities
- Condition of infant
- Blood type of mother and infant

A. *Vital signs*
   1. *Tachycardia and tachypnea* are abnormal and are usually secondary to intravascular volume depletion or fever. An investigation of volume depletion should include an immediate CBC, urine specific gravity, evaluation of

intake and output, and a physical examination to determine the site of blood loss. Fever may be due to infection or allergic reaction or may be transiently elevated without pathologic significance. The appropriate evaluation of each possibility is indicated. *Unexplained tachycardia and tachypnea should prompt an immediate evaluation for pulmonary embolism.*

2. *Bradycardia* of 40 to 50 is normal and may represent cardiac response to the marked reduction in blood flow to the placental site. If the patient is symptomatic, an ECG should be obtained to rule out heart block.

3. *Hypertension* may persist in patients who were preeclamptic or chronically hypertensive during pregnancy. A sudden increase in blood pressure should prompt an immediate investigation of preeclampsia, which may ensue postpartum.

4. *Decreased blood pressure* (hypotension) when combined with tachycardia and tachypnea may indicate either severe intravascular volume depletion or pulmonary embolism.

5. *Postpartum febrile morbidity* is defined as a temperature greater than 100.4 F (38 C) on any 2 of the first 10 postpartum days, excluding the first 24 hours. A slight temperature elevation no higher than 100.4 F may be noted during the first 24 hours after delivery. The cause is unknown. Febrile morbidity should be thoroughly evaluated.

B. *Character and amount of lochia.* A uterine discharge normally persists until the first menstrual period. *Lochia rubra* is a blood-stained discharge containing sloughed decidua that is present for three to four days after delivery. *Lochia serosa* is pale red, serosanguineous, and watery and occurs for the next four to five days. After the tenth day, a yellow drainage, *lochia alba*, will be present; this contains a high concentration of leukocytes.

1. *Heavy vaginal bleeding* usually indicates retained placental fragments or uterine atony.

2. *Foul-smelling, purulent lochia* usually indicates endometritis or a retained vaginal sponge.

C. *Bowel function.* If a bowel movement has not occurred by the third postpartum day, a mild laxative or enema should be administered. Symptomatic hemorrhoids may be treated with sitz baths or analgesic sprays and creams as used for episiotomy pain.

D. *Urinary function.* Urinary frequency is often the result of the normal postpartum diuresis. Dysuria usually indicates urinary tract infection. Inability to urinate after multiple catheterizations should be evaluated by a thorough examination of the vagina and urethra. Common causes of urinary retention requiring specific treatment include vaginal hematoma, periurethral hematoma, and retained vaginal sponge.

E. *Breasts.* Breast pain unrelieved by routine symptomatic measures should be evaluated for the presence of mastitis or galactocele. Colostrum will be secreted by the breasts for the first week after delivery. A slow conversion to mature milk will then occur. The majority of medications administered to the lactating mother will be excreted in the breast milk. If specific drug therapy is indicated and the infant may be seriously affected, the breasts may be pumped and the milk discarded. Breast-feeding may be resumed after discontinuation of the drug.

F. *Uterus.* Primarily through a decrease in the size of individual cells, the uterus begins to lose mass soon after delivery. Twenty-four hours after delivery, the uterus will involute at a rate of 2 to 4 cm per day, finally descending into the true pelvis approximately two weeks after delivery. Failure to involute at this rate suggests retained placental fragments or distended bladder. Uterine tenderness associated with fever and foul-smelling vaginal discharge indicates probable endometritis. *After-birth pains* are due to uterine contractions, most commonly occurring in multiparous patients. Mild analgesics are useful in controlling pain.

G. *Perineum.* For the first two to three days after delivery the perineum may be edematous, especially if an episiotomy is present. Excessive pain and swelling of this area should be evaluated promptly, as it may indicate infection or hematoma formation. Though deep infection of an episiotomy is uncommon, incision and drainage may be required. Small hematomas of the episiotomy are common and usually resolve completely with conservative local care. Large or expanding hematomas will require surgical evacuation and ligation of bleeding vessels.

H. *Extremities.* The lower extremities should be examined for signs of thrombophlebitis: local tenderness, swelling, and palpable veins.

I. *Condition of the infant.* The condition of the infant should be checked daily *before* making postpartum rounds. If abnormalities exist, the physician will be prepared to give medical interpretation and psychologic support to the mother.

J. *Blood type of mother and infant.* Rho (D) immunoglobulin, RhoGAM, has been shown to be effective in preventing the postpartum formation of antibodies to Rho (D) factor in Rho (D)-negative and D^u-negative women who have delivered an Rho (D)-positive or D^u-positive infant. RhoGAM is a sterile, concentrated IgG immunoglobulin containing anti-Rho (D). After intramuscular administration of RhoGAM to the mother, passive immunity is established, suppressing the maternal immunologic response to fetal red blood cells. Effectiveness in preventing sensitization is approximately 98 percent.

  1. *Indications for RhoGAM*

    a) RhoGAM should be administered to all Rho (D)-negative and D^u-negative mothers not previously sensitized to the Rho (D) factor who deliver an Rho (D)- or D^u-positive infant.

    b) RhoGAM should also be administered to patients when the Rh factor of the fetus has not been determined, as in ectopic pregnancy and abortion.

  2. *Contraindications to RhoGAM*

    a) RhoGAM should not be administered to patients

already immunized to the Rho (D) factor as detected by a positive indirect Coombs test.

  b) RhoGAM should not be administered to patients whose infants have a positive direct Coombs test due to anti-Rho (D).

  c) RhoGAM should never be administered to the infant.

3. *Dosage*

  a) One vial of RhoGAM will completely suppress immunity to 15 ml of Rh-positive fetal red blood cells. In a normal term delivery, one vial will be sufficient to suppress immunity.

  b) In cases where a large fetomaternal hemorrhage is suspected — after cesarean section, placental abruption, or manual removal of the placenta — additional RhoGAM should be administered.

  c) The magnitude of the fetomaternal transfusion can be calculated, using the acid elution test of Kleihauer-Betke. One vial of RhoGam should be administered for every 15 ml of fetal red blood cells detected.

DISCHARGE FROM THE HOSPITAL

If no intrapartum or postpartum complications occurred, most patients can be discharged from the hospital 48 to 72 hours after delivery.

A. *Discharge examination.* A thorough physical examination should be performed, paying specific attention to the breasts, uterus, episiotomy site, and lower extremities.

B. *Discharge instructions.* Patients should be specifically counseled in the following areas:

  1. *Hygiene.* Hygienic practices initiated in the hospital should be continued at home, specifically breast and perineal care. Bathing and showering are permissible.

  2. *Activity.* The patient may maintain a relatively normal activity level when at home. She may experience easy fatigability the first two weeks.

  3. *Diet.* A normal diet should be resumed, but the patient

should be warned against voluntary weight-loss programs until the end of the puerperium.

4. *Sexual intercourse.* Because of the possibility of uterine infection and disruption of the episiotomy, sexual intercourse should be discouraged until complete healing and involution of the genital organs have occurred.

5. *Resumption of menses.* The first menstrual period occurs about six to eight weeks after delivery. Resumption of menses is variable in lactating women and often will not occur until discontinuation of breast-feeding.

6. *Contraception*

7. *Complications.* The patient should be instructed to immediately report any of the following:
   a) *Vaginal bleeding* (retained products of conception, subinvolution)
   b) *Fever* (endometritis, mastitis, episiotomy infection)
   c) *Foul-smelling vaginal discharge* (endometritis, episiotomy infection, retained vaginal sponge)
   d) *Urinary retention* (vaginal hematoma, retained vaginal sponge)
   e) *Urinary frequency and dysuria* (urinary tract infection)
   f) *Lower-extremity pain and edema* (thrombophlebitis)
   g) *Breast pain and swelling* (mastitis)

8. *Discharge medications*
   a) *Iron (ferrous sulfate),* one tablet per day for one month
   b) *Vitamins (multivitamin),* one tablet per day for one month
   c) *Laxatives-stool softeners,* as needed
   d) *Analgesics,* as indicated

POSTPARTUM OFFICE EXAMINATION

The follow-up postpartum office visit is usually scheduled for approximately six weeks after delivery, and earlier if specific problems require close follow-up.

A complete physical examination should be performed. Pelvic examination should reveal complete involution of the reproductive organs.

Contraceptive counseling should be undertaken.

BIBLIOGRAPHY

Anderson PO: Drugs and breast feeding. Semin Perinatol 3:20, 1979

Bowman JM: Suppression of Rh isoimmunization: a review. Obstet Gynecol 52:385, 1978

Newton M, Bradford W: Postpartum blood loss. Obstet Gynecol 17:229, 1961

O'Leary J, et al.: Detection of postpartum pulmonary emboli by lung scan. Obstet Gynecol 30:721, 1967

15

Medical and Surgical Complications of Pregnancy

Section 1
Cardiovascular Diseases

Jeffrey C. King, M.D.

PRACTICE PRINCIPLES

Although the incidence of heart disease has declined dramatically over recent years, it remains one of the four major causes of maternal mortality. Most women with known cardiac disease withstand pregnancy with little morbidity; however, pregnancy-induced cardiovascular alterations can predispose patients to cardiac failure and death. It is essential for the physician to understand the normal changes in the cardiovascular system caused by pregnancy and how these may affect the mother and fetus.

The primary cause of cardiac disease has changed progressively from rheumatic fever to suspected congenital cardiac defects. The advances in cardiovascular surgery and improved general health care made survival into the reproductive age the rule rather than the exception. While a significant decrease in maternal mortality has been noted for all cardiac patients, the outcome of pregnancy for both the mother and fetus is directly related to the functional capacity of the heart.

PHYSIOLOGIC CHANGES

A. *Heart rate.* A gradual rise of 10 to 15 beats per minute (bpm) occurs during pregnancy. *At term, heart rates greater than 85 to 90 bpm require an explanation other than pregnancy.* It is interesting to note that twin gestations result in a greater increase in heart rate than in singletons: 40 and 21 percent, respectively, above nonpregnant rates. Within the puerperium (six weeks postdelivery), the heart rate will return to baseline.

B. *Stroke volume.* During the first half of pregnancy an increase to about 95 ml per beat occurs. Following this peak, there is a progressive decline to 70 ml per beat at term, which is approximately equal to nonpregnant volumes.

C. *Cardiac output.* The arithmetical product of heart rate and stroke volume, cardiac output begins to increase prior to the end of the first trimester and reaches values of 40 to 50 percent above normal by about 24 weeks. This increase is then maintained without further increase until term. Cardiac outputs must be measured at rest with the patient in the lateral recumbent position to avoid aortic or vena caval compression by the gravid uterus.

D. *Blood volume.* An increase of 20 percent occurs during the first half of pregnancy. Between 20 and 32 weeks there is an additional 20 percent rise. Following 32 weeks there is no apparent change in blood volume. Although an increase in red cell mass will occur, the plasma volume expansion is usually greater, resulting in "anemia of pregnancy."

E. *Arterial blood pressure.* Both systolic and diastolic pressure show a *slight fall* during pregnancy. Despite the rise in cardiac output, mean arterial pressure (MAP)* declines until midpregnancy and then rises toward nonpregnant values near term. This decline is caused by a more significant drop in diastolic pressure, leading to a rise in pulse pressure.

F. *Vascular resistance.* This measure falls during pregnancy not only because of the pregnant uterus, but also because of changes in the pulmonary vascular bed. From animal studies, it appears that arteriolar reactivity is significantly reduced during normal pregnancy.

ALTERATIONS DURING LABOR AND DELIVERY

A. Uterine contractions lead to a rise in central venous pressure caused by an increase in venous return to the heart. A rise in cardiac output is noted during the *first stage of labor,* but the exact extent depends on the method of analgesia employed, i.e., small rise with epidural block. There is a balance between blood loss at delivery and the "expansion" of blood volume caused by the decrease in uterine size and its associated uterine venous plexus.

B. *During the second stage,* maternal bearing-down efforts can result in marked alteration of hemodynamic status. While these changes are easily tolerated by the normal parturient, *patients with severe heart disease should avoid bearing down because of its effect on venous return.*

MANAGEMENT GUIDELINES

A team approach using obstetrician and cardiologist familiar with the hemodynamic changes of pregnancy is essential. Early consultation during labor with the anesthesiologist and neonatologist is equally important in providing optimal care. It should be remembered that newborn congenital heart lesions occur in 2 to 5 percent of patients with preexisting congenital defects, corrected or uncorrected.

*MAP = 1/3 pulse pressure (systolic − diastolic) + diastolic pressure.

A. *Prenatal care*
   1. *Diet.* Adequate nutritional intake is extremely important. Obviously, excessive weight gain places undue stress on the cardiovascular system. Eliminating table salt and avoiding high-salt food will result in a diet providing approximately 2 gm of sodium per day. Further restriction is unnecessary. Dietary consultation should be encouraged.
   2. *Activity.* Patients with cardiac lesions are known to be less tolerant during pregnancy. Therefore, physical exertion should be restricted if symptoms develop. However, some mild forms of activity (walking if symptoms are absent) should be encouraged.
   3. *Drugs.* Digitalis and quinidine are safe during pregnancy. However, oral anticoagulants and diuretics should be discouraged. The use of propranolol needs further study because of its assumed relationship to growth retardation, preterm labor, and fetal hypoglycemia. Heparin is the anticoagulant of choice during pregnancy because it does not cross the placenta and its half-life is extremely short.
B. *Management in labor*
   1. *Spontaneous labor* at term should be allowed for all cardiac patients with the exception of those who are unstable. General anesthesia or segmental epidural analgesia is *usually* well tolerated.
   2. Patients should undergo *forcep delivery or vacuum extraction* during second stage to prevent prolonged bearing down and its associated hemodynamic changes.
   3. The function of the maternal cardiovascular system should be *monitored continuously* during labor and the early postpartum period. Some centers have suggested that Swan-Ganz catheters are necessary to optimize maternal care.
   4. *Antibiotics* to prevent endocarditis should be used in patients with valvular abnormalities, congenital abnormalities, or a prosthetic valve. Protection against gram-

negative organisms is mandatory. Intravenous aqueous penicillin G, 2 million units, and gentamycin (or tobramycin), 1.5 mg/kg (not more than 80 mg), given during the active phase of labor and repeated every eight hours until two doses postdelivery is adequate. Patients allergic to penicillin should receive vancomycin, 1 gm IV over one hour as a substitute.

SPECIFIC CARDIAC LESIONS

A. *Congenital heart disease*
   1. *Patent ductus arteriosis.* This is an extremely uncommon finding in pregnancy; however, in uncorrected cases, the risks of heart failure or infection of the duct are great. Patients who have undergone surgical correction prior to pregnancy have an unremarkable gestation.
   2. *Coarctation of the aorta.* Although rare, most women with coarctation have successful pregnancies. Coarctation involves a narrowing of the aorta just distal to the left subclavian artery. The diagnosis is made by the findings of systolic hypertension in the arms and diminished femoral pulses. Rupture and/or dissection of the aorta and infection at the coarctation are the major risks. A bicuspid aortic valve is often associated with this lesion. Up to a 3.5 percent maternal mortality has been noted in complicated coarctation by some investigators, but pregnancies following successful correction are generally unremarkable.
   3. *Eisenmenger's syndrome.* This condition is not surgically correctable and is characterized by *severe pulmonary hypertension secondary to high pulmonary vascular resistance*. The increased resistance is the result of shunting between the ventricles or atria or at the aortopulmonary level. Complications such as hemoptysis, pulmonary infarction, congestive failure, syncope, and arrhythmias can develop early and lead to substantial morbidity.

Maternal mortality of 25 to 35 percent is seen depending on the degree of pulmonary hypertension. Syncope resulting from an arrhythmia is the usual cause of death. Fetal survival is usually less than 50 percent. *Pregnancy is contraindicated.* Because these patients are at increased risk of intrapulmonary thrombosis, a 10-day regimen of heparin postpartum is advised.

4. *Marfan's syndrome.* Aortic dissection and rupture secondary to medial cystic degeneration are associated with this rare condition. *Since pregnancy is associated with a high mortality rate, it is contraindicated.* If pregnancy occurs, termination should be offered. If the patient refuses, or presents late in pregnancy, β-blockers such as propranolol should be started on a prophylactic basis to decrease cardiac work and stroke volume.

5. *Mitral valve prolapse (Barlow's syndrome).* This abnormality of the posterior leaflet of the mitral valve is *found in 5 to 10 percent of young women.* The diagnosis is made when a mid-to-late systolic click associated with a late systolic murmur is heard on examination. In most cases the pregnancy is unremarkable. However, if significant regurgitation occurs, treatment of congestive heart failure may become necessary. Presently, there is much controversy concerning the necessity of antibiotic prophylaxis.

6. *Idiopathic hypertrophic subaortic stenosis (IHSS).* Recognized as an autosomal dominant abnormality, IHSS can result in significant obstruction of the aortic outflow tract. This condition may result in snycope, congestive failure, pain, and sudden death. The diagnosis is made by echocardiography, which shows a thickened ventricular septum and abnormal systolic anterior mitral valve motion. Hypovolemia must be avoided; therefore, excessive blood loss and epidural analgesia are not tolerated. Antibiotic prophylaxis is controversial.

7. *Primary pulmonary hypertension. Pregnancy is contraindicated,* since maternal mortality rates of greater than 50 percent have been reported. Hypotension must be

avoided, and a lateral Sims' delivery should be encouraged. Graded elastic stockings should be used to increase venous return to the heart.

B. *Acquired cardiac lesions*

1. *Mitral stenosis is the most common acquired lesion encountered during pregnancy.*

   a) The *functional defect* is restriction of blood flow between the left atria and ventricle during diastole. When the left atrial pressure is greater than 25 Torr, transudation of fluid into the lung occurs. Generally, the valve area must be less than 2 cm^2 for pulmonary edema to occur.

   b) If a woman with significant mitral stenosis becomes *pregnant,* symptoms should be controlled by attempting to limit activity, treatment of arrhythmias, avoidance of hypovolemia, and aggressive treatment of fluid overload. Sims' delivery position is encouraged because of the necessity of maintaining cardiac output.

   c) *Surgical intervention* should be reserved for those patients unresponsive to usual measures. Mitral valve commissurotomy is associated with a 1 percent maternal mortality, and it must be remembered that it is only palliative, not corrective. Valve replacement may be considered under exceptional circumstances and preferably after the first trimester.

2. *Aortic stenosis* is associated with a maternal mortality of 35 percent. Generally, patients do well as long as the gradient between aorta and left ventricle is less than 100 mm Hg. The pregnancy must be watched closely because of progressive changes in cardiac disease during pregnancy. Women with known severe aortic stenosis have done well intrapartum, but risks are significantly increased during the first days postdelivery. Hypovolemia must be avoided to prevent circulatory collapse.

3. *Cardiomyopathy of pregnancy*

   a) The exact *etiology* is unknown, but recent interest concerns a possible immunologic basis for the disease.

The *main finding* is myocardial failure with associated pulmonary edema. It is most commonly found in black, multiparous patients over 30 years of age who are carrying a multiple gestation or have hypertension. It is associated with a *15 to 50 percent maternal mortality* and usually becomes evident in the post-delivery period. No history of previous cardiac disease is usually found.

   b) Treatment consists of attempting to prevent worsening congestive failure. Fifty percent of survivors have some type of residual damage, i.e., cardiomegaly. This residuum has been shown to shorten life expectancy significantly and to predispose to recurrence of congestive failure.

4. *Myocardial infarction.* This is *truly a rare condition,* with a rate of 1 per 10,000 deliveries. However, with the increased use of β-mimetics to inhibit preterm labor, many centers are reporting that pain and cardiac findings occur more frequently. The overall mortality is 29% but this is dependent on the duration of the pregnancy and when symptoms first present. Management of an acute infarction is unchanged from the nonpregnant patient.

C. *Previous valve replacement*

1. The most common surgically corrected valvular lesions involve the *mitral* or *aortic* valve. Once corrected, these prosthetic valves predispose patients to the formation of microthrombi and thromboembolic disease. Therefore, continuous *anticoagulation* is prescribed. Oral anticoagulants (coumadin) have been associated with the development of morphologic abnormalities of the fetus. Recently, porcine heterografts have been used because they do not require continuous anticoagulation. However, the life span of these grafts appears to be shortened when placed in a high-pressure system such as the left side of the heart.

2. *Aortic valve prosthesis* allows the normal increases in cardiac output to occur during pregnancy. Therefore, pregnancy is usually well tolerated. If anticoagulants are

not used during pregnancy, they should be started postpartum for at least two weeks to prevent thromboembolic disease. Of course, antibiotic prophylaxis is essential to prevent prosthetic valve endocarditis, which is associated with a mortality rate of greater than 50 percent.

3. *Mitral valve prosthesis* is often more detrimental to successful pregnancy. In spite of a corrected lesion, cardiac and congestive heart failure may occur. Since the valve is usually replaced only after significant enlargement of the left atrium has occured, microthrombus formation and embolism are everpresent risks. Anticoagulants are usually prescribed.

VENOUS DISEASE

A. *Between 5 and 30 percent of pregnant women manifest a venous disorder during pregnancy.* Approximately 10 to 20 percent develop varicose veins or hemorrhoids, and pedal edema is common. However, thrombophlebitis is the major complication of venous disease. The result of many factors, the least of which is the increased venous pressure in the lower extremities during pregnancy, the various diagnostic tests have many inaccuracies.

B. *Varicose veins*
   1. This abnormality is often familial and can become evident as early as 12 weeks' gestation. Usually the patient will complain of heaviness or discomfort only while walking. If the vulva is involved, perineal pressure is common. This abnormality of the venous system may progress to venous stasis with skin ulceration, bleeding, or persistent edema.
   2. Since this condition is benign, its presence in no way affects fetal outcome. Varicosities may become significantly larger with subsequent pregnancies and may progress to superficial thrombosis.

3. *Management*
   a) *Pressure gradient elastic support* stockings or panty hose (Jobst) should be used during pregnancy. Patients may require remeasurement during pregnancy as their weight progressively changes. Vulvar varicosities may be treated by perineal pressure using large sanitary napkins held in place by an athletic supporter.
   b) Obviously, *attempts to decrease lower extremity venous pressure should be employed.* Frequent rest periods in the lateral recumbent position throughout the day are necessary. The legs should be elevated during sleep by placing six-inch blocks under the footboard.
   c) *During delivery,* the stirrups must be thickly padded to prevent acute angulation of the knee. *Patients must be encouraged to ambulate soon after delivery to prevent thrombosis.* Suppression of lactation by estrogens and the use of birth control pills should probably be avoided.

C. *Superficial thrombosis*
   1. This condition usually involves the saphenous venous system, but deep vein thrombosis is possible. The diagnosis is made by the complaint of pain and the finding of a firm, nodular mass following the course of the vein. There is no effect on the fetus.
   2. *Management.* Fortunately, superficial thrombi rarely embolize. Therefore, management consists of warm packs and elevation of the involved leg. Analgesics may be helpful to reduce tenderness. Estrogens should be avoided.

D. *Deep vein thrombosis (DVT)*
   1. This condition can result in significant morbidity and even mortality if pulmonary embolism occurs. The diagnosis is often difficult because of the physiologic changes already mentioned.
   2. *Signs and symptoms of DVT*
      a) Pain and tenderness of the entire involved limb

    b) Asymmetric limb (usually more than 2 cm greater in circumference than the uninvolved leg)

    c) Localized warmth may be present

    d) Dependent cyanosis may occur

    e) Homan's sign is variably present

3. DVT frequently occurs during the *puerperium*. Patients undergoing operative deliveries or those of advanced age or with varicosities or lactation suppression caused by high doses of estrogens are most susceptible. When fever presents postpartum, careful evaluation for the development of DVT versus endomyometritis or urinary tract infection is mandatory.

4. *Diagnosis*. There is much controversy concerning the optimal diagnostic tool for DVT. The methods include: venography, ^{125}I fibrinogen scanning, impedance plethysmography, and Doppler studies. All the techniques have advantages and disadvantages. The method depends on the equipment available and the experience of hospital personnel.

5. *Management*

    a. Once the diagnosis of DVT has been made, the mainstay of treatment is *anticoagulation*. Complete anticoagulation should be achieved by continuous infusion or pulse-dose heparin.

        (1) Most centers feel that continuous infusion provides smoother control of partial thromboplastin times (PTT). The theraputic range is 2 to 2.5 times control values.

        (2) Initial anticoagulation is achieved by IV push heparin (75 to 100 units/kg), followed by a continuous infusion of 15 to 20 units/kg/hour. Heparin should be mixed only with normal saline, as some studies have suggested that dextrose solutions interfere with its activity. Generally, only a six- to eight-hour dose should be hung at any time to prevent accidental overdosage.

        (3) Continuous heparin should be used for at least

10 to 14 days to prevent propagation of the clot and to assist in clot lysis. Subcutaneous heparin, 5,000 to 10,000 units every 12 hours, is usually continued for at least three weeks. Therapy may be extended if the patient has had recurrence, embolization, or iliofemoral thrombosis. If the patient has not been receiving prophylactic heparin, this should be instituted during labor, delivery, and the early puerperium.

b) *Additional treatment* during the acute phase consists of *bed rest* and leg elevation. The foot of the bed should be elevated by blocks. Once pain has resolved, ambulation should be encouraged. Obviously, sitting for long periods of time must be avoided.

c) The use of anti-inflammatory agents, aspirin or indomethacin, is usually not indicated; although, many feel that the antiplatelet effect of aspirin makes treatment with subcutaneous heparin more effective.

d) It is important to remember that heparin is a large molecule with negative charge. Therefore, it does not cross the placenta. It is the anticoagulant of choice for conditions requiring anticoagulation during pregnancy. Heparin prevents the conversion of fibrinogen to fibrin by inhibiting thrombin formation. While it does enter breast milk in small quantities, breakdown by newborn gastric enzymes makes it innocuous for the baby.

BIBLIOGRAPHY

Hull R, Delmore T, Carter C, et al.: Adjusted subcutaneous heparin versus warfarin sodium in the longterm treatment of venous thrombosis. N Engl J Med 306:189, 1982

Kahler R: Cardiac disease. In Burrow GN, Ferris TF (eds): Medical Complication During Pregnancy. Philadelphia, Saunders, 1975

Szekely P, Snaith L: Cardiac disorders. Clin Obstet Gynecol 4:265, 1977

Ueland K (ed): Cardiovascular diseases in pregnancy. Clin Obstet Gynecol 24:691, 1981

Ueland K: Dangerous cardiovascular lesions in pregnancy. In Sciarra J (ed): Gynecology and Obstetrics. Hagerstown, Md., Harper & Row, 1981

Section 2
Hypertensive Disease
Jeffrey C. King, M.D.

PRACTICE PRINCIPLES

The problem of hypertension concurrent with or complicating pregnancy has challenged all personnel involved with obstetrical care for years. The effect of hypertension manifests itself as a wide spectrum of pathologic changes in multiple organ systems. The intention of this section is to classify the various hypertensive disorders and to provide a logical approach to their management. The indications for contraception or sterilization in these patients will be explored as well as the effects of hypertension on the fetus and neonate.

CLASSIFICATION

A. *Hypertensive disorders of pregnancy* are a variety of conditions that have as their common denominator hypertension or elevated mean arterial pressure (MAP).* Most investigators consider a *blood pressure or MAP greater than 130/80 and 95 mm Hg,* respectively, to be abnormal. Because it is both confusing and misleading, the term "toxemia" is mentioned only to condemn its use as a description of this disease.

*MAP = 1/3 pulse pressure (systolic − diastolic) + diastolic pressure.

B. *Classification*
  1. Pregnancy-induced hypertension
     a) Preeclampsia
        (1) Mild
        (2) Severe
     b) Eclampsia
  2. Chronic hypertension (any cause and preceding pregnancy)
  3. Chronic hypertension (any cause) with superimposed pregnancy-induced hypertension
     a) Superimposed preeclampsia
     b) Superimposed eclampsia
  4. Gestational or transient hypertension

DEFINITIONS

A. *Pregnancy-induced hypertension (PIH)*
  1. *Preeclampsia — mild*
     a) The diagnosis of preeclampsia is usually based on the *development of hypertension plus proteinuria and/or edema after the 20th week of gestation.* It occurs almost exclusively in primigravidas, particularly those less than 20 or greater than 35 years of age. If preeclampsia develops prior to the 20th week, conditions such as multiple gestation or molar pregnancy must be ruled out. The disease is occasionally seen in the multipara with underlying vascular or renal disorders.
     b) *Diagnostic criteria*
        (1) *Hypertension.* 140/90 or an increase of 30 mm Hg systolic or 15 mm Hg diastolic over base-line values. Blood pressure meeting the criteria must be observed on at least two occasions, six or more hours apart with the patient at rest.
        (2) *Proteinuria.* 500 mg or more of protein in a 24-hour urine collection or a dipstick measurement of 2 + or greater in a random urine specimen. The degree of proteinuria may vary greatly over any

24-hour period. If membranes have ruptured, a catheterized specimen is often necessary to exclude amniotic fluid, which may give a falsely elevated dipstick reading.

   (3) *Edema.* Lower-extremity edema is a common physical finding during normal pregnancy. When associated with preeclampsia, significant edema usually refers to the hands or face (nondependent). A useful clinical indication is the patient's complaint that her rings have become too tight.

2. *Preeclampsia — severe*
   a) The *diagnosis* of severe preeclampsia is made when *one or more* of the following is present:
      (1) Blood pressure of at least 160 mm Hg systolic or 110 mm Hg diastolic on two occasions at least six hours apart with the patient at bed rest
      (2) Proteinuria of at least 5 gm/24 hours, or 3 + to 4 + by dipstick
      (3) Oliguria (24-hour urinary output less than 500 ml)
      (4) Cerebral or visual disturbance (i.e., altered consciousness, blurred vision, scotomata, or headache)
      (5) Pulmonary edema or peripheral cyanosis
      (6) Usually, if the diagnosis of severe preeclampsia is suspected, an interval of six hours is not mandatory prior to initiation of therapy.
   b) Additional signs and symptoms suggestive, but not diagnostic, of advancing preeclampsia include:
      (1) Epigastric or right upper quadrant pain — probably a result of subcapsular hemorrhage in the liver leading to stretching of Glisson's capsule
      (2) Thrombocytopenia and/or altered liver function tests

3. *Eclampsia.* Eclampsia is the most severe extension of preeclampsia. It is characterized by the development of grand mal type seizures. In about one-third of cases, the seizures first appear before labor, one-third develop during the labor and delivery process, and one-third

occur postpartum. Seizures that occur more than 48 hours postpartum are usually not caused by eclampsia, but are more likely to result from an underlying lesion of the central nervous system.

B. *Chronic hypertension*

1. The *diagnosis* of chronic hypertension can be made on either a history of hypertension (140/90 or greater) prior to the 20th week of pregnancy and/or persistence of hypertension for more than 6 weeks (puerperium) postpartum.

2. *Clinical findings* suggestive of underlying chronic hypertension include:

   a) Presence of any chronic disease, i.e., diabetes, connective tissue disease, renal, etc.

   b) Funduscopic exam revealing hemorrhage and exudates

   c) BUN above 20 mg/100 ml or serum creatinine above 1 mg/100 ml

3. Chronic hypertension *may be due to a wide variety of disease or congenital abnormalities.* Conditions such as renal vascular disease, low- or high-renin hypertension, coarctation, pheochromocytoma, glomerulonephritis, polycystic kidney disease, systemic lupus erythematosus, nephrotic syndrome, and diabetic nephropathy must be considered as a cause for chronic hypertension.

4. *Abruptio placentae* has been found to occur in up to 10 percent of chronically hypertensive pregnant women. In addition, the fetus is at significant risk for *intrauterine growth retardation* and sudden, unexplained *intrauterine death.*

C. *Chronic hypertension with superimposed preeclampsia*

1. *Acute aggravation of existing hypertension with rapid development of edema and proteinuria* is chronic hypertension with superimposed PIH. Unfortunately, this condition often develops prior to the 30th week of gestation and may progress quickly to eclampsia.

2. To be sure of the diagnosis, the patient should present with accelerated hypertension plus proteinuria and/or

edema. Studies have suggested that 5.7 to 82 percent of patients with chronic hypertension will develop superimposed preeclampsia during pregnancy.

D. *Gestational or transient hypertension.* This condition describes patients who manifest transient elevations of blood pressure during labor, delivery, or in the early postpartum period. Associated signs of proteinuria and edema are absent. This may represent a mild varient of PIH or early, essential hypertension.

EVALUATION

A. *History*
   1. Each patient must be carefully evaluated with regard to past medical and obstetric history. Obviously, information concerning blood pressures prior to and during early pregnancy is essential to determine if significant elevation has occurred. At each visit, the patient must be questioned for the development of headaches, visual disturbances, and nondependent edema.
   2. A history of preeclampsia/eclampsia should place the obstetrician on guard. Certain medical disorders such as chronic renal disease, pheochromocytoma, systemic lupus erythematosus, or primary aldosteronism increase the chances of a poor pregnancy outcome.
B. *Physical examination*
   1. *Weight.* Normal weight gain is one pound per week during the second and third trimester. Rapid increases in weight must be investigated.
   2. *Funduscopic examination.* With preeclampsia, arteriolar spasm "boxcar effect" may be seen. Vascular changes (arteriovenous nicking, "silverwire" arteries, hemorrhages, exudates) are usually seen when chronic hypertension is present.
   3. *Cardiovascular examination.* Usually normal unless congestive heart failure is present.

4. *Abdominal examination.* Usually normal unless hepatic tenderness is found. Ascites is extremely rare, and if present, alternative conditions should be considered.

5. *Extremities.* The amount and extent of both dependent and nondependent *edema* must be documented. *Deep tendon reflexes* (DTRs) should be checked in the upper and lower limbs for symmetry and briskness. DTRs are often brisker in preeclampsia — a sign of neuromuscular irritability. The skin must be examined for evidence of *ecchymoses and/or purpura* (signs of thrombocytopenia).

C. *Laboratory studies*

1. *Complete blood count (CBC).* During the development of PIH, plasma volume is often decreased, resulting in elevation of the hematocrit compared to values earlier in pregnancy.

2. *Blood urea nitrogen and serum creatinine level*

3. *24-Hour urine collection for creatinine clearance and total protein*

4. *Coagulation status.* Evaluated by platelet count and fibrinogen level. Usually these studies become abnormal before alterations of prothrombin time (PT), partial thromboplastin time (PTT), or fibrin split products (FSP) are seen. The obstetrician must remember that elevated FSP are seen in approximately 15 percent of normal pregnancies. Therefore, the presence of FSPs alone does not indicate coagulopathy.

5. *Follow-up studies* depend on the severity and progression of the disease. Accurate fluid intake and output is essential. Patients should be weighed at least twice a week.

MANAGEMENT

A. *Preeclampsia — mild.* The initial treatment for a parturient with mild preeclampsia is hospitalization for rest and observation. Some practitioners may elect to follow mild preeclampsia on an outpatient basis with return visits at least twice a week.

1. *Bed rest with bathroom privileges only.* Patients should be encouraged to remain in the lateral recumbent position not only to increase uterine blood flow, but also to reduce lower-extremity venous pressure increased because of the enlarged uterus, in an attempt to mobilize peripheral edema.

2. *Sedation.* The use of sedatives may become necessary to help allay anxiety and to allow compliance with inactivity. Phenobarbital, 30 to 60 mg p.o. q6h, is usually sufficient. Caution must be exercised, because phenobarbital has been shown to have an adverse effect on the release of surfactant from the fetal Type II alveolar cells.

3. *Fetal surveillance*
   a) *Sonography* should be performed to evaluate fetal well-being and confirm gestational age. Estimates of fetal weight, amount of amniotic fluid, and placental maturation are frequently helpful.
   b) *Estriol determinations* should be started on a daily basis to evaluate placental function (controversial).
   c) *NST/CST* antepartum fetal heart rate monitoring is very useful in evaluating fetal status and placental reserve.
   d) *Fetal Movements.* Patient perception of fetal movements during specific times of the day has been shown to be quite predictive of fetal health. Absence of movement for greater than 12 hours must be investigated immediately.

4. *Lack of improvement or worsening condition.* If after 72 to 96 hours, the patient's condition does not improve, as manifested by onset of diuresis with decreasing weight, edema, and blood pressure, delivery should be considered. In addition, if the condition significantly worsens by any criteria, accelerating hypertension or progression to severe preeclampsia, delivery is indicated.

5. *Delivery.* Mode of delivery, vaginal versus cesarean,

depends on gestational age, fetal condition, fetal presentation, cervical examination (Bishop score), and maternal condition. Attempts at vaginal delivery by oxytocin induction of labor with direct fetal monitoring should be made if at all possible.

6. *Conduct of labor/delivery.* During spontaneous or induced labor in a patient with diagnosed preeclampsia, magnesium sulfate should be started. While the mechanism whereby magnesium sulfate prevents convulsion is not completely understood, the principal anticonvulsant effect is the result of peripheral neuromuscular blockade. Hypermagnesemia impairs acetylcholine release by the motor nerve impulses and decreases the sensitivity of the motor end plate to acetylcholine.

7. *Administration of magnesium sulfate.* Mix 20 gm magnesium sulfate [$MgSO_4 \cdot 7H_2O$ (USP)] in 1,000 ml of 5 percent dextrose in water. An initial loading dose of 4 gm (200 ml) should be given intravenously over 20 minutes. Thereafter, an infusion pump system should administer 1 to 2 gm magnesium sulfate/hour (50 to 100 ml). A Foley catheter should be placed to ensure correct intake and output measurement. If urinary output is less than 30 ml/hour, the magnesium dosage must be decreased to prevent toxicity. Magnesium levels may be helpful, but therapeutic levels (6 to 8 mEq/liter) are usually present if the DTRs are present but slightly hypoactive. DTRs must be monitored and charted hourly. Respiratory depression occurs when DTRs are absent and magnesium levels reach 10 to 15 mEq/liter. Calcium gluconate, 10 ml of 10 percent solution (1 gm), may be given as a *slow* IV push to correct magnesium overdosage. *Magnesium infusion should be continued for at least 24 hours postpartum to prevent convulsions.*

8. *Anesthesia/analgesia.* During labor, pain relief may be achieved by intravenous narcotics or segmental epidural after adequate (500 ml Ringer's lactate) preloading. Paracervical blockade is contraindicated. Pudendal block

or local infiltration of the perineum is sufficient for most vaginal deliveries. Cesarean section should be performed under balanced general anesthesia or segmental epidural. The use of epidural analgesia during labor and delivery for a patient with PIH is controversial.

B. *Preeclampsia—severe*

1. *General principles.* All of the above-mentioned modes of therapy are employed with addition of antihypertensive medication. Usually when severe preeclampsia occurs, conservative measures to prolong pregnancy are unsuccessful and delivery is indicated.

2. *Management of hypertension*

   a) *Magnesium sulfate* does have a mild, transient antihypertensive effect as a result of splanchnic vasodilation. However, when the diastolic blood pressure exceeds 110 mm Hg, *the antihypertensive drug of choice is hydralazine*. The goal of therapy is to protect the mother's heart and brain long enough to accomplish delivery. *Diastolic blood pressure should be lowered to 90 to 100 mm Hg.*

   b) Patients with a diastolic pressure of greater than 110 mm Hg should receive 5 mg hydralazine IV with blood pressure monitored every 5 minutes; an additional 10 mg may be injected IM as needed. The blood pressure is again monitored every 5 minutes.

   c) Each 20 minutes, the need for additional antihypertensive medication is assessed. Rarely is a dose greater than 50 mg necessary to achieve diastolic pressures of 90 to 100 mm Hg. This plan of management is repeated whenever diastolic blood pressure rises to 110 mm Hg or greater. Blood pressure lowered to less than 90 mm Hg may cause significant abnormalities of fetal heart rate monitoring.

3. *Cardiovascular management.* The use of central pressure monitoring can be extremely helpful in determining the amount and type of fluids necessary to restore maternal circulating volume. While central venous pressure (CVP)

may be sufficient in most cases, Swan-Ganz catheters to monitor pulmonary artery pressure, wedge pressure, and cardiac output may be necessary in the seriously ill patient.

4. *Anesthesia/analgesia.* Labor pain should be managed by intravenous narcotics. Vaginal delivery can usually be accomplished using pudendal block, local infiltration, or supplemental nitrous oxide. Cesarean section should be performed under balanced general anesthesia. Conduction anesthesia (epidural) is considered contraindicated by some authorities.

C. *Eclampsia*

1. *Initial therapy*

   a) *Principles*

      (1) Maintain airway and oxygenation

      (2) Avoid maternal injury

      (3) Stop seizure

   b) A padded tongue blade should not be forced between the patient's teeth if they are already closed. Attempts to do so may result in dental injury to the patient or finger injury to the personnel.

   c) The mouth and oropharynx should be suctioned frequently, if possible, to prevent aspiration pneumonia. Following maternal stabilization, a chest x-ray should be obtained. As the seizure resolves, an oral airway should be inserted until the mother regains complete consciousness.

   d) Treatment of the actual convulsion is controversial. A loading dose of magnesium sulfate (4 gm) IV, diazepam (5 to 10 mg) IV, or sodium amytal (up to 250 mg) IV may be given.

   e) Additional treatment has been outlined above (Section B, Preeclampsia, severe).

2. *Delivery.* Delivery *should not* be accomplished immediately following a maternal seizure. Stabilization of maternal blood pressure and neuromuscular status must be achieved over the next two to four hours. Only at this

point can active management of labor and delivery be considered. Full assessment of fetal well-being is mandatory.

3. *Further management.* Obviously, magnesium sulfate must be continued for at least 24, but up to 36, hours postpartum. Attention to blood pressure, blood loss at delivery, cardiac filling pressures, and urinary output is critical. Fluid therapy may consist of balanced salt, blood (for hypovolemia), and/or fresh frozen plasma (for correction of coagulopathy).

D. *Chronic hypertension*

1. *General principles.* The patient with chronic hypertension is at risk for worsening hypertension and fetal intrauterine growth retardation. Medication should be used to control diastolic blood pressure in the range of 80 to 90 mm Hg. In addition, patients should be counseled regarding increased amounts of rest in the lateral recumbent position. A high-protein diet (1 gm/kg body weight) is encouraged. At 22 to 24 weeks a three-hour glucose tolerance test should be performed, and if negative, a repeat study at 30 to 32 weeks is indicated. Serial sonography beginning in the early second trimester will assist in the determination of fetal growth parameters.

2. *Medication*

a) *Hydrochlorothiazide*

(1) A diuretic that is usually used in combination with methyldopa or hydralazine, it initially causes a decrease in intravascular and extracellular volume. In addition, a fall in cardiac output and decrease in peripheral resistance is noted. The change in blood volume is transient.

(2) *Dosage* is 25 to 50 mg p.o. daily. The most frequent maternal side effects are hypokalemia and hyperuricemia. Thrombocytopenia and hyponatremia have been reported in the neonate.

(3) Most patients should not be started on a diuretic for control of hypertension during pregnancy.

However, many feel that patients, adequately controlled by diuretic alone prior to pregnancy, may continue this therapy during pregnancy.

b) *Methyldopa* (Aldomet)

(1) The primary mechanism of action of this drug is interference with chemical neurotransmitters at the postganglionic nerve endings. The drug causes depletion of norepinephrine and acts as a false neurotransmitter. This results in lowered peripheral arteriolar resistances and both systolic and diastolic blood pressure. While a decrease in cardiac output is noted, the drug is not thought to decrease uterine blood flow.

(2) Dosage is usually begun at 250 mg p.o. every eight hours, but may be increased to a maximum of 2 gm per day. Full effect of a particular dosage requires 72 hours.

(3) A positive Coombs reaction occurs in up to 20 percent of patients on methyldopa for more than six months. Rare side effects include hemolytic anemia and abnormal liver function tests.

c) *Hydralazine*

(1) This drug causes a reduction in arteriolar resistance, as seen by a greater decrease in diastolic than systolic blood pressure. Compensatory tachycardia is often noted.

(2) Dosage is 25 to 50 mg p.o. every six hours.

(3) Maternal side effects include headache, palpitations, nausea, and diarrhea. A false-positive lupus erythematosus (LE) cell preparation may be seen, which is completely reversible with discontinuation of the drug.

d) *Other.* Propranolol, diazoxide, sodium nitroprusside, and the new combination β-blocking agents may be required in unusual circumstances.

3. *Fetal surveillance.* Weekly nonstress tests should be started at 34 weeks' gestation. In many centers, such

evaluation is begun at fetal viability. The patient is encouraged to monitor fetal movements, and absence of movement for more than 12 hours mandates further investigation.

4. *Delivery.* If blood pressure is inadequately controlled or fetal maturity is reached (lecithin/sphingomyelin greater than 2.0), delivery is indicated. If the cervix is favorable (Bishop score of 6 or more), induction of labor with oxytocin infusion and direct fetal monitoring should be undertaken, Cesarean section becomes necessary when the vaginal delivery cannot be accomplished safely.

E. *Chronic hypertension with superimposed PIH.* These pregnancies should be monitored and managed using any and all of the above-mentioned therapies. It must be remembered that these patients are often the most severely ill and intensive care is mandatory.

F. *Gestational or late hypertension.* This problem is always transient but must be carefully observed for progression into clinical preeclampsia. Since it resolves, usually within 7 to 10 days, following delivery, expectancy is the indicated management.

CONTRACEPTION/STERILIZATION

A. *General considerations.* In general, if a patient develops PIH in her first pregnancy, the likelihood of having at least one additional pregnancy complicated by hypertension is approximately 25 to 35 percent. Fortunately, the hypertension does not usually recur in each subsequent pregnancy, and when it does recur, severe hypertension develops in only 8 percent of pregnancies and eclampsia rarely develops. If severe, life-threatening complications such as congestive heart failure occur in a first pregnancy, future childbearing should be restricted.

B. *Contraception.* The question of oral contraceptive use following PIH is controversial. Blood pressure has been noted to increase during the first year of oral contraceptive use in patients following PIH as compared to controls. The systolic pressure has a mean increase of 6.6 mm Hg with a diastolic mean increase of 2.6 mm Hg. The occurrence of PIH does not preclude the use of oral contraceptives in young primiparous patients provided a low-dose contraceptive steroid is administered. Patients must be followed carefully, first at three-month intervals. Then, if stable, every six months.

C. *Sterilization*. This should be recommended only when medical conditions preclude future pregnancies.

1. Intrinsic cardiac disease characterized by cardiac enlargement, ischemia, strain, or failure
2. Chronically impaired renal function
3. Fresh retinal disease related to the hypertensive condition
4. Severe hypertension (persistent diastolic pressure greater than 120 mm Hg with therapy)
5. Superimposed severe PIH in a chronically hypertensive patient
6. Chronic severe irreversible disease process

BIBLIOGRAPHY

Berkowitz R: Anti-hypertensive drugs in the pregnant patient. Obstet Gynecol Surv 35:191, 1980

Chesley L; Hypertension in pregnancy: definitions, familial factor, and remote prognosis. Kidney Int 18:234, 1980

Ferris TF: Toxemia and hypertension. In Burrown GN, Ferris TF (eds): Medical Complications During Pregnancy. Philadelphia, Saunders, 1975

Gant N (ed): Pregnancy-induced hypertension. Semin Perinatol 2:1, 1978

Gant N, Worley R: Hypertension in Pregnancy Concepts and Management. New York, Appleton-Century-Crofts, 1980

Perkins R: Management of the hypertensive pregnant patient. Clin Perinatol 7:313, 1980

Pritchard J: Management of preeclampsia and eclampsia. Kidney Int 18:259, 1980

Rafferty T, Berkowitz R: Hemodynamics in patients with severe toxemia during labor and delivery. Am J Obstet Gynecol 138:263, 1980

Rubin P: Beta-blockers in pregnancy. N Engl J Med 305:1323, 1981

Symonds EM (ed): Hypertensive states in pregnancy. Clin Obstet Gynecol 4:529, 1977

Welt S, Crenshaw MC: Concurrent hypertension and pregnancy. Clin Obstet Gynecol 21:619, 1978

Section 3
Renal Disease
Jeffrey W. Ellis, M.D.

INFECTION

A. *Asymptomatic bacteriuria*
   1. *Definition.* The presence of significant bacteriuria, greater than 100,000 colonies/ml urine, without clinical symptoms of urinary tract infection.
   2. *Incidence*
      a) Nonpregnant: 2 percent of women.
      b) Pregnant: 4 to 12 percent of women.
      c) Incidence is increased in association with low socioeconomic class, sickle cell trait, and diabetes mellitus.
   3. *Clinical significance.* Approximately 40 percent of patients will develop acute symptomatic urinary tract infection.
   4. *Diagnosis*
      a) The findings of greater than 100,000 colonies of bacteria/ml urine on culture correlates with urinary tract infection in 80 percent of cases. Two positive cultures correlates 93 percent and three positive cultures 95 percent.
      b) Pyuria does not differentiate between true infection and contamination.

5. *Treatment*
   a) Antibiotic treatment should be delayed until bacterial sensitivities are obtained.
   b) Standard dosages of antibiotics should be administered for 10 to 14 days. Some controversy exists regarding the duration of therapy.
   c) Care must be taken not to administer antibiotics with potential fetal effects.
6. *Follow-up evaluation*
   a) A urine culture should be repeated following therapy to ensure sterile urine.
   b) Urine cultures should then be repeated every four to six weeks thereafter.

B. *Cystitis.* Symptomatic infection of the bladder commonly occurs in women with previous asymptomatic bacteriuria. Symptoms include dysuria, frequency, and urgency. Urinalysis will reveal pyuria and possibly hematuria. The diagnosis is confirmed by urine culture revealing more than 100,000 colonies/ml urine. *Since the patient is symptomatic, it will generally be necessary to initiate antibiotic treatment before antibiotic sensitivities are available.* A broad-spectrum penicillin or sulfonamides may be administered. Follow-up cultures should be obtained as when evaluating asymptomatic bacteriuria.

C. *Acute pyelonephritis*
1. *Incidence*
   a) Women with sterile urine on initial evaluation: 3 percent.
   b) Women with untreated bacteriuria: 40 percent.
2. *Etiology.* Pregnancy leads to urine stasis as a result of ureteral compression and decreased ureteral tone. Pyelonephritis generally results from an ascending infection from an infected lower urinary tract.
3. *Symptoms*
   a) Initial symptoms usually occur after the 20th week of pregnancy.

b) The onset of signs and symptoms is generally abrupt.

c) Fever and costovertebral pain are the most common initial symptoms.

d) Nausea and vomiting are less common symptoms.

e) Symptoms of lower urinary tract infection, dysuria, frequency, and urgency occur with variable frequency.

4. *Diagnosis*

a) Differential diagnosis includes labor, placental abruption, and chorioamnionitis.

b) The diagnosis of pyelonephritis is confirmed by positive urine culture. Urinalysis will reveal pyuria and possibly hematuria.

c) Physical examination will reveal fever and marked costovertebral angle tenderness. Abdominal palpation will be normal.

5. *Treatment*

a) Hospitalization is required for adequate treatment of the infection and management of associated problems such as vomiting and dehydration.

b) Broad-spectrum antibiotics should be administered parenterally as soon as the diagnosis is made. Antibiotics may be changed according to subsequent sensitivity reports.

c) After approximately 48 to 72 hours, oral antibiotics may be administered to complete a 14 day course of therapy.

d) Urinary tract obstruction should be considered if improvement does not occur after 72 hours.

6. *Follow-up evaluation*

a) Following therapy, monthly urine cultures should be obtained.

b) After the puerperium, the patient should undergo a complete urologic evaluation, since urologic abnormality may be discovered in 30 percent of the patients.

GLOMERULONEPHRITIS

A. *Acute.* This is a rare complication of pregnancy. Symptoms occur approximately two weeks after a group A β-streptococcal infection and include hematuria, proteinuria, oliguria, and hypertension. These symptoms may be indistinguishable from pregnancy-induced hypertension. The diagnosis is confirmed by an elevated antistreptolysin O titer. Management is expectant with prompt recovery of normal maternal renal function the rule.

B. *Chronic.* In most cases, the etiology of this condition is unknown, though some patients may develop it after acute glomerulonephritis. Symptoms include proteinuria, hypertension, and impaired renal function. Women with normal renal function and no hypertension will generally have an uncomplicated pregnancy. There is some increased risk of developing superimposed preeclampsia. Impaired renal function and hypertension result in a poor maternal and fetal prognosis. Prenatal care includes frequent office evaluations with monthly renal function studies. Hypertension is treated with standard medications, including methyldopa and thiazide diuretics. Appropriate fetal monitoring is mandatory.

ACUTE RENAL FAILURE

A. *Incidence.* 1/2000 to 5000 pregnancies.

B. *Etiology.* Acute renal failure may occur as a result of a variety of conditions that acutely decrease renal blood flow to the point of ischemia. The following complications of pregnancy have been associated with acute renal failure.

    1. *Hemorrhage.* Placenta previa, abruptio placentae, postpartum hemorrhage

    2. *Sepsis.* Septic abortion, chorioamnionitis

    3. *Intravascular hemolysis.* Disseminated intravascular coagulation associated with abruptio placentae, retained

dead fetus, sepsis, preeclampsia, amniotic fluid embolism, and transfusion reaction

C. *Symptoms.* This condition is characterized by acute oliguria and markedly impaired renal function.

D. *Pathology*
   1. *Acute tubular necrosis* occurs in the majority of patients.
   2. *Acute cortical necrosis* is generally associated with preeclampsia and abruptio placentae.
   3. *Acute fatty liver* of pregnancy is a rare disorder characterized by jaundice and severe impairment of hepatic function. This condition is often fatal due to combined hepatic and renal failure.
   4. *Idiopathic postpartum renal failure* is rare and generally follows a normal pregnancy. This condition is associated with uremia, severe hypertension, and microangiopathic hemolytic anemia. This condition is often fatal, and survivors generally have severely impaired renal function.

E. *Treatment.* Management of the patient with acute renal failure should be conducted only by physicians experienced with this condition. Careful central monitoring with frequent evaluation of blood chemistry is mandatory. In some cases, dialysis will be necessary.

URINARY CALCULI

A. *Incidence.* Renal and ureteral calculi have been associated with 0.03 to 0.35 percent of pregnancies.

B. *Symptoms*
   1. In most cases, the pregnancy is uneventful.
   2. Acute symptoms may include renal colic, acute ureteral obstruction, and acute pyelonephritis.
   3. The course of stone formation is not affected by pregnancy.

C. *Diagnosis*
   1. Urinary calculi should be considered in the differential diagnosis of acute abdominal pain with or without fever.

2. Urinalysis will generally reveal hematuria and pyuria in cases of associated infection.
3. An intravenous pyelogram may be necessary to establish the diagnosis.
4. If a urinary stone is discovered, the patient should be evaluated for primary hyperparathyroidism.

D. *Treatment*
1. In most cases, the stone will be passed spontaneously.
2. Surgical removal may be necessary if ureteral obstruction occurs.

RENAL TRANSPLANTATION

Successful term pregnancy after renal transplantation has been reported by several authors. Numerous maternal and fetal complications have been reported, including maternal death, severe hypertension, graft rejection, septicemia, fetal growth retardation, and premature delivery. Prospective parents should be carefully informed of these complications.

Davison and associates have suggested that the following criteria should be met before a woman with a renal transplant considers pregnancy:

1. Good general health for at least two years prior to transplantation
2. Stature compatible with good obstetric outcome
3. No proteinuria
4. Absence of graft rejection
5. No evidence of pelvicaliceal distention on recent intravenous pyelogram
6. Serum creatinine of 2 mg/100 ml or less
7. Drug therapy:
    Prednisone, 15 mg/day or less
    Azothioprine, 3 mg/kg/day or less
8. No significant hypertension

BIBLIOGRAPHY

Coe FL, Parks JH, Lindheimer MD: Nephrolithiasis during pregnancy. N Engl J Med 298:324, 1978

Cunningham FG: Acute pyelonephritis of pregnancy; A clinical review. Obstet Gynecol 42:112, 1973

Davison J: Planned pregnancy in a renal transplant patient. Br J Obstet Gynaecol 83:518, 1976

Davison J, Lindheimer M: Renal disease in pregnant women. Clin Obstet Gynecol 21:411, 1978

Harkins JL, et al.: Acute renal failure in obstetrics. Am J Obstet Gynecol 118:331, 1974

Lindheimer M, Katz A: Kidney Function and Disease in Pregnancy. Philadelphia, Lea & Febiger, 1977

McGeown M: Renal disorders and renal failure. Clin Obstet Gynaecol 4:319, 1977

Strong DW, et al.: The management of ureteral calculi during pregnancy. Surg Gynecol Obstet 146:604, 1978

Yacur H, et al.: Renal disease in pregnancy. Med Clin North Am 61:1, 1977

Section 4
Endocrine Disease
Jeffrey C. King, M.D.

PRACTICE PRINCIPLES

Pregnancy involves profound alterations of maternal neuroendocrine function and metabolism. The evaluation and treatment of endocrine disease in pregnancy depends on an appreciation of the effects of these changes on mother and baby, as well as the superimposed effects of endocrine disease.

DIABETES MELLITUS

A. *Introduction*
   1. Prior to the discovery of insulin, the occurrence of pregnancy in a diabetic not only was an unusual event but also frequently resulted in fatal consequences for the mother and fetus. By definition, *diabetes refers to those conditions in which there is a relative or absolute lack of functional insulin.* This results in hyperglycemia, glycosuria, increased protein and fat catabolism, and a tendency to develope ketoacidosis. Long-standing diabetes may result in vascular disease, leading to hypertension or heart disease, retinopathy, nephropathy, or neuropathy.

2. The *incidence* of diabetes during pregnancy varies between *1 and 5 cases per 1000 pregnancies*. Fortunately, aggressive management of this condition has reduced the *perinatal mortality* from 65 percent (early 1900s) to 4 percent and the *maternal mortality* from 30 percent (early 1900s) to 0.5 percent, which is still 20 times that of the general obstetric population.

3. *A team effort is necessary in order to achieve optimal maternal and fetal outcome.* Consultation among the obstetrician, pediatrician, maternal-fetal medicine specialist, neonatologist, and internist is essential for supervision of diabetic control, assessment of fetal welfare, and timing of delivery.

B. *Diagnosis*

1. *Symptomatic patients* will occasionally present a history of *polydipsia, polyphagia, polyuria,* weight loss, blurring of vision, or significant orthostatic changes in blood pressure. *One must be cautioned because many of these symptoms are compatible with normal pregnancy.*

a) *Asymptomatic patients* require laboratory confirmation by either fasting blood sugar (FBS) and two-hour postprandial blood sugars or glucose tolerance test (GTT). *Most centers accept a standard three-hour GTT having two or more abnormal values as criteria for the diagnosis of diabetes.* After the patient has been placed on a diet containing at least 300 gm of carbohydrate per day for three days, the test is administered. Following an overnight fast an FBS is obtained. Then a 100-gm liquid glucose solution is given, and blood specimens are drawn at one, two, and three hours. Values exceeding the following are considered abnormal:

	Plasma	Whole Blood
FBS	105	90
1 hour	190	165
2 hour	165	145
3 hour	145	125

C. *Screening*
  1. *Indications for screening during pregnancy* (FBS and two-hour postprandial or GTT).
     a) Previous perinatal loss
     b) Previous macrosomic infant (greater than nine pounds)
     c) Glycosuria. While this may be normal because renal tubular reabsorption does not increase proportionately to the increases in glomerular filtration rate, persistent glycosuria demands investigation.
     d) Family history of diabetes
     e) Maternal age greater than 35 years
     f) Obesity. Twenty percent overweight or greater than 90 kg
     g) History of congenital malformation
     h) Presence or history of hydramnios
  2. Some authorities recommend screening all pregnant patients with an FBS and two-hour postprandial during the late second trimester and prior to GTT for patients with the risk factors mentioned above.
D. *Classification.* The scheme of Priscilla White is generally used.

  • Class A. Appearing during pregnancy, not requiring insulin (abnormal GTT and normal FBS)
  • Class B. Overt Diabetes, onset after age 20, duration less than 10 years
  • Class C. Overt diabetes, onset before age 20, duration 10 to 20 years
  • Class D. Onset before age 10 or duration more than 20 years, benign retinopathy
  • Class E. Calcified pelvic vessels (this category no longer used)
  • Class F. Diabetic nephropathy—reduced creatinine clearance and proteinuria in excess of 100 mg/100 ml urine
  • Class R. Proliferative retinopathy
  • Class RF. Nephropathy plus retinopathy

- Class H. Cardiac disease
- Class T. Status post-renal-transplant

E. *Physiology*. Pregnancy can be described as a state of "accelerated starvation" because of low blood glucose, low serum insulin, and a tendency toward ketosis in the fasting state. When fed, the mother has impaired glucose tolerance, hyperglycemia, increased insulin levels, and decreased sensitivity to insulin at the cellular level. The placental hormones (human placental lactogen, estrogen, and progesterone) and the increased levels of cortisol exert an anti-insulin effect.

As pregnancy progresses, insulin requirements change dramatically. During the first trimester, the fetus "extracts" glucose and amino acids; this results in insulin requirements of approximately two-thirds the prepregnancy levels. Later, as the placental hormones and their effect rise, requirements increase by 50 to 100 percent of prepregnancy doses.

F. *Maternal effect*

1. *The major dangers encountered by the diabetic parturient* during the third trimester are related to a ketoacidosis and postpartum hypoglycemia.

   a) The development of *ketoacidosis* has been associated with a maternal mortality rate of 5 to 15 percent and a perinatal mortality rate of 30 to 70 percent. This condition occurs most frequently in very late pregnancy, when the insulin requirements are changing fairly rapidly.

   b) *Hypoglycemia* may occur postdelivery, when the effect of placental hormones is falling.

2. The exact effect of pregnancy on diabetic nephropathy, retinopathy, and neuropathy is questionable. Many believe that "tight" physiologic control of blood sugars will retard progression of disease; however, others have shown that outcomes are not affected if control is loose. It is essential to point out that studies showing loose control to be as good as tight control had, as their objective, the attainment of tight control in all patients.

3. Approximately 20 to 30 percent of Class A diabetics will develop permanent diabetes within five years.

G. *Fetal effect*. Perinatal morbidity and mortality
   1. During the last trimester, *perinatal mortality* results from:
      a) Prematurity as a result of unnecessary preterm delivery
      b) Functional immaturity of various organ systems
      c) Both of the above
      d) Traumatic vaginal delivery of a macrosomic infant
      e) Unexpected, sudden intrauterine death
   2. The effect of diabetes on *respiratory distress syndrome* (RDS) has been noted by many studies. (Stekbens found that when corrected for gestational age and mode of delivery, infants of diabetic mothers were 5.6 times more likely to develop RDS than controls.)
   3. *Macrosomia and related birth trauma* (fractured clavicle, humerus, or skull, and brachial plexus injuries) are seen most frequently in Classes A to C.
   4. Patients in classes D to T have vascular disease and are therefore more likely to produce *intrauterine growth retardation* (IUGR) and its sequela of placental insufficiency and perinatal asphyxia.
   5. Approximately 10 to 15 percent of infants of diabetic mothers have some *congenital malformation*. The most common anomalies are cardiac (transposition, ventricular septal defect), caudal regression syndrome, genitourinary (agenesis, duplication), gastrointestinal (anal/rectal atresia), and anencephaly. Some believe that tight control during the period of conception and early embryonic life may decrease fetal anomaly rates. But others believe that hypoglycemic episodes may, in and of themselves, be teratogenic.
   6. Following delivery, *short-term neonatal morbidity* is seen frequently: hypoglycemia (30 percent), hypocalcemia (10 to 15 percent), and hyperbilirubinemia (30 to 40 percent).

H. *Management*. The physician must be concerned with regulation of maternal glucose, assessment of fetal well-being, and monitoring the extent of pulmonary maturation.

1. Class A
   a) *Education* of the patient is most important. The patient must feel that she has been made a member of the "team" and that her input is necessary.
   b) *Diet* should contain 30 to 35 cal/kg actual body weight in order to achieve a physiologic weight gain of 25 pounds during pregnancy. The diet should be broken down into 20 percent protein (1 to 1.5 gm/kg), 35 percent fat (90 gm), and 45 percent carbohydrates.
   c) *Accurate dating and serial observation of fetal growth by sonography are essential.*
   d) *Biweekly visits with FBS until 36 weeks, then weekly.* Approximately 10 percent of Class A patients will become overt diabetics requiring insulin during pregnancy. Patients should record daily double-voided morning urine specimens for sugar and acetone. The presence of acetone requires an increase in caloric intake.
   e) Since uncomplicated Class A patients do not have an increased perinatal mortality until 40 weeks, fetal surveillance should be withheld until then (see below).
2. Other classes
   a) Basic management as in Class A patients.
   b) Baseline *diagnostic studies* should be obtained in early pregnancy: creatinine clearance, protein excretion, ophthalmologic consultation for funduscopic exam, and electrocardiogram.
   c) *Calories* should be provided on the following schedule: breakfast (25 percent), lunch (30 percent), dinner (30 percent), bedtime snack (15 percent). The bedtime snack is most important when an evening dose of intermediate insulin is necessary.
   d) Double-voided urine specimens should be checked for sugar and acetone prior to each meal. Results should be recorded.
   e) *The goal of therapy is a FBS of less than 100 and a postprandial blood sugar of less than 150.*

f) *Insulin management*
   (1) Most overt diabetics who receive more than 40 units of insulin/day require split-dosage (A.M. and early P.M.). Usually two-thirds of the total daily dose in a ratio of 2:1, NPH to regular, is given prior to breakfast. A predinner injection of one-third of the daily dose in a ratio of 1:1, NPH to regular, is also necessary. These ratios are rough guidelines; actual dosage and distribution depends on patient control.
   (2) *Oral hypoglycemic agents have no place in the management of diabetes during pregnancy.*
g) *Patients must be seen weekly* to assess the development of hypertension, hydramnios, IUGR, or changing insulin requirements. Falling insulin requirements suggest dropping levels of placental hormones and the possibility of fetal compromise. Maternal perception of decreased fetal movement may also indicate fetal distress.
h) *Biochemical surveillance* with unconjugated plasma estriol should be obtained weekly beginning at 30 weeks and increased to daily determinations at 34 weeks for Classes B and C. Classes D through T should have daily values from 32 weeks.
i) *Biophysical surveillance* should include ultrasonography at three- to four-week intervals to document fetal growth, amount of amniotic fluid, and placental morphology. Antepartum heart rate testing (nonstress test) should be twice weekly from 34 weeks for Classes B and C, from 32 weeks for Classes D through T. If the NST is nonreactive, a contraction stress test (CST) is mandatory. Daily assessment of fetal activity should be started at 30 weeks. Marked changes in fetal movement should be investigated by an NST at least.
j) *Outpatient management should be attempted for as long as possible during pregnancy.* However, if worsening maternal condition, suspicion of fetal compromise, or noncompliance is noted, immediate

hospitalization and intensive surveillance are mandatory.

I. *Delivery*

1. *Delivery should be accomplished when fetal lung maturation is attained.* Amniocentesis should be performed at 37 weeks for lecithin/sphingomyelin ratio (L/S) and phosphatidyl-glycerol (PG). An L/S ratio of greater than 2.0 and a PG greater than 2 percent assure fetal lung stability.

2. *The mode of delivery* (vaginal versus cesarean) depends on the status of the cervix and the well-being of the fetus. If these factors are favorable, an attempt at induction of labor with direct fetal monitoring is indicated. However, if fetal status is questionable or the cervix is firm, cesarean section should be performed.

3. *If during the course of the third trimester, biochemical or biophysical tests suggest fetal jeopardy, delivery must be considered.* An assessment of pulmonary maturation is the next step. An L/S ratio indicative of maturity should prompt delivery. A test indicative of immaturity requires careful evaluation of all maternal and fetal interactions. Delivery may still be indicated despite an immature value.

4. *Management of insulin requirements during labor and/or delivery* can be intermittent subcutaneous injection or continuous intravenous infusion. One-third to one-half of the prepregnancy dose of insulin given as *regular* insulin may be given on the morning of induction. If the patient is to undergo a cesarean section, this dose is administered following the operation. Alternatively, a continuous infusion delivery of 1 to 2 units/hour may be started, up to two days prior to delivery, with reduction of 0.5 units/hour at night to prevent maternal hypoglycemia. Each of these methods requires careful and frequent monitoring of maternal glucose levels. This can be accomplished easily with a glucose reflectance meter (Ames dextrometer).

5. *Management following delivery is aimed at preventing*

hypoglycemia. Reduction in insulin dosage is necessary because of the rapid fall in placental hormones. Since requirements are changing rapidly, no attempt should be made at tight control but rather at keeping blood sugars less than 250 mg/100 ml.

J. *Ketoacidosis*

  1. The *development* of ketoacidosis during pregnancy is associated with *a fetal loss of up to 70 percent.* The rising insulin resistance during pregnancy makes the parturient at high risk for ketosis. *Various stimuli can result in ketoacidosis:* infection, failure to meet rising insulin needs, and stress of any sort.

     a) *Symptoms* include polydipsia and polyuria due to rising glucose levels, which result in an osmotic diuresis and dehydration. Nausea and vomiting will contribute to fluid loss and dehydration.

     b) *Physical findings* are those of depressed sensorium, acidotic breathing, signs of dehydration and hemoconcentration, and the fruity breath odor of ketones.

     c) *Laboratory evaluation* shows a grossly elevated glucose level, serum bicarbonate is usually less than 15 mEq/liter, urinary ketone levels arc high, and serum ketones may be absent to high.

  2. *Management* depends on the severity of the condition. Obviously, *underlying disease must be treated concurrently* (e.g., antibiotics for pyelonephritis). Severe cases may require admission to an intensive care setting, whereas mild forms may be treated on the antepartum/high-risk floor.

     a) Attention to *hydrational status* is important, since these patients are often depleted to the equivalence of 1 to 3 liters of saline. This should be administered over 6 to 12 hours to correct the deficit, then normal daily requirements should be infused. In many centers it is felt that this condition warrants placement of central pressure monitoring (CVP or Swan-Ganz) to prevent acute overload.

b) *Sodium bicarbonate.* One or two ampules should be placed in the first liter of IV fluid if pH is less than 7.25 or bicarbonate is less than 10 mEq/liter. The management of acidosis and hyperglycemia causes an intracellular shift of potassium. Therefore, *10 mEq of KCl should be administered IV each hour, starting at the fourth hour of therapy. A baseline ECG is necessary to evaluate potassium status.*

c) An indwelling urinary catheter is helpful in monitoring output and urinary spillage of sugar and ketones. Serum glucose should be watched hourly with the use of a reflectance meter. Electrolytes, BUN, creatinine, and pH should be repeated at two- to six-hour intervals as determined by clinical status.

d) *Mild ketoacidosis* (blood sugar, 200 to 600; serum ketones, low values; bicarbonate, greater than 16) can be treated with 10 units regular insulin by IV push every hour.

e) *Moderate disease* (blood sugar, 300 to 800; serum ketones, low to moderate; bicarbonate, 10 to 15) requires 15 units, IV push, and a constant infusion delivering 6 to 10 units of regular insulin per hour.

f) *Severe disease* (stupor; blood sugar above 500; serum ketones, moderate to high; becarbonate, less than 10) is serious. Initially, 25 units of regular insulin is given by IV push, followed by an infusion system to delivery 10 to 20 units per hour. *It is mandatory that these management protocols be continued for at least 24 hours following the clearance of serum ketones to prevent recurrent ketoacidosis.*

THYROID DISEASE

A. Because of the various effects of pregnancy on the patient, the diagnosis and management of thyroid disorders during pregnancy is quite challenging. The usual signs and symptoms of a hypermetabolic state (warm skin, palpitations, increase in gland size, and heat intolerance) normally may occur during pregnancy. Pregnancy causes an alteration in the *total thyroxine* (T_4) and triiodothyronine resin uptake (T_3RU) due to elevation of *thyroxine-binding globulin* (TBG). Finally, the treatment of thyroid abnormalities is complicated by the fetus, which may be jeopardized by antithyroid medication or surgery. The use of radioactive iodine during pregnancy is contraindicated.

B. *Thyroid physiology in pregnancy*

1. At least two biologically active hormones are secreted by the thyroid: *T_4* and *triiodothyronine* (T_3). Most of the T_3 is formed from the conversion of T_4. *Reverse T_3* (rT_3) is also formed by peripheral deiodination of T_4, but rT_3 does not appear to have biologic activity.

2. *T_3 and T_4 are bound to proteins, mainly TBG.* Serum levels of TBG double by the end of the first trimester and then rise slowly to term. The effects of increased levels of TBG are as follows:

   a) Total T_4 may be elevated but rarely exceeds 15 μg/dl for a euthyroid patient.

   b) Free T_4 is unchanged by pregnancy.

   c) T_3RU is slightly below normal nonpregnant values. T_3RU refers to the percentage radioiodine-labeled T_3 that is absorbed onto a resin after incubation with the patient's serum and attachment to unoccupied TBG binding sites.

3. Endogenous or exogenously administered thyroid hormones do not cross the placenta in significant amounts. Long-acting thyroid stimulator (LATS) and antithyroid medications cross without difficulty. The actual onset of fetal synthesis of thyroid hormones is between 10 and 12 weeks.

4. While free T_4 is unchanged by pregnancy and can be used to determine a euthyroid state, it is not always necessary to perform direct assay. A free thyroxine index (FT_4I)

may be calculated that correlates well with actual free T_4 values:

$$FT_4I = T_3RU \text{ patient}/T_3RU \text{ normal mean}$$

Elevated levels are consistent with hyperthyroidism; low values indicate hypothyroidism (Table 15–1).

C. *Hyperthyroidism*

1. The *incidence* of hyperthyroidism in pregnancy is about *0.2 percent*. The *most common cause of hyperthyroidism is Grave's disease*. Other conditions such as multinodular goiter, toxic adenoma, hydatidiform mole, subacute thyroiditis, or thyrotoxicosis fictitia may also result in hyperthyroidism. Fertility is generally not affected when mild to moderate hyperthyroidism occurs.

2. *Diagnosis*

   a) The *clinical diagnosis* during pregnancy is difficult. Usually, the presence of tachycardia (pulse greater than 100) and failure to gain weight or actual weight loss are signs suggestive of thyrotoxicosis. Eye signs — such as exophthalmos, lid lag, lid retraction, and chemosis — may be helpful.

   b) *The diagnosis is confirmed by* an elevated FT_4I, free T_4, T_3RU, and total T_4. In patients who present clinical signs of hyperthyroidism but whose thyroid studies are normal, total T_3, and FT_3I should be assayed. Rarely, T_3 hyperthyroidism may be discovered.

3. *Maternal effect.* In the absence of thyroid storm, the mother is at little increased risk from hyperthyroidism.

4. *Fetal effect.* The fetus is at a small increased risk of perinatal mortality and a definite increase in the incidence of low birth weight.

5. *Management.* Surgery (subtotal thyroidectomy) and medical management with antithyroid drugs are the options of therapy.

TABLE 15–1. SUMMARY OF THYROID FUNCTION TESTS DURING PREGNANCY

Patient	Total T_4	Free T_4	FT_4I	Total T_3	FT_3I	T_3RU	TSH	LATS
Nonpregnant normal	Normal	Normal	Normal	Normal	Normal	Normal	Normal	Negative
Pregnant normal	Increased	Normal	Normal	Slight increase	Normal	Decreased	Normal	Negative
Pregnant hyperthyroid	Increased	Increased	Increased	Normal to slight increase	—	Increased	Normal	Often positive
Pregnant hypothyroid	Decreased	Decreased	Decreased	Normal to slight decrease	—	Decreased	High	Negative

a) *Surgical intervention* has as its major risk, injury to the recurrent laryngeal nerve, hypoparathyroidism, thyroid storm, or initiation of labor. Therefore, most recommend medical management. However, surgery is indicated if the disease cannot be controlled, poor patient compliance is noted, or a large obstructing goiter exists.

b) *Medical management*

   (1) Obtain LATS value as an aid to neonatal management since it crosses the placenta easily.

   (2) Begin *thiourea therapy* (*propylthiouracil or methimazole*). Both drugs are equally effective in blocking the synthesis of thyroid hormones; however, most prefer propylthiouracil, because methimazole has been associated with a few cases of scalp defects in the offspring of treated mothers. Since these drugs easily cross the placenta, observation for fetal goiter or hypothyroidism is necessary.

   (3) *Initial dose of propylthiouracil* is 100 to 150 mg every eight hours. Since the plasma half-life of T_4 is seven days, laboratory assessment of the effect from a particular dose should be delayed at least one week. *Most patients show signs of improvement within two to four weeks.* The most sensitive indicators of euthyroid status are increase in body weight and resolution of tachycardia. Repeat values should be obtained at one- to two-week intervals to assess maternal thyroid status. When the total T_4 is 13 to 15, FT_4I is normal, and symptoms are controlled, the dosage should be reduced as much as possible. Many patients can be completely removed from therapy by 34 weeks if treatment has been ongoing for the previous 12 weeks. If a relapse occurs, the dose is increased to that noted above.

   c) *Thiourea complications*
     (1) *These medications produce adverse reactions in about 5 to 7 percent of patients.* Most commonly, skin rash, pruritis, fever, and nausea occur. Since there is little cross-reactivity, the physician should use the alternate drug.
     (2) *Agranulocytosis* is a rare (0.3 to 0.6 percent) complication. It occurs after one to two months of therapy and is usually associated with fever and sore throat; therefore, patients should be instructed to discontinue their medication and obtain a leukocyte count if symptoms occur.
     (3) Long-term follow-up of both infants and mothers exposed to thiourea medication has not revealed any mental or physical deficits.
     (4) During labor, vaginal examination for flexion attitude of the fetal head is essential to determine if a large fetal goiter is present.

D. *Hypothyroidism*
  1. This is a *rare condition during pregnancy.* Usually patients with hypothyroidism are infertile. *The most common etiologies* of primary hypothyroidism include Hashimoto's thyroiditis, antithyroid drug therapy, and destruction of the gland (by iodine-131 or surgery).
  2. *Diagnosis*
    a) *Early symptoms* are quite variable and nonspecific. Malaise, lethargy, cold intolerance, weight gain, dry skin, hair loss, and paresthesias may occur. Loss of hair at the lateral aspect of the eyebrows is often noted. A slow relaxation phase for deep-tendon reflexes may be found.
    b) *The diagnosis is confirmed* by the presence of low total T_4, free T_4, and T_3RU. The TSH level is well above normal.
  3. *Management.* Treatment consists of thyroid preparations in sufficient amount to achieve clinical and biochemical euthyroidism. L-Thyroxine, 0.2 mg/day, is considered a

replacement dose. This medication will result in a steady-state serum concentration of both T_4 and T_3. Thyroid-stimulating hormone levels may require up to eight weeks to return to baseline following the initiation of therapy.

4. *Prognosis.* With hormonal replacement, outcome for mother and fetus is good.

PARATHYROID DISEASE

A. *Calcium metabolism in pregnancy.* In the absence of major changes in the mass of calcium in the skeleton, extracellular calcium concentration is determined by a balance between calcium absorption from the gut and its excretion into the urine and feces. The skeleton acts as a surface to provide about 300 mmol of calcium exchange between blood and bone each day. This exchange is regulated by parathyroid hormone (PTH), which shifts calcium into the blood, and by calcitonin, which inhibits this shift.

During pregnancy, calcium levels, especially free calcium, are maintained within a rather narrow range but show a slight downward trend. It is felt that this change is due primarily to hemodilution. There is a progressive rise in PTH levels during pregnancy in an attempt to correct the slight drop in calcium. However, there is also a modest rise in calcitonin levels. The exact reason for this elevation is unknown.

B. *Hyperparathyroidism*
   1. This is an exceedingly *rare* condition. Patients are generally asymptomatic, although when *symptoms* are present, they may include polydipsia, polyuria, constipation, nausea/vomiting, or those of nephrolithiasis. Profound hypercalcemia may result in stupor or coma.
   2. The *diagnosis* is made on persistently elevated serum calcium levels, particularly free calcium, and increased PTH values.
   3. *Effects* on mother and baby. The effect on the mother is

minimal, with labor and delivery being generally uncomplicated. However, fetal outcome is significantly altered. Persistent maternal hypercalcemia leads to persistent fetal hypercalcemia, since calcium is actively transported across the placenta, and fetal levels are 1 to 2 mg/dl higher than maternal levels. Following delivery, when the maternal supply of calcium is removed, profound neonatal hypocalcemia may occur between 5 and 14 days postpartum. This can result in a neonatal tetany that is usually self-limited; recovery often occurs without treatment.

4. If the diagnosis of hyperparathyroidism is made during pregnancy, the treatment of choice is maternal parathyroidectomy. This should be accomplished early enough during pregnancy so that maternal and fetal calcium levels fall to within the normal range and allow the atrophy of the fetal parathyroid glands to resolve prior to delivery. Neonates should be treated with prophylactic calcium following delivery to prevent tetany. Unfortunately, most cases of maternal hyperparathyroidism are detected postpartum, when the patients are fully recovered and after the occurrence of neonatal tetany.

C. *Hypoparathyroidism*

1. The most common cause of hypoparathyroidism is iatrogenic, secondary to thyroid or parathyroid surgery, when the glands are removed or their blood supply compromised.

2. This condition is even rarer than hyperparathyroidism. *Symptoms* include weakness, paresthesias, muscle cramps, and fatigue. Occasionally, maternal tetany, laryngospasm, or generalized convulsions may occur if calcium levels are extremely low. However, the most common cause of tetany during pregnancy is alkalosis secondary to hyperventilation.

3. The diagnosis is made by persistently low serum calcium values, especially free calcium, and inappropriately low PTH levels.

4. Treated hypoparathyroidism appears to have no deleterious effects on the pregnancy. On the contrary, untreated disease may result in neonatal hyperparathyroidism. Fortunately, this "congenital" disease is self-limited.

   a) Maternal treatment of this condition consists of providing 2 gm elemental calcium per day orally plus 50,000 to 100,000 units of vitamin D per day orally. Calcium values should be checked frequently and the vitamin D dose adjusted accordingly. Vitamin D does cross the placenta and whether it is a teratogen is questionable.

   b) Breast-feeding should be discouraged because human milk contains up to 400 mg of calcium per liter. Replacement of this amount of calcium loss is difficult.

ADRENAL DISEASE

A. *Introduction.* The diagnosis of adrenal disease is often complicated because the signs and symptoms mimic normal pregnancy. Plasma levels of cortisol rise progressively during pregnancy, reaching a peak at delivery of two to three times normal. This increase is primarily due to the rise in cortisol-binding globulin. Plasma levels of catecholamines are unchanged by pregnancy.

B. *Adrenocortical insufficiency*

1. The signs and symptoms of Addison's disease are unchanged by pregnancy. Weakness, fatigue, weight loss, nausea/vomiting, anorexia, hypotension, and increased skin pigmentation may occur. However, these findings may also occur during normal pregnancy. Persistent, unexplained nausea, vomiting, and weight loss may be the most sensitive indicators of adrenal insufficiency.

2. The diagnosis is made when plasma cortisol levels are found to be low for pregnancy. However, the values may be within the normal range for nonpregnant patients. An

adrenocorticotropic hormone (ACTH) stimulation test may also be performed. A baseline serum cortisol is drawn and 25 units of ACTH are administered intramuscularly. A repeat cortisol is obtained one hour later. Normally, the baseline value is doubled.

3. With proper treatment, maternal and fetal prognosis is good. The neonate should be watched for the rare condition of depressed adrenal function secondary to maternal therapy. Parturients with untreated or undiagnosed Addison's disease tend to tolerate pregnancy without difficulty. However, they may present with acute adrenal insufficiency postpartum due to their inability to mount an adrenal response to the stress of delivery.

4. Maintenance replacement with adrenocortical hormones is necessary. Prednisone, 5 mg p.o. each morning and 2.5 mg p.o. each evening, is sufficient. The addition of 0.05 to 0.1 mg of 9-fluorohydrocortisone daily is necessary because of its salt-retaining effect. This dose may be altered if significant edema or hypertension develops. Delivery, whether by cesarean or the vaginal route, is a major stress. Therefore, sufficient additional steroids must be administered to prevent acute adrenal crisis. Following delivery, dosage may be decreased by 50 percent per day until maintenance levels are reached.

C. *Cushing's syndrome.* This is a rare disorder of steroid overproduction from adrenal tumor or from adrenal hyperplasia secondary to elevated ACTH secretion. Since patients are usually infertile, this condition is very rare in pregnancy. Endocrine consultation is advised prior to attempting suppression.

D. *Pheochromocytoma*

1. Tumors of the chromaffin tissue located most often in the adrenal medulla can produce catecholamine excess.

2. Diagnosis

a) *Hypertension* is a mandatory finding for diagnosis. While it may be constant with wide fluctuations, it may also be intermittent. Additional symptoms such as sweats, palpitations, and tremulousness may also be found.

b) The diagnosis can be made based on elevated plasma catecholamines. Previously, 24-hour urine collections for vanillylmandelic acid, metanephrines, and catecholamines were necessary. Obtaining these was often complicated by the necessity of introducing medical treatment, which interfered with the determinations.

3. Prognosis. Fetal and maternal mortality approaches 50 percent. The usual cause of death is hemorrhage in the tumor or in the brain, or cardiovascular collapse.

4. Management. Immediate surgical removal is curative; however, some have proposed that the mother should be treated with adrenergic-blocking agents until fetal maturity is attained. At that point, cesarean section and resection could be performed.

BIBLIOGRAPHY

Burrow GN: Adrenal, pituitary and parathyroid disorders. In Burrow GN, Ferris T, (eds): Medical Complications During Pregnancy. Philadelphia, Saunders, 1975

Burrow GN: Hyperthyroidism during pregnancy. N Engl J Med 298:150, 1978

Distler W, Gabbe SG, Freeman RK, et al.: Estriol in pregnancy. V. Unconjugated and total plasma estriol in the management of pregnant diabetic patients. Am J Obstet Gynecol 130:424, 1978

Gabbe SG: Congenital malformations in infants of diabetic mothers. Obstet Gynecol Surv 32:125, 1977

Gabbe SG, Mestman JH, Freeman RK, et al.: Management and outcome of pregnancy in diabetes mellitus, Classes B to R. Am J Obstet Gynecol 129:723, 1977

Kreisberg RA: Diabetic ketoacidosis: new concepts and trends in pathogenesis and treatment. Ann Intern Med 88:681, 1978

Merkatz IR, Adam PA (eds): Diabetes in pregnancy. Semin Perinatol 2:287, 1978

Mestman JH: Management of thyroid diseases in pregnancy. Clin Perinatol 7:371, 1980

Montoro M, Collea JV, Frasier D, Mestman JH: Successful outcome of pregnancy in women with hypothyroidism. Ann Intern Med 94:31, 1981

Reeve J: Calcium metabolism. In Hytten G, Chamberlain D (eds): Clinical Physiology in Obstetrics. London, Blackwell, 1980

Rogge PT: Endocrine complications. In Niswander K (ed): Manual of Obstetrics. Boston, Little, Brown, 1980

Seeds AE (ed): Diabetes in pregnancy. Clin Obstet Gynecol 24:1, 1981

Stekbens JA, Baker GL, Kitchell M: Outcome at ages 1, 3, and 5 years of children born to diabetic women. Am J Obstet Gynecol 127:408, 1977

Section 5
Pulmonary Disease
Michael Parsons, M.D.

MECHANICAL AND HORMONAL CHANGES
Significantly alter the respiratory state in pregnancy.

A. *Hyperemia, edema, and increased secretion* may cause nasal obstruction or epistaxis.
B. *Elevation of diaphragm*
C. *Alterations in physiologic measurements*
   1. *Increased.* Tidal volume, inspiratory capacity, minute ventilation, and alveolar ventilation
   2. *Decreased.* Functional residual capacity, residual volume, expiratory reserve volume, and total lung capacity
   3. *No change.* Respiratory rate, forced vital capacity (FVC), FEV (forced expiratory volume) or FEV_1 (forced expiratory volume in one second), arterial pH

DYSPNEA OF PREGNANCY

A. The majority of women possess a *sensation of increased breathing effort,* mostly in the first half of pregnancy.
B. *Suggested mechanisms*
   1. Extra stretching of muscles from increased tidal volume, causing a sensation of overbreathing

2. A greater response to P_{CO_2} levels resulting from increased progesterone levels

ACUTE RESPIRATORY DISEASE

A. *Upper respiratory tract infections*
   1. *The vast majority are mild and of viral etiology* (rhino-, adeno-, parainfluenza virus).
   2. *Complications*
      a) Sinusitis
      b) Otitis media
      c) Bronchitis
      d) Pneumonia
   3. *Treatment*
      a) Bed rest
      b) Hydration
      c) Antipyretics (acetaminophen [Tylenol])
      d) Antibiotics are not routine
B. *Acute bronchitis*
   1. *Etiology*
      a) Upper respiratory tract infection
      b) Chemical and physical irritants
      c) Aspiration
      d) Associated with mucosal edema
   2. *Treatment*
      a) Expectorants
      b) Inhalants, steam
      c) Bronchodilators
      d) Antibiotics if needed
      e) Postural drainage
C. *Asthma*
   1. *Incidence.* 0.2 to 1.3 percent of pregnancies
   2. *Effect of pregnancy on asthma*
      a) Variable responses
         (1) Mild asthma may remain the same, improve, or worsen.

(2) Severe asthma has a greater tendency toward exacerbation.

(3) Subsequent pregnancies tend to have similar effects on asthma.

b) Possible influences improving asthmatic status

(1) Increased corticosteroid levels

(2) Increased progesterone levels

(3) Increased serum cyclic — AMP

(4) Decreased cell-mediated immunity

c) Possible influences worsening asthmatic status

(1) Antigenically via fetus

(2) Nasal congestion

(3) Decreased functional residual volume

(4) Decreased cell-mediated immunity leading to viral infections

(5) Dyspnea of pregnancy increasing anxiety

3. *Effect of asthma on pregnancy.* There is a twofold increase in perinatal deaths, an increase in prematurity, IUGR, and neurologically abnormal infants, primarily in severe asthmatics.

4. *Evaluation of the asthmatic patient*

a) *History*

(1) Events leading to attack

(2) Duration of symptoms

(3) Medications

(4) Allergies

(5) Symptoms

b) *Examination*

(1) Vital signs. Rectal temperature more accurate

(2) Auscultation for wheezing

(3) Check for pulsus paradoxus (abnormal if inspiration decreases blood pressure more than 12 mm Hg)

c) *Laboratory studies*

(1) CBC

(2) Sputum. Gram stain for neutrophils vs. eosinophilsand for bacteria

(3) FEV. Before treatment for an attack, FEV is usually less than 1500 cc. If treatment is successful, FEV will increase by more than 500 cc.

(4) Arterial blood gases

(5) Chest x-ray if febrile

5. *Treatment*

a) *Oxygen* by nasal cannula at 3 liters/minute initial rate

b) *Hydration* (100 to 200 ml/hour)

c) *Epinephrine*

(1) 0.3 ml of 1:1000 dilution subcutaneously every 15 to 20 minutes

(2) *Toxicity*. Hypertension, cardiac arrhythmia

d) *Theophyllines*

(1) Inhibits phosphodiesterase (enzyme that breaks down adenyl cyclase) to control bronchospasm.

(2) Loading dose: 6 mg/kg in 100 ml D5/W over 20 minutes

(3) Maintenance: 0.9 mg/kg/hour

(4) Oral dose. 2 to 4 mg/kg q6h

(5) Therapeutic level: 10 to 20 mg/ml

(6) Toxicity. Nausea and vomiting, abdominal pain, tachycardia, headache, cardiac arrhythmia

e) β-*Agonist agents*.Stimulate the production of cyclic AMP, which inhibits mediator release from cells.

(1) *Terbutaline*. 2.5 mg p.o./b.i.d. to 5 mg p.o./t.i.d.

(2) *Metaproterenol* (Alupent). 10 to 20 mg p.o./q.i.d. or spray, 2 to 3 times inhalation q3–4h

(3) Side effect. Tremor

f) *Intermittent positive pressure breathing* to deliver drugs and help patients take deeper breaths

g) *Corticosteroids* if not responding to initial therapy.

(1) *Hydrocortisone*. Loading dose, 7 mg/kg; maintenance, 100 to 300 mg q4–6h, decrease to 50 to 100 mg q6h over next 24 hour; then change to prednisone, 1 mg/kg/24 hour p.o.

h) Antibiotics if indicated

i) If the P_{CO_2} is greater than 35 mm Hg or arterial pH less than 7.35, consider transfer to an intensive care setting. If the PO_2 is less than 60 mm Hg, the fetus may be in jeopardy.

j) At delivery, regional anesthesia is preferable to general, but if necessary, halothane is the best general anesthetic because of its bronchodilation effect.

k) Drugs not used: tetracycline, medications with iodine, prostagladins.

6. *Chronic asthma.* The goals of therapy are: relief of bronchospasm, reduction of secretions, prevention and treatment of infections, and avoidance of irritants.

D. *Pneumonia*

1. *Incidence.* 1 percent of patients with acute respiratory disease

2. *Effect on pregnancy*

a) Spontaneous abortion occurs in 17 to 57 percent of pregnancies with pneumonia in the first 20 weeks of pregnancy.

b) Premature labor occurs in 60 percent of pregnancies between the 25th and 36th weeks.

c) Pneumonia is the second most common cause of nonobstetrical maternal deaths following cardiac disease.

3. Organisms commonly involved include *Streptococcus pneumonia, Mycoplasma*, influenza virus.

4. *Treatment*

a) Antibiotics, based on Gram stain of sputum, with changes as indicated based on culture and sensitivity results

b) Oxygen

c) Hydration

d) No sedatives

e) Prevent premature labor

E. *Amniotic fluid embolism*

F. *Tuberculosis*

1. *Incidence.* 1.6 to 3 percent of patients with acute respiratory disease

2. *Mortality.* 10/100,000 live births

3. *Pathophysiology*
   a) Airborne bacilli to alveoli, where tubercles are formed; leads to casseous necrosis and fibrosis
   b) Positive skin test 4 to 12 weeks following infection
4. *Presentation*
   a) Positive tuberculin test
   b) Positive chest x-ray
   c) Fever, cough, hemoptysis, malaise, weight loss, night sweats
   d) Pleuritic chest pain
5. *Diagnosis*
   a) Sputum Gram stain
   b) Biopsy
   c) If positive tuberculin test, obtain chest x-ray (posteroanterior and lateral) with abdomen shielded. The Mantoux test is preferable to the Tine test
6. *Effect on pregnancy*
   a) Pregnancy is unaffected if adequate treatment is administered.
   b) Rarely, congenital tuberculosis can affect the newborn. The route of infection to the infant is transplacental or aspiration/swallowing of bacilli in utero. The infant mortality is 40 percent (including the untreated).
7. There is no effect of pregnancy on tuberculosis.
8. *Management*
   a) Admit for work-up and notify U.S. Public Health Service.
   b) *If in labor*
      (1) Isolate mother in labor, delivery, and postpartum.
      (2) Isolate newborn.
   c) *Medications*
      (1) *Isoniazid (INH)* is the safest, most used, and least expensive drug, given in an oral dose of 300 mg/day. It is associated with maternal hepatitis. There are no effects on the fetus. *Pyridoxine* (50 mg p.o. q.d.) should be used to prevent neuropathy.

    (2) *Ethambutol* in an oral dose of 15 to 25 mg/kg/day. Toxic effect is retrobulbar neuritis. No effect on the fetus.

    (3) *Rifampin* in an oral dose of 600 mg/day. Toxic doses cause changes in liver function and thrombocytopenia. Probably safe for the fetus.

    (4) *Streptomycin* in an IV dose of 1 gm q.d. for three months. Fetal effect is ototoxicity in 1 of 6 cases.

  d) *Common treatment is isoniazid and ethambutol* (with rifampin if third drug is needed). Treatment regimens have been for one to two years, but shorter regimens (six to nine months) are being tried.

  e) Treatment is needed for active disease, disease not previously treated, recent conversion, contacts of patients with tuberculosis.

  f) *Treatment for infant*

    (1) Isoniazid (if sensitive) and immunize with isoniazid-resistant BCG

    (2) Patients with active tuberculosis who have been treated for three weeks may have contact with infant receiving INH.

CHRONIC RESPIRATORY DISEASE

A. *Smoking*
1. Frequency. 50 percent of pregnant women smoke
2. Pulmonary function
  a) Decreased FEV
  b) Increased airway resistance
3. Effect on pregnancy
  a) Increased abnormal bleeding
  b) Increased abruptio placenta
  c) Increased placenta previa
  d) Increased fetal morbidity and mortality
    (1) Infants weigh 200 gm less than average

    (2) Nicotine decreases fetal pH

    (3) Carbon dioxide crosses the placenta and has a high affinity for hemoglobin.

B. *Kyphoscoliosis*
  1. Chronic disease with acute changes during pregnancy
  2. Frequency. 0.8 to 6/10,000 pregnancies
  3. Causes include tuberculosis, rickets, polio, trauma, idiopathic factors
  4. Respiratory compromise
     a) Compression of lungs
        (1) Atelectasis
        (2) Emphysema
     b) Decreased FVC
     c) Increased perinatal mortality and increased prematurity, stillbirths
  5. Treatment
     a) Monitor maternal and fetal status
     b) Oxygen
     c) Antibiotics if indicated
     d) Digitalis if indicated

C. *Sarcoidosis*
  1. Systemic granulomatous disease
  2. Frequency. 0.02 to 0.05 percent of pregnancies
  3. Physiologic changes
     a) Decreased FVC and total lung capacity
     b) Normal FEV/FVC ratio
  4. Influence on pregnancy
     a) No damage is caused by sarcoidosis itself.
     b) Severe disease may cause decreased pulmonary or cardiac function, which may lead to deleterious effects in pregnancy.
  5. Influence of pregnancy on sarcoidosis
     a) Course unaffected or improved during pregnancy.
     b) Clinical exacerbation may occur three to six months postpartum.
  6. Effect of sarcoidosis on newborn
     a) No effects on newborn

       b) No increase in anomalies or stillbirths

       c) No placental transfer

       d) May be familial tendency

   7. Management

       a) Treat if there is progressive symptomatic pulmonary disease with dyspnea or x-ray evidence of progression. Also treat if other systemic effects.

       b) Prednisone

          (1) 30 to 40 mg/day p.o. for four to six weeks, then taper and continue for 9 to 12 months.

       c) Other medications

          (1) Antimalarials

          (2) Immunosuppression

   8. No specific contraindications to labor

D. *Mediastinal emphysema* (pneumomediastinum)

   1. Most commonly occurs in asthmatic patients in first and second stages of labor

   2. Pathophysiology

       a) Rupture of distal alveoli allows air to escape to perivascular tissue and to the mediastinum.

       b) With air in mediastinum, obstruction to venous inflow may occur.

   3. Symptoms

       a) Chest pain

       b) Dyspnea, mild

       c) Dysphagia

   4. Signs

       a) Mediastinal crunch (Hamman's sign), crepitus with heart beat

       b) Subcutaneous emphysema in 30 percent

       c) Pneumothorax

       d) Vessel compression

       e) Temperature elevation

       f) Increased pulse

       g) X-ray air halo around heart.

   5. *Treatment.* Consultation with cardiovascular surgery. Chest tube and respiratory support if indicated.

BIBLIOGRAPHY

Burrow GN, Ferris TF (eds): Medical Complications During Pregnancy. Philadelphia, Saunders, 1975

Fishburne JI: Physiology and disease of the respiratory system in pregnancy. Reprod Med 22:4, 1979

Gluck JC: The effects of pregnancy on asthma: a prospective study. Ann Allergy 37:164, 1976

Hageman J: Congenital tuberculosis: critical reappraisal of clinical findings and diagnostic procedures. Pediatrics 66:980, 1980

Hague WM: Mediastial and subcutaneous emphysemia in a pregnant patient with asthma. Br J Obstet Gynecol 87:440, 1980

Hernandez E: Asthma in pregnancy. Curr Concepts Obstet Gynecol 55:790, 1980

Manual of Medical Therapeutic, 23rd ed. Washington University School of Medicine, St. Louis, 1980

Medical Disorders in Pregnancy. Clin Obstet Gynecol 4:287, 1977

Pritchard TA, McDonald PC: Williams Obstetrics, 16th ed. New York, Appleton-Century-Crofts, 1980, pp 240–241

Snider DE: Treatment of tuberculosis during pregnancy. Am Rev Respir Dis 122:65, 1980

Warkany J: Antituberculous drugs. Teratology 20:133, 1979

Weinstein AM: Asthma and pregnancy. JAMA 241:1161, 1979

Section 6
Hematologic Disease
Bruce A. Work, Jr., M.D.

PHYSIOLOGIC CHANGES IN PREGNANCY

A. *Blood volume*
1. Forty-five percent increase by term
2. Thirty-three percent increase in erythrocytes (by increased production, thus increased mean corpuscular volume as young cells)
3. Forty to sixty percent increase in plasma volume, hence decrease in hemoglobin and hematocrit (average, 10 percent)

B. *Iron requirements*
1. *Total for pregnancy: approximately one gm*
   a) Fetus and placenta: 300 mg
   b) Normal losses: 200 mg
   c) Increased erythrocytes: 500 mg
2. *Average daily requirement: 5 mg* (range, 3 to 7 mg)
3. Plasma iron decreases and iron-binding capacity increases

C. *Leukocytes.* Ranges: 5000–12,000/mm^3 (up to 25,000/mm^3 or more in labor). Gradual decline over pregnancy of all elements.

D. *Coagulation factors*
1. Fibrinogen: average 450 mg/dl (range, 300 to 600 mg/dl)

2. Increase: Factors VII, VIII, IX, X
3. Decrease: Factors XI, XIII
4. Platelets: range, 75,000–324,000/mm^3. Gradually decrease over course of pregnancy
5. Prothrombin time and partial thromboplastin times: shortened slightly
6. Plasminogen: marked increase
7. Clot dissolution or fibrinolytic activity: prolonged

ANEMIAS

A. *Definition.* Hemoglobin, less than 10 to 11 gm/dl; hematocrit, less than 30 to 33 percent
B. *Approach* to anemias associated with pregnancy
   1. Careful history for associated causes such as chronic renal disease, twins, etc.
   2. Bleeding history, family history of hematologic disorders, prior diagnosis of anemia
   3. Complete blood count with evaluation of smear and reticulocyte percentage, red cell indices, serum iron and iron-binding capacity, sickle cell screen when indicated. Bone marrow rarely needed
C. *Nutritional deficiency anemias*
   1. *Iron*
      a) *Diagnosis*
         (1) Microcytosis (MCV < 80 fl./RBC)
         (2) Hypochromia (MCH < 27 pg/RBC and MCHC < 32 gm/100 cells)
         (3) Serum iron low (< 60 μg/ml)
         (4) Iron-binding capacity. High (> 300 μg/ml)
         (5) Transfusion saturation. ≤ 15 percent
         (6) No stainable iron in bone marrow
         (7) Response to iron therapy
      b) *Treatment*
         (1) Requires 150 to 200 mg/day *orally* (ferrous sul-

fate, 325-mg tablet with 60 to 65 mg of available iron per tablet taken 1 tablet t.i.d. or equivalent)

    (2) *Parenteral* with iron-dextran IM or IV following manufacturers' recommendation

    (3) *Transfusion* for indication of bleeding in labor or anticipated surgery

  c) *Perinatal impact*

    (1) Increased premature labor

    (2) Increased intrauterine growth retardation

    (3) Fetal iron deficiency anemia

  2. *Folic acid or folate*

    a) *Diagnosis*

      (1) Hypersegmentation of neutrophils (lobe average > 3.7)

      (2) Macrocytosis (MCV > 95 fl/RBC)

      (3) Megaloblasts and nucleated erythrocytes in buffy coat

      (4) Increased urinary form in isoglutamic acid —not universally accepted

    b) *Treatment*. Folate, 400 μg to 1 mg, is present in most perinatal vitamin preparations (may complicate seizure control with phenytoin)

    c) *Perinatal impact*. Same as iron deficiency

D. *Other anemias*

  1. *Hereditary spherocytosis*

    a) *Diagnosis*

      (1) Spherocytes in peripheral smear

      (2) Anemia

      (3) Increased erythrocyte osmotic fragility

      (4) Hemolysis

    b) *Treatment*

      (1) Splenectomy

      (2) Folate therapy

    c) *Perinatal impact*. No increase

  2. *Acquired hemolytic anemia*

    a) *Diagnosis*

      (1) Anemia

(2) Positive direct (Coombs) antiglobulin test
  b) *Treatment.* Depends on cause
  c) *Perinatal impact.* Proportional to severity of anemia
3. *Glucose-6-phosphate dehydrogenase (G6PD) deficiency*
  a) *Diagnosis*
    (1) Anemia
    (2) Demonstration of G6PD deficiency in RBCs
  b) *Treatment.* Discontinue offending drug
  c) *Perinatal impact.* Minimal
4. *Aplastic anemia*
  a) Diagnosis. All elements deficient, including marrow
  b) Treatment. Steroids and deliver
  c) Perinatal impact. Indeterminate

HEMOGLOBINOPATHIES

A. *Major types involving amino acid chains*
  1. Sickle cell anemia (HbS-S)
  2. Sickle cell — hemoglobin C disease (HbS-C)
  3. Sickle cell — thalassemia disease (HbS-Thal)
  4. Sickle cell trait — (HbS-A)
B. *Diagnosis*
  1. Positive screening test and anemia
  2. Positive sodium metabisulfate test (reducing agent)
  3. Hemoglobinelectrophoresis
    a) HbS-S. 90 to 95 percent HbS
    b) HbS-C. 45 to 55 percent each of HbS and HbC
    c) HbS-Thal. 60 to 75 percent HbS, 5 to 15 percent HbF, 3 to 5 percent HbA_2, 5 to 15 percent HbA
    d) HbS-A. up to 40 percent HbS
C. *Therapy*
  1. Oxygen, bed rest, analgesia, possible alkali therapy
  2. Transfusion as needed (role of prophylactic transfusion not established); attempt to maintain:
    a) Hematocrit: 30 to 35 percent
    b) Hemoglobin A: 40 to 90 percent

    3. Folic acid without iron (assess each individual for iron deficiency)

D. *Perinatal impact*
    1. *HbS-S.* Abortion, 22 percent; fetal death, 19.2 percent; perinatal mortality, 10.2 percent
    2. *HbS-C.* Abortion, 12 percent; fetal death, 8.9 percent; perinatal mortality, 2 percent.
    3. *HbS-Thal.* Variable dependent on percent of HbS
    4. *HbS-A.* Same as general population

E. *Maternal impact.* The well-known complications of HbS-S and catastrophic events of HbS-C lead to approximately 2.2 percent mortality for both together in collected series.

F. *Hemoglobinopathies involving polypeptide chains — thalassemia*
    1. *Alpha.* Rare, Bart hemoglobin; very lethal.
    2. *Beta.* Homozygous (Cooley anemia.) Marked hypochromia and microcytosis, bizarre erythrocytes; HbF, 40 to 70 percent; only therapy is transfusion, prognosis is very guarded.
    3. *Beta-heterozygous.* Mild hypochromic, microcytic anemia (HbA_2 3.5 percent; HbF, 2 to 5 percent; HbA decreased). Urinary tract infections and hyperemesis are common. Minimal perinatal mortality, except as related to infection impact.

HEMORRHAGIC CONDITIONS

A. *von Willebrand's disease*
    1. Primary *risk* is postpartum hemorrhage due to factor VIII deficiency.
    2. *Therapy* is factor VIII-rich cryoprecipitate as needed.

B. *Thrombocytopenia*
    1. Normal platelets concentration is 150,000 to 400,000/mm³, but 50,000/mm³ should give no spontaneous bleeding, which occurs at levels of 20,000 to 30,000/mm³.

2. *Causes.* Decreased production associated with leukopenia and anemia in addition to thrombocytopenia
   a) Tumor replacement of marrow
   b) Vitamin B_{12} or folate deficiency
   c) Bacterial and viral infection
   d) Cytotoxic drugs such as chloramphenicol and alcohol
3. *Causes of increased platelet destruction with anemia or leukopenia*
   a) Drugs
   b) Immunologic, i.e., systemic lupus erythematosus
   c) Disseminated intravascular coagulation as part of infection, abruptio placentae, dead fetus syndrome, amniotic fluid embolus, hydatid mole, saline-induced abortions, and liver damage
   d) Infection
   e) Preeclampsia/eclampsia (whether cause or effect is uncertain)
4. *Immunologic (autoimmune) thrombocytopenic purpura (ITP)*
   a) *Diagnosis.* Decreased platelets, purpura, shortened platelet life span, demonstrable IgG antibody, megakaryocytes in serum, bleeding time prolonged, and poor clot retraction. Normal prothrombin and partial thromboplastin time as well as coagulation time.
   b) *Therapy*
      (1) Steroids (prednisone, 40 to 80 mg/day); consider splenectomy
      (2) Platelet therapy for surgery or life-threatening hemorrhage
      (3) It is possible to have transient thrombocytopenia of the newborn. Use scalp blood platelet count to decide route of delivery. If maternal and/or fetal platelets are greater than $100,000/mm^3$, vaginal delivery is allowable.
      c) *Perinatal impact.* Abortion, 5 to 33 percent. Perinatal mortality, 13 to 25 percent

5. *Thrombotic thrombocytopenic purpura (TTP)*
   a) *Diagnosis.* Thrombocytopenia, fever, neurologic abnormalities, renal compromise, and microangiopathic hemolytic anemia
   b) *Significance.* Rare, often fatal in pregnancy
   c) *Therapy*
      (1) Disappointing
      (2) Heparin, steroids, antiplatelet agents, exchange transfusions, plasma transfusions, and plasmapheresis have been tried
   d) *Perinatal impact.* Significant in poor outcome

ISOIMMUNIZATION AND HEMOLYTIC DISEASE OF THE NEWBORN (HDN)

A. *Cause* is maternal antibody production, resulting in hemolytic disease of the newborn. *Most common* causes of HDN are fetomaternal ABO incompatibility and fetomaternal Rho (D) incompatibility [ABO: Rho (D) = 2:1]. These account for 98 percent of HDN. Rho(D) HDN is usually more severe; ABO requires less treatment. ABO and Rh *together* produce less severe Rh disease, perhaps because of the rapid loss of Rh antigen due to prompt hemolysis as a result of ABO reaction; this results in *less* sensitization and thus less HDN.
B. *ABO incompatibility* usually involves maternal type O with anti-A and anti-B (IgGs) in low titer and fetal type A (B less common)
   1. *Diagnosis*
      a) Anemia (fetal)
      b) Positive direct (Coombs) antiglobulin test; can have negative Coombs and jaundice is less
   2. *Therapy for the newborn*
      a) Phototherapy previously
      b) Exchange transfusion (rare)

3. *ABO incompatibility is less severe than Rh*
    a) Adult expression of A and B is less until age two to four; antigenic stimulation is therefore less.
    b) A and B antigens are found in all tissues and compete for maternal antibody with fetal RBCs. Can absorb antigen from gut as early as six months of age, giving anti-A and anti-B.
C. *Rh sensitization* is usually Rho (D)
    1. *Cause*
        a) Exposure in pregnancy to fetal RBCs at delivery, abortion, ectopic, fetomaternal bleeding in pregnancy
        b) Mismatched transfusion
    2. *Detection and evaluation*
        a) Early prenatal visit typing for ABO and Rh with antibody screen
        b) If serum negative (regardless of Rh type), repeat at 28 to 32 weeks. If negative then give Rho immune globulin (use debated by some as not all fetuses are Rh positive)
        c) If serum positive, identify father's Rh, and identify and titer maternal antibody(s).
        d) Amniocentesis for significant titer (generally 1:8 or 1:16) beginning at 28 weeks if no indication for performing earlier.
        e) Management by interpretation of spectrophotometric analysis of optimal density at 450 mμ (Liley's zones, Fig. 15–1):
            (1) Consistent *low zone* (Zone 1-Liley). No intervention, delivery at term
            (2) *Midzone* (Zone 2-Liley). Preterm delivery with evidence of pulmonary maturity and exchange transfusion for neonate
            (3) *High zone* (Zone 3-Liley). Immediate delivery with evidence of pulmonary maturity and intrauterine transfusion for immature fetuses
        f) Amniocenteses usually every two weeks

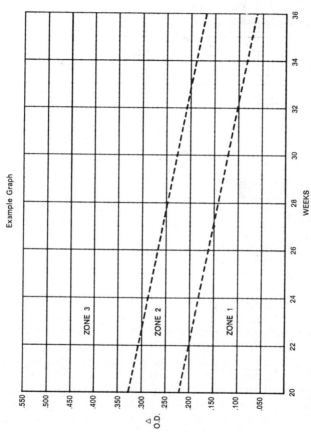

Figure 15–1. Change in optical density (Δ O.D.) plotted against weeks of gestation, with the three clinical zones described by Liley shown. (From Pritchard JA, MacDonald PC: Williams Obstetrics, 16th ed. New York, Appleton-Century-Crofts, 1980, p 967.)

BIBLIOGRAPHY

Blatner P, Hanna D, Nitowsky HM: Pregnancy outcome in women with sickle cell trait. JAMA 238:1392, 1977

Dufour DR, Monoghan WP: ABO hemolytic disease of the newborn: a retrospective analysis of 254 cases. Am J Clin Pathol 73:369, 1980

Horger EO (ed): Obstetric hematology symposium. Clin Obstet Gynecol 22:785, 1979

Levin J, Algazy KM: Hematologic disorders. In Burrow GN, Ferris TF (eds): Medical Complications During Pregnancy. Philadelphia, Saunders, 1975, pp 689–737

Milner PF, Jones BR, Döbler J: Outcome of pregnancy in sickle cell anemia and sickle cell-hemoglobin C disease. Am J Obstet Gynecol 138:293, 1980

Perkins RP: Thrombocytopenia in obstetrics syndromes. Obstet Gynecol Surv 34:101, 1979

Pitkin RM, White DL: Platelet and leukocyte counts in pregnancy. JAMA 242:2696, 1979

Pritchard JA, MacDonald PC (eds): Williams Obstetrics, 16th ed. New York, Appleton-Century-Crofts, 1980, pp 233–237, 712–730

Queenan JT: Modern Management of the Rh Problem. Hagerstown, Md., Harper & Row, 1977

Sheehy TW, Plumb JT: Treatment of sickle cell disease. Arch Intern Med 137:779, 1977

Sicmanza BJ, et al.: Thalassamia minor. NY State J Med 78:1691, 1978

Section 7
Dental Disease
Trusten P. Lee, D.D.S.

PRACTICE PRINCIPLES

Routinely, dentists see a small percentage of pregnant patients, primarily because physicians are lax in insisting that prenatal care include a dental visit for information and preventive care. The need for perinatal dental care is underscored by two myths that are nevertheless widely believed: (1) that a tooth is lost with each child born, and (2) that the mother's teeth lose their calcium content to the fetus, become "soft" teeth and therefore more subject to decay. Neither is true, but there are reasons why patients come to accept them. Of course, these misconceptions are not inevitable, and new parents may be properly informed when dentist and physician provide a comprehensive care plan that includes routine dental care.

DENTAL COUNSELING

Prenatal dental counseling stresses preventive care and timely treatment. Since prenatal parents are very receptive to new knowledge, it is the professional's best opportunity to introduce the new family to necessary dental health habits. It is through this creation of parental role models that the professional can most contribute to the mother's dental health, as well as that of the developing child. The physician can be helpful in encouraging the parents to practice preventive care from the onset of pregnancy and into the first year or two of the child's development. This is especially important to the newborn, since a dentist rarely sees or has any opportunity to administer preventive care to the child before the complete set of deciduous teeth is present. The amount of care needed at this first visit is often, unfortunately, substantial.

DENTAL COMPLICATIONS OF PREGNANCY

A. During pregnancy, the mother may develop dental complications unique to the changing conditions caused by the pregnancy. The patient should be made aware of these possible complications and advised about how to minimize their risk or prevent their occurrence.

B. *Pregnancy gingivitis*
   1. Gingivitis usually appears in increasing intensity from the second month of pregnancy through the eighth month. This condition is noted by red, inflamed, and/or bleeding gingiva caused by the mother's decreasing resistance to common plaque, bacteria, and calculus accumulations, despite continuation of her previously established hygiene regimen. This redness and bleeding will appear at the margin of the soft tissue and the tooth. The papilla between the teeth may also be swollen and red and bleed easily on touching or cleaning.
   2. Women experience increasing susceptibility to gum disease during puberty, menstruation, oral contraceptive use, and particularly, pregnancy. The dental myths mentioned earlier no doubt find some of their origin in this common phenomenon. Several studies have attributed this change in immunity to an increase in the gingiva's blood vessel size and permeability caused by the patient's fluctuating levels of progesterone and estrogen.
   3. Meticulous oral hygiene care prevents plaque and calculus buildup, which virtually eliminates these gingival conditions.

C. *Pregnancy tumor*
1. Occasionally, pregnancy gingivitis may appear as an inflammatory growth, most likely in the papilla area between the teeth. Close examination will confirm that the "pregnancy tumor," as it is most commonly referred to, is merely a *pyogenic granuloma* caused by some local irritant.
2. This lesion can be removed through surgery with little or no complications. Its return is prevented by removal of the source of irritant and proper oral hygiene.

D. *Tooth mobility and gingival pocket depth.* Patients may complain that their teeth are loose, and in fact they may be. This mobility may be accompanied by increased pocket depth. This condition will usually return to its pre-pregnancy state after delivery.

E. *Syphilis* contact during pregnancy manifests in the malformation of the fetus's permanent dentition as notched or screwdriver-shaped incisors and malformed molars. Every precaution should be taken, and the mother should be forewarned of the impending consequences to the child resulting from this infection.

F. *Drugs*
1. All drug usage should be minimized.
2. *Tetracycline drugs* pose the greatest hazard to the fetus's dentition. Even though prescribed in small maternal doses, this drug is capable of discoloring the fetus's developing deciduous dentition, especially when administered after the fourth month in utero. Both deciduous and permanent teeth are endangered when tetracycline is consumed by children under seven years of age. Tetracycline should not be administered during pregnancy unless no other drug substitutions are available and abstinence would jeopardize the mother's health.
3. *Analgesias* suggested for limited use during pregnancy include aspirin and acetaminophen with codeine. Lidocaine with 1/100,000 epinephrine is the most acceptable choice for local anesthetic when treating the pregnant patient. Total dosages above 300 mg are generally

not advisable. General anesthetics, intravenous seda-
tions, and nitrous oxide should be used only in consultation with the patient's obstetrician.
4. The safest and most effective form of antibiotic at this
time is penicillin.

DENTAL CARE

A. *The dental visit*
1. Dental care should start as early as possible to enhance
successful treatment and avoid the need for extensive or
traumatic procedures later in pregnancy. When care is
not received during pregnancy, the new mother will tend
to postpone treatment indefinitely owing to her ever-
increasing responsibilities and new demands on her time.
Eventually she will be forced into the dental office
exhibiting severe problems. These often could have been
managed earlier in a conservative manner, but subsequently require extensive treatment that is often a
compromise, i.e., extraction, periodontal surgery, root
canal treatment, etc.
2. Generally, all radiography is kept to a minimum during
pregnancy. However, should films be needed to complete
necessary treatment, proper precautions (high-speed
film, filtration, collimation, and protective lead apron)
should be taken to guarantee the safety of the patient and
baby. Radiation studies involving use of a lead apron
result in negligible gonadal exposure. Nevertheless, use
of radiography should be limited.
3. Preventive care is stressed and periodontal conditions are
monitored.
4. Only emergency treatment is recommended during the
first trimester because of the high incidence of abortion
and the risk of damage to the fetus's developing organs.
(Most dentists are reluctant to treat during this period for
fear of being implicated, justly or not, in any resulting
complications.)

5. Most dental care (especially if extensive or "elective") is administered during the *second trimester,* when the incidence of spontaneous abortions is lowest, and after consultation with the physician.
6. In the *third trimester,* the risk of premature labor and the increasing discomfort of the mother limits care to moderate, less extensive treatment and emergency care.

B. *After delivery.* The mother can help ensure proper dental development in the newborn by:
1. Providing a good oral hygiene role model.
2. Decreasing or eliminating the use of pacifiers, particularly those coated with sweet substances.
3. Resisting the temptation to sweeten or season natural foods or commercially prepared baby foods for her child. This habit merely satisfies the parent's desensitized palate while developing needless sugar and salt addiction in the newborn.
4. Discouraging bedtime bottles. Liquids, with the exception of water, foster maximum decay when they continually seep into the child's mouth and remain there for indefinite periods of time. This condition is called "baby bottle mouth" and is recognized by large-scale decay, especially in the front teeth.
5. Rubbing gauze gently over the child's gums to break up the oral flora of the mouth and assist in eruption of the child's dentition during teething.
6. Providing unsweetened snacks for the child, preferably after meals instead of between meals.
7. Requesting her dentist's fluoride recommendations for her area and following his advice.
8. Arranging the child's first dental examination between the second and third birthdays.

BIBLIOGRAPHY

Cohen DW, Shapiro J, Friedman L, Kyle GC, Franklin S: A longitudinal investigation of the periodontal changes during pregnancy and fifteen months post-partum. J Periodontol 42:653, 1971

Holm-Pederson P, Loe H: Flow of gingival exudate as related to menstruation and pregnancy. J Periodontal Res 2:13, 1967

Jones JH, Mason DK (eds): Oral Manifestations of Systemic Disease. Philadelphia, Saunders, 1980, pp 314–315, 476–477, 521–522

Lindhe J, Bjorn AL: Influence of hormonal contraceptives on the gingiva of women. J Periodontal Res 2:1, 1967

Loe H: Periodontal changes in pregnancy. J Periodontal 36:209, 1965

Moffitt JM, Cooley RO, Olsen NH, Hefferren JJ: Prediction of tetracycline-induced tooth discolouration. J Am Dental Assoc 88:547, 1974

Nowak AJ, Casamassimo PS, McTigue DJ: Prevention of dental disease from nine months in utero to eruption of the first tooth. J Am Soc Psychosom Dent Med 6(5):6, 1976

O'Neil TCA: Plasma female sex-hormone levels and gingivitis in pregnancy. J Periodontol 50:279, 1979

Poma PA, Zajdzinski CV, Rana N, et al.: Oral cavity evaluation a part of prenatal care. Ill Med J 155:85, 1979

Pregnancy and dental treatment, part I. Dentists Med Dig 2(6):1, 1980

Pregnancy and dental treatment, part II. Dentists Med Dig 2(7):4, 1980

Pregnancy and dental treatment, part III. Dentists Med Dig 2(8):4, 1980

Rood JP: Local analgesia during pregnancy. Dent Update 8:483, 1981

Silness J, Loe H: Periodontal disease in pregnancy, III. Response to local treatment. Acta Odontol Scand 24:747, 1966

Sutcliff P: A longitudinal study of gingivitis and puberty. J Periodontal Res 7:52, 1972

Wood NK (ed): The Complete Book of Dental Care. New York, Hart Publishing, 1978

Wood NK (ed): Treatment Planning a Pragmatic Approach. St. Louis, Mosby, 1978

Yaffe G. Drug use during pregnancy. Drug Ther 8:137, 1978

Section 8
Gastrointestinal Disease
Michael Parsons, M.D.

CHANGES DURING PREGNANCY

A. *Anatomic.* Uterine enlargement leads to displacement of abdominal organs.
B. *Physiologic*
   1. Increased appetite
   2. Decreased taste sensation
   3. Pica (compulsive ingestion of various materials such as starch, earth or clay, ice)
   4. Oral fissures, gingivitis, caries
   5. Ptyalism (excessive salivation)
   6. Decreased esophageal sphincter tone
   7. Possible decreased motility of small intestine, colon
   8. Decreased serum amylase and lipase levels
   9. Decreased gastric and gallbladder emptying
   10. Decreased gastric acid secretion

NAUSEA AND VOMITING

A. *Incidence.* Very common; used as a symptom in the diagnosis of pregnancy
B. *Morning sickness.* Starts at first missed menstrual period, peaks at 10 weeks, and is usually mild

C. *Suggested etiologies*
   1. hCG levels correspond to peak times of nausea
   2. Estrogen-nausea seen with exogenous estrogen
   3. Allergic reaction to fetoplacental unit
   4. Psychosomatic component
D. *Hyperemesis gravidarum* is intractable vomiting in pregnancy and is often associated with psychological problems.
   1. *Incidence.* 0.35 percent of pregnancies
   2. *Complications*
      a) Aspiration pneumonia (Mendelson syndrome)
      b) Gastroesophageal mucosal tears (Mallory-Weiss syndrome)
      c) Esophageal rupture
      d) Electrolyte disturbance
      e) Dental caries
      f) Weight loss
      g) Dehydration
      h) Ketosis
      i) Electrocardiographic changes (usually secondary to hypokalemia)
   3. *Diagnosis*
      a) Persistent vomiting
      b) Dehydration
      c) Postural changes in blood pressure and pulse
      d) Acetone on breath
      e) Laboratory values
         (1) Increased hematocrit and blood urea nitrogen (BUN)
         (2) Increased serum and urinary osmolality
         (3) Aceturia
         (4) Decreased urine volume
         (5) Hypernatremia, hypokalemia, hypochloremia
E. *Treatment*
   1. *Conservative*
      a) Small meals; separate solids and liquids at separate meals
      b) Avoid irritating foods
      c) Give assurance to patient

    d) Medication if necessary. *Bendectin* (one tablet b.i.d. or t.i.d.) is effective, and no teratogenic effects have been demonstrated

  2. *For intractable vomiting*
    a) Hospitalize
    b) IV fluids
    c) NPO, then slowly start with liquids
    d) Monitor potassium and BUN levels
    e) Sedation
    f) Parenteral vitamins
    g) Antiemetics
    h) Psychiatric consultation

F. If management to prevent systemic alterations and complications, such as ketotic state, is successful, there should be no increased incidence of maternal or neonatal mortality, malformations, or preeclampsia

GASTROESOPHAGEAL REFLUX

A. *Incidence.* Up to 50 percent of pregnancies, usually occurring in third trimester
B. *Etiology*
  1. Decreased lower esophageal sphincter tone may be due to progesterone levels.
  2. Hiatal hernia (from the decreased tone, upward displacement of abdominal organs, and gastric atony) may be responsible in 10 to 20 percent of cases.
C. *Complications*
  1. Esophagitis (very rare)
    a) Bleeding
    b) Perforation
    c) Stricture
  2. Does not alter the course of pregnancy and is not detrimental to the fetus
D. *Therapy*
  1. Gravity. Elevate head of bed
  2. Small, frequent meals

   3. Loose clothes
   4. Medications
      a) Antacids, 15 to 30 ml p.o. at bedtime or p.r.n.
         [Mg(OH)$_2$ and Al(OH)$_3$ combination]
      b) Cimetidine is not approved during pregnancy
      c) Do not use anticholinergics, because they further
         impair resting tone of the esophageal sphincter

CONSTIPATION

A. *Definition*
   1. Excessively dry stool
   2. Less than 50 mg/day of stool
   3. Infrequent bowel movement (less than every other day)
B. There is no evidence that pregnant women suffer from
   increased constipation, but these following factors have been
   suggested to aggravate its occurrence:
   1. Progesterone. Decreases colon function
   2. Mechanical pressure of uterus on colon
   3. Decreased exercise
   4. Decreased fluid intake
C. *Treatment*
   1. Increase fiber in diet (bran, roughage)
   2. Fluids
   3. Medications (magnesium hydroxide, hydrophilic colloid)

PEPTIC ULCER

A. *Incidence.* Very rare in pregnancy
B. *Effect of pregnancy on peptic ulcer*
   1. Overall improvement in 88 percent; usually becomes
      asymptomatic perhaps due to histaminase produced by
      the placenta
   2. Recurrence postpartum
      a) 50 percent by three months

    b) 90 percent by two years

    c) Increased recurrence if breast-feeding

  3. Reason for improvement

    a) Decreased gastric acid during midpregnancy

    b) Decreased gastric pepsin production in early and midpregnancy

    c) Decreased plasma histamine

    d) Effect of estrogen and progesterone may be beneficial

C. *Complications.* Perforation and hemorrhage are rare. An exception is in severe preeclampsia, when gastromucosal lesions may result.

D. *Diagnosis*

  1. Radiographic evidence with the use of barium.

  2. Fiberoptic endoscopy is diagnostic and is the preferred method of diagnosis in pregnancy.

E. *Treatment*

  1. Goal is to *neutralize gastric hydrochloric acid*

    a) No evidence that bland diet helps, but avoidance of irritating foods seems to do so.

    b) Avoidance of cigarettes and alcohol

    c) $Mg(OH)_2$ and $Al(OH)_3$ antacids. Overuse can lead to phosphate depletion and mobilization of calcium and phosphate from bone.

    d) Anticholinergics contraindicated

    e) The safety of cimetidine (a histamine H_2-receptor antagonist) in pregnancy has not been established.

  2. *If hemorrhage occurs,* treat as any active ulcer.

    a) *Moderate.* Nasogastric suction and ice-water lavage

    b) *Severe.* Replacement of blood and possible surgery

PANCREATITIS

A. *Incidence.* 0.1 to 0.01 percent (more often in primigravidas in the third trimester)

B. *Etiology*

  1. Biliary disease

  2. Alcohol abuse

3. Drug use — thiazides
4. Idiopathic

C. Physiologic changes in normal pregnancy important in diagnosis and treatment
1. Decreased serum amylase and lipase early in pregnancy
2. Gradual rise of serum lipids during pregnancy
   a) Starting at third month
   b) Peaks at 33rd week
3. Increased incidence of gallstones in pregnancy
4. Possible duodenal stasis caused by progesterone (which would add to pancreatic duct reflux)
5. Increased intraabdominal pressure

D. *Diagnosis*
1. Signs and symptoms. Same as in nonpregnant state
   a) Pain. Severe, constant, and epigastric; radiates to back in 90 percent.
   b) Nausea and vomiting
   c) Fever in 60 percent
   d) Decreased bowel sounds (ileus)
   e) Ascites, pleural effusion
2. Laboratory studies
   a) Serum amylase level increased two to three times at 2 to 12 hours after onset; but may be normal in severe hemorrhagic pancreatitis
   b) Increased serum lipase level
   c) Hyperglycemia
   d) Hypocalcemia (less than 7.0 mg/dl)
   e) Anemia if hemorrhagic pancreatitis
   f) Leukocytosis
   g) Increased sedimentation rate

E. *Cause in pregnancy*
1. Similar to nonpregnant
2. No effect on fetus unless serious complications result such as ketoacidosis

F. *Therapy*
1. Same as nonpregnant
2. Empiric treatment
   a) Nasogastric suction until no pain and no nausea

      (1) Remove gastric acid
      (2) Prevent ileus
   b) No role for anticholinergics
   c) Bed rest
   d) Analgesics
   e) Fluid replacement
   f) Antibiotics if temperature greater than 102 F
   g) Observe for hyperglycemia and frank diabetes
  3. If poor response, surgical drainage may be needed

GALLBLADDER DISEASE IN PREGNANCY

A. *Cholelithiasis*
  1. There is an increased incidence of cholelithiasis in women, especially during pregnancy.
   a) Women have increased cholesterol saturation and a decreased bile salt pool.
   b) Women have impaired gallbladder contraction, especially during pregnancy.
  2. Hormones of pregnancy may decrease muscle response of the gallbladder and decrease contraction in response to cholecystokinin.
   a) Leaves high residual volume of bile
   b) May be related to increased formation of cholesterol stones
  3. Signs and symptoms. Similar to nonpregnant state
   a) Epigastric pain or right subcostal pain with possible radiation to the scapula area
   b) Nausea with possible vomiting
   c) Occasional icterus
  4. Diagnosis
   a) Becomes more difficult as pregnancy advances
   b) Ultrasound to detect stones
  5. Development of cholecystitis
   a) Unusual in pregnancy
   b) Biliary colic, temperature elevation to 101 F, leukocytosis, possible elevated liver function tests.

6. Therapy
   a) Conservative. Intravenous fluids, n.p.o., analgesics (not morphine), nasogastric suction, and antibiotics if indicated
   b) If worsening condition or if no response within 12 to 36 hours, consider operation
      (1) Cholecystostomy
      (2) Cholecystectomy
      (3) Exploration of common bile duct

APPENDICITIS IN PREGNANCY

A. *Incidence.* 0.1 to 0.18 percent of pregnancies
   1. Pregnancy does not predispose to appendicitis.
   2. Incidence is equal in all three trimesters
B. *Diagnosis*
   1. Error in 20 to 40 percent of cases operated
   2. Similar presentation as nonpregnant
      a) Nausea and vomiting
      b) Anorexia
      c) Elevated temperature
      d) Lab values not reliable (white cell count is normally elevated in pregnancy)
      e) Initial symptoms resemble those in the nonpregnant, including periumbilical pain. The pain is located towards right middle to upper abdomen as pregnancy advances, because the uterine enlargement displaces the appendix upward and to the right.
      f) Uterus may cause a mechanical separation of the appendix from the peritoneal surface leading to decreased symptoms.
      g) Increased cortisol may inhibit the inflammatory response and decrease resistance to infection.
      h) Complications of appendicitis may be worse in pregnant state due to:
         (1) Abnormal position of appendix

(2) Increased vascular engorgement
(3) Decreased efficiency of omental function due to enlarged uterus
  i) To differentiate extrauterine from uterine or tubal pathology, mark the point of maximal tenderness and have patient turn so that the uterus will fall away from the hand marking the point. If the pain persists in the same area, it is more likely due to an extrauterine lesion.
C. *Effect of appendicitis on the pregnancy*
1. Postoperative abortion is less than 5 percent.
2. If peritonitis develops, overall fetal loss is 8 to 10 percent.
D. *Treatment*
1. Appendectomy
2. Avoid retraction and manipulation of the uterus during surgery
3. Antibiotics if indicated
4. Tocolytic agents if indicated

ILEOJEJUNAL BYPASS

A. An operative technique to reduce the active surface of the intestine for weight reduction. This method of weight control is used increasingly and several pregnancies have been completed postbypass with varying success.
B. Complications
1. Abnormalities of liver function and amino acid metabolism are noted, usually evident within six months of bypass.
  a) SGOT, alkaline phosphatase, bilirubin, prothrombin time may be abnormal
  b) Hypoalbuminemia and decreased amino acids
    (1) Return to normal at 12 to 36 months after bypass
    (2) Seems to affect fetal development leading to intrauterine growth retardation, prematurity, fetal distress, neonatal mortality and mental retardation

    c) Increased incidence of hypertension and electrolyte
       imbalance

    d) Patients who weigh more than 300 pounds before
       operation or who lose 120 pounds after operation
       have a greater incidence of dysmature and hypoxic
       infants

2. Patient may need parenteral nutrition, either supplemental or total, if extremely poor gastrointestinal tract function results.

3. Other complications: Diarrhea, hypokalemia, hypocalcemia, nephrolithiasis, cholelithiasis.

BIBLIOGRAPHY

Biggs JSG: Treatment of gastrointestinal disorders of pregnancy. Drugs 19:70, 1980

Burrow GN, Ferris TF (eds): Medical Complications During Pregnancy. Philadelphia, Saunders, 1975

Frisenda R: Acute appendicitis during pregnancy. Am Surg 45:503, 1979

Manual of Medical Therapeutics, 23rd ed. Washington University School of Medicine, St. Louis, 1980, pp 261–278

McKay AJ: Pancretitis, pregnancy, and gallstones. Br J Obstet Gynecol 87:47, 1980

Medical Disorders of Pregnancy. Clin Obstet Gynecol 4:297, 1977

Pritchard JA, MacDonald PC (eds): Williams Obstetrics, 16th ed. New York, Appleton, 1980

Woods JR: Influence of jejunoileal bypass on protein metabolism during pregnancy. Am J Obstet Gynecol 130:9, 1978

Section 9
Hepatic Disease
Ana Tomasi, M.D.

EVALUATION OF THE LIVER IN PREGNANCY

A. *Physical examination.* The liver is difficult to palpate toward term, since the enlarging uterus displaces the liver upward, backward, and to the right. A readily palpable liver in the third trimester nearly always has pathologic significance.

B. *Laboratory examination.* Most liver tests show some deviations from the accepted "normal" nonpregnant subjects. The most valuable tests to assess liver function in pregnancy are those that remain normal (e.g., serum transaminases, 5-nucleotidase, γ-glutamyl transpeptidase, the Isoenzyme V of lactic dehydrogenase, and prothrombin time—(Table 15–2).

C. In rare instances, *liver biopsy* may be indicated and does not have an increased risk during pregnancy.

JAUNDICE IN PREGNANCY

A. The *incidence* is 0.06 percent, 1/1500 gestations, but varies according to different countries from 1/300 to 1/5,000.

TABLE 15-2. MORPHOLOGIC, FUNCTIONAL AND BIOCHEMICAL CHANGES DURING NORMAL PREGNANCY

NO CHANGES

Erythrocyte volume/kg body weight	Total plasma volume
Total intravascular albumin volume	Total erythrocyte volume
Haptoglobin	Cardiac output
β_{1c}-globulin	Serum and urinary aldosterone
Cryoglobulin	Basal metabolic rate
Serum transaminases	Blood pH
Serum 5-nucleotidase	Total white cell count
Serum γ-glutamyl transpeptidase	Segmented and nonsegmented granulocytes
Serum lactic dehydrogenase V	Myelocytes and metamyelocytes
Oral galactose tolerance test	Erythrocyte sedimentation rate
Liver blood flow	Serum alpha and beta globulins
	Ceruloplasmin
	Serum copper
	a_1-Antitrypsin
	Transferrin
	a_2-Macroglobulin
	Hemopexin
	Prothrombin
	Fibrinogen
	Coagulation factors VII, VIII, IX, X
	Plasminogen
	Total serum lipids

MINOR NONSPECIFIC CHANGES

Liver displacement by enlarging uterus
Liver histology
Total serum lactic deyhdrogenase

PROGRESSIVE DECREASE TOWARD TERM

Hemoglobin
Hematocrit
Erythrocyte count/mm^3

Arterial P_{CO_2} concentration
Arterial HCO_3 concentration
Total serum protein concentration
Serum albumin concentration
Prealbumin
Orosomucoid
Serum gamma globulin
IgG
Plasma lysolecithin
Serum cholinesterase
Serum tirbutyrinase
IV bilirubin tolerance test
Maximal bromsulfalein excretory capacity (T_m)

PROGRESSIVE INCREASE TOWARD TERM

Spider nevi and palmar erythema
Total body water
Total blood volume

α- and β-Lipoproteins
Serum triglycerides
Serum cholesterol
Phospholipids (except lysolecithine)
Serum alkaline phosphatase
Serum leucine aminopeptidase
Serum ornithyl carbamyl-transferase
Bromsulfalein retention
Hepatic bromsulfalein storage capacity

OCCASIONAL INCREASE NOT DEPENDENT ON STAGE OF GESTATION

Urinary bile pigments
Serum bilirubin
Serum turbidity and flocculation tests

ERRATIC BEHAVIOR, BOTH ABNORMALLY LOW AND HIGH LEVELS

Serum iron

(From Haemmerly UP: Jaundice during pregnancy. In Schiff L (ed): Disease of the Liver. Philadelphia, Lippincott, 1975, pp 1336–1353.)

B. *Etiology*
 1. Forty percent are due to *infectious hepatitis,* 20 percent to
    intrahepatic cholestasis.
 2. *Rare cause* of jaundice during pregnancy are *gallstones*
    and *hemolysis* (Tables 15–3 and 15–4).

TABLE 15–3. JAUNDICE DURING PREGNANCY (ICTERUS GRAVIDARUM)

A. Jaundice in pregnancy (synonyms; icterus in graviditate, concomitant jaundice, coincidental jaundice, ictere intercurrent)
 1. Usual forms of jaundice that occur also in nonpregnant persons
    a) Hepatic parenchymal disease (especially viral hepatitis)
    b) Intrahepatic cholestasis (i.e., drug jaundice)
    c) Extrahepatic cholestasis (i.e., common duct stones)
    d) Congenital "idiopathic" hyperbilirubinemias
    e) Hemolytic disorders
 2. Jaundice in typical medical complications of pregnancy
    a) Jaundice in severe pyelonephritis
    b) Jaundice in pyelonephritis and tetracycline toxicity
    c) Delayed chloroform poisoning
    d) Jaundice after (criminal) abortions (*Clostridium perfringens* septicemia, quinine toxicity, etc.)
B. Jaundice of pregnancy (synonyms; icterus e graviditate, icterus graviditatis, icterus peculiar to pregnancy, ictère lié à la grossesse)
 1. Idiopathic jaundice of pregnancy
    a) Intrahepatic cholestasis of pregnancy ("jaundice of late pregnancy," "recurrent jaundice of pregnancy")
    b) Acute fatty metamorphosis of pregnancy ("obstetric acute yellow atrophy")
 2. Jaundice as a complication of another disease linked to pregnancy
    a) Jaundice in hyperemesis gravidarum
    b) Jaundice in severe toxemia of pregnancy
    c) Jaundice with hydatidiform mole
    d) Jaundice in megaloblastic anemia of pregnancy
    e) Jaundice in hemolytic anemia of pregnancy
C. Nonclassified cases

(From Haemmerly: Disease of the Liver. Philadelphia, Lippincott, 1975. By permission.)

TABLE 15-4. RECURRENT JAUNDICE DURING PREGNANCY

A. Recurrent jaundice in pregnancy
   1. Recurrent jaundice recurring also in nonpregnant persons
      a) Recurrent viral hepatitis or exacerbation of anicteric chronic hepatitis
      b) Recurrent jaundice in primary biliary cirrhosis
      c) Recurrent posthepatitic hyperbilirubinemia
      d) Recurrent common bile duct obstruction due to gallstones
      e) Recurrent exacerbations of familial nonhemolytic jaundice
      f) Recurrent hemolytic jaundice
   2. Recurrent jaundice due to medical complications of pregnancy
      a) Recurrent jaundice in severe pyelonephritis
B. Recurrent jaundice of pregnancy
   1. Recurrent idiopathic jaundice of pregnancy
      a) Recurrent intrahepatic cholestasis of pregnancy
   2. Recurrent jaundice as complication of disease linked to pregnancy
      a) Recurrent jaundice in hyperemesis gravidarum
C. Recurrent jaundice during pregnancy due to different diseases causing jaundice during pregnancy
   Example: Hepatitis in one, hemolytic jaundice in the other gestation
D. Nonclassified cases of recurrent jaundice during pregnancy

(From Haemmerly UP: Jaundice during pregnancy. In Schiff L (ed): Disease of the Liver. Philadelphia, Lippincott, 1975, pp 1336–1353)

HEPATITIS IN PREGNANCY

A. Although hepatitis is the most common cause of jaundice during pregnancy, pregnant women are not more susceptible than the general population. It occurs in all trimesters and is not necessarily more severe than in the nonpregnant women. Jaundice and associated symptoms are often mild.

B. Mortality is 1.8 percent, although it may reach 50 percent in underdeveloped countries. Gamma globulin prophylaxis during hepatitis epidemics has been recommended by WHO.

C. Spontaneous or elective abortions in severe cases with or without coma do not ameliorate the course of the disease. Premature delivery occurs in 40 to 90 percent of jaundiced mothers. Babies of mothers with hepatitis do surprisingly well.

D. *Hepatitis B*
   1. Frequency. HB Ag in 1 percent adults in the United States.
   2. *Transmission* to the infant is possible if acute hepatitis B develops during pregnancy, particularly near the time of delivery or in the first two weeks postpartum. The mode of transmission is by oral contamination of the baby by the mother's blood or feces during delivery or perhaps postpartum. Very few cases of transplacental transmission have been proven. HB Ag is said to be undetectable in mother's milk.
   3. *Diagnosis of hepatitis B* (Table 15–5)
   4. *Management of hepatitis B* (Table 15–6)

E. *Other types of hepatitis*
   1. *Hepatitis A* (infectious hepatitis) has not been found to be associated with fetal or newborn disease. Pregnant women with short-duration exposure should be given 1SG, 0.02 to 0.05 ml/kg, to modify the disease. For prolonged exposure, the dose of 1SG should be 0.06 to 0.14 mg/kg to provide protection for five to six months.
   2. *Non-A/B hepatitis* has become the most frequent cause of transfusion-related hepatitis. Recent studies suggest that the course is similar to that of hepatitis B, and management should be similar to that described for hepatitis B.

INTRAHEPATIC CHOLESTASIS OF PREGNANCY

A. This is the second most common cause of jaundice in pregnancy, having an incidence of 1/200 to 1/8000 pregnancies. No single feature is diagnostic. It is extremely benign

TABLE 15–5. DIAGNOSIS OF HEPATITIS B

Mother	Newborn
Clinical Signs	
Blood or secretion exposure Incubation usually 50 to 180 days Fever, headache, dark urine, jaundice, hepatomegaly	Most asymptomatic, about 10 percent icteric at 3 to 4 months of age Rarely death
Laboratory Tests	
Hepatitis B surface antigen (HBsAg) in blood SGPT increased Hepatitis Be antigen (HBeAg) in blood indicates increased risk for transmission to the child	Persisting HBsAg in blood Some increase in SGPT Repeat biopsies show unresolved hepatitis for many months

TABLE 15–6 MANAGEMENT OF HEPATITIS B

Mother	Newborn
Treatment	
Increased rest, symptomatic treatment High-protein, low-fat diet Needle precautions and sterile technique, but not isolation	Increased rest, symptomatic treatment No specific treatment Needle precautions and sterile technique, but not isolation
Prevention	
Minimize exposure Definite exposure: HB1G (0.05 to 0.07 ml/kg) and repeat in 25 days. If HB1G not available, use 1SG	Minimize exposure Mother with hepatitis B during pregnancy and HBsAg positive at term: HB1G on day of birth (0.13 ml/kg). If HB1G not available, use 1SG, 0.5 ml/kg.

for both mother and child and is without residual liver damage, although it leads to an increased incidence of gallstones. There is a marked tendency to recurrence with subsequent pregnancies.

1. The predominant symptom is pruritus, often violent, involving the trunk, extremities, and palmar and plantar surfaces. It is especially noticed at night. Pruritis disappears rapidly after delivery.
2. Jaundice reaches a plateau and remains mild for the rest of the pregnancy.
3. General well-being is unimpaired except for the lack of sleep. Urine is dark and the stools are light. After delivery, pruritus disappears within two days, although it may rarely last up to four weeks.

B. *Biochemical changes*
   1. Serum bile acids are increased 10- to 100-fold. CA: CDCA:DCA ratios change. The cholic acid comprises 90 percent of total bile acids. Total serum bilirubin is below 5 mg/dl, and direct bilirubin constitutes the major fraction. Urobilinogen and bilirubinuria may be present. Serum alkaline phosphatase is elevated moderately. Serum cholesterol is elevated (600 mg/dl), but is also increased in normal pregnancy. Prothrombin time is prolonged and factors II, VII, IX, X are decreased. Cryoglobulin may be increased up to six times. Gamma-glutamyl transpeptidase and serum transaminase are also elevated. The biliary system is unobstructed. Liver structure is normal; there is only mild focal irregular intrahepatic cholestasis; not all lobules are involved.

C. *Prognosis* is good, with no obstetric complications during labor and delivery. Premature delivery occurs in 33 percent of cases. The babies are not jaundiced, but some have a prolonged PT.

D. *Treatment*
   1. Restrictive diet and bed rest are not indicated.
   2. *Cholestyramine* is the drug of choice in a dosage of 12 to 18 mg/daily; after one to two weeks, the dosage can be

decreased. Pruritus will be relieved but does not disappear completely.
3. Vitamin K supplementation.
4. Therapeutic abortion will stop the process, but should not be recommended.

BIBLIOGRAPHY

Haemmerly UP: Jaundice during pregnancy. In Schiff L (ed): Disease of the Liver. Philadelphia, Lippincott, 1975, pp 1336–1353

Heikkinen J, et al.: Changes in serum bile acid concentrations during normal pregnancy, in patients with intrahepatic cholestasis of pregnancy and in pregnant women with itching. Br J Obstet Gynecol 88:240, 1981

Lber FL: Jaundice in pregnancy—a review. Am J. Obstet Gynecol 91:721, 1965

Samsoie G, et al.: Studies in cholestasis of pregnancy. Acta Obstet Gynecol Scand 56:31, 1977

Thomassen PA: Urinary bile acids in late pregnancy in recurrent cholestasis of pregnancy. Eur J Clin Invest 9:425, 1979

Section 10
Infectious Diseases

Gayle Wager, M.D.

PRACTICE PRINCIPLES

Numerous infectious diseases may occur in the pregnant woman. Several of these may lead to serious neonatal complications. Immunization in the United States has substantially reduced the incidence of many of these diseases. It is imperative that the obstetrician be aware of the clinical presentations and effects of these diseases.

HERPESVIRUS (HSV)

A. *General principles*
1. Fetal and neonatal infection is generally via ascending infection or passage of the infant through an infected birth canal.
2. The distinction between HSV type 1 and HSV type 2 is not of great clinical importance, since there is no difference in neonatal outcome.
3. When infants are infected, 99 percent will manifest symptoms. Two-thirds will have disseminated infection, and one-third will have localized infection.
4. The role of transplacental antibodies is uncertain.

B. *Maternal clinical manifestations*
1. Vesicular lesions may occur on the cervix, vagina, and vulva. The lesions will eventually break down and become ulcerated.
2. *Primary infection.* A wide range of symptoms may occur, including fever, malaise, anorexia, and local lymphadenopathy. Primary infection may be associated with viremia and meningitis.
3. *Recurrent infection.* Symptoms are generally less severe, manifesting with only local genital involvement.
4. Acute urinary retention may occur with urethral involvement.

C. *Diagnosis*
1. *Virus isolation from lesions.* Vesicles contain the highest titer of virus during the first 24 to 48 hours. Viral culture may be obtained by breaking open a vesicle and culturing the drainage.
2. *Cytologic examination.* A Pap smear of the suspected lesion may identify multinucleated giant cells.
3. *Serologic testing* is rarely useful.

D. *Treatment of maternal symptoms*
1. Specific therapies have not been effective. Numerous agents are currently under evaluation.
2. Local symptomatic treatment may include warm sitz baths, local anesthetics, and analgesics.
3. The following treatments are not recommended: ointments and salves, photoinactivation using vital dyes, topical ether, bacille Calmette-Guérin vaccination.

E. *Obstetric management*
1. Any patient with an active genital lesion at the onset of labor should be delivered by cesarean section.
2. Patients with a history of recurrent genital herpes lesions should have weekly cervical cultures starting at 36 weeks' gestation.
3. Patients with a negative cervical culture within one week of the onset of labor and with no evidence of active genital lesions may be considered for vaginal delivery.

4. Patients with an active genital lesion or a positive culture within one week of the onset of labor should be delivered by cesarean section if the membranes are intact. If the membranes have been ruptured for more than four hours, some authors feel that delivery should occur by the vaginal route. Others recommend cesarean section regardless of the duration of membrane rupture.
5. With appropriate precautions to avoid contact with active lesions, and with careful handwashing, breast-feeding may be allowed.

F. *Neonatal clinical manifestations.* A wide range of signs and symptoms may occur: jaundice, hepatosplenomegaly, disseminated intravascular coagulation, seizures, irritability, temperature instability, skin vesicles, conjunctivitis, lethargy, poor feeding, vomiting.

G. *Neonatal diagnosis* is based on clinical suspicion, cytology, and virus isolation.

H. *Neonatal treatment.* No effective therapy is available. Several agents are currently under investigation.

RUBELLA

A. *General principles*
   1. Transmission to the fetus is transplacental.
   2. The effects of rubella virus on the fetus depend to a large extent on the gestational age at the time of infection. Generally, the earlier in gestation the fetus is exposed, the more severe the manifestations.
   3. Risks of fetal infection during the first 8 weeks of gestation is 40 to 60 percent; from 8 to 12 weeks, 30 to 35 percent; and from 12 to 16 weeks, 10 percent.
   4. Delayed manifestations of rubella have been observed as late as schoolage. Careful follow-up and examination of the child should extend over several years.
   5. Susceptible women may be vaccinated in the immediate postpartum period. Pregnancy should be avoided for three months after vaccination.

    6. If vaccine is inadvertently administered to a pregnant woman, pregnancy termination should be offered. To date, no infant with congenital rubella syndrome has been born to a woman vaccinated while pregnant. The risk remains, however, since virus has been isolated from aborted tissue.

B. *Maternal clinical manifestations*

    1. A nonconfluent maculopapular rash begins on the face and moves down the trunk to finally affect the extremities. The rash is generally present for three to five days.

    2. Prodromal symptoms include malaise, fever, and anorexia.

    3. Lymphadenopathy is generally present, involving the posterior auricular, posterior cervical, and suboccipital chains.

    4. Complications include conjunctivitis and arthritis involving the fingers, wrists, and knees.

C. *Diagnosis*

    1. Serologic testing using hemagglutination inhibition is the most commonly used technic. A fourfold or greater increase in titer indicates infection.

    2. A specific rubella IgM antibody identification is available in reference laboratories.

    3. Viral isolation may be obtained through throat culture. Amniotic fluid culture may reveal virus.

D. *Treatment of maternal symptoms*

    1. There is no specific therapy. Immune serum globulin is not recommended.

    2. Symptomatic relief may be obtained with bed rest, analgesics, and antipyretics.

E. *Neonatal clinical manifestations*

    1. *Head.* Microcephaly, mental retardation, seizure disorders, degenerative brain disease

    2. *Eyes.* Glaucoma, cataracts, microphthalmia, retinopathy, cloudy cornea, myopia

    3. *Thorax.* Patent ductus arteriosis, pulmonic stenosis, my-

ocarditis, cardiac malformations (atrial or ventricular septal defects).

    4. *Miscellaneous.* Deafness, pneumonitis, low birth weight, thrombocytopenic purpura, hepatitis, interstitial nephritis, diabetes mellitus, dysgammaglobulinemia

F. *Neonatal diagnosis* is based on clinical suspicion, persistence or rise of serum antibody titer beyond three months of age, specific rubella IgM antibody identification, and virus isolation.

G. *Neonatal treatment*
    1. No specific treatment is available.
    2. Infected infants can shed virus from the nasopharynx up to one year of age.

TOXOPLASMOSIS

A. *General principles*
    1. Maternal infection may be acquired by ingestion of raw meat or by close contact with infected cats.
    2. Transmission to the fetus is primarily transplacental.
    3. Direct person-to-person transmission does not occur.
    4. The incidence of congenital infection depends on the trimester during which maternal infection occurred.
    5. Incidence of fetal infection. First trimester, 15 percent; second trimester, 25 percent; third trimester, 60 percent. Overall, one-third of infants born to mothers who acquired toxoplasmosis during pregnancy will be infected.
    6. Spontaneous abortion, stillbirth, or prematurity may occur.
    7. Pathologic examination of the placenta may identify *Toxoplasma gondii* cysts.
    8. Most infected infants are asymptomatic at birth.

B. *Maternal clinical manifestations*
    1. May be completely asymptomatic
    2. A mononucleosis-like illness may develop

C. *Diagnosis*
   1. Serologic testing. Seroconversion: an eightfold increase in titer by the Sabin-Feldman dye test; a fourfold increase in titer by indirect immunofluorescence, complement fixation, hemagglutination.
   2. Histologic identification of cysts in the placenta.
D. *Maternal treatment*
   1. Pyrimethamine, 25 mg/day orally for 28 days, and sulfadiazine, 1 gm orally four times a day for 28 days.
   2. Do not use pyrimethamine during the first trimester.
   3. Do not use sulfadiazine during the third trimester.
   4. Monitor drug toxicity with a complete blood count and platelet count every other week.
   5. The exact regimen for optimal results has not been established.
E. *Neonatal clinical manifestations.* These may be extremely variable and include: chorioretinitis, seizures, microcephaly, intracranial calcification, abnormal CSF, hepatosplenomegaly, jaundice, fever, thrombocytopenia, interstitial pneumonitis, nephritis, focal adrenal necrosis.
F. *Neonatal Diagnosis* is based upon identification of specific IgM antibodies and by recovery of the organism.
G. *Neonatal Treatment.* Pyrimethamine and sulfadiazine.

CYTOMEGALOVIRUS (CMV)

A. *General principles*
   1. Infection may occur in utero by transplacental transmission or during passage through an infected birth canal. Infants have also acquired CMV via transfusion with infected blood.
   2. Primary maternal infection is associated with a high intrauterine infection rate.
   3. Virus may be shed from the urine, cervix, or nasopharynx for months to years after primary infection.

B. *Maternal clinical manifestations*
   1. May be completely asymptomatic
   2. A mononucleosis-like illness may develop.
C. *Diagnosis*
   1. Viral isolation from the urine or cervix
   2. Serologic testing. A greater than fourfold increase in titer with paired sera (IHA, ELISA, FA, CF)
   3. Up to 60 percent of the general population may have antibodies to CMV
D. *Maternal treatment.* No specific treatment is available.
E. *Neonatal clinical manifestations*
   1. May be asymptomatic
   2. Jaundice, hepatosplenomegally, petechial rash, microcephaly, motor disability, chorioretinitis, periventricular calcification, mental retardation
F. *Neonatal diagnosis* is based on virus isolation and demonstration of IgM specific antibody.
G. *Neonatal treatment.* No specific treatment is available.

RUBEOLA (Measles)

A. *General principles*
   1. In utero infection may occur by transplacental passage of the virus.
   2. The incidence of spontaneous abortion and premature labor is increased.
B. *Maternal clinical manifestations*
   1. A maculopapular rash begins on the face and moves down the trunk to affect the extremities.
   2. Koplik spots may be present on the oral mucosa.
   3. Additional symptoms include fever, malaise, cough, and keratoconjunctivitis.
   4. Encephalitis and myocarditis are rare complications.
   5. A secondary bacterial pneumonia may occur.

C. *Diagnosis*
1. Identification of virus by immunofluorescence or by culture.
2. Serologic testing using either hemagglutination inhibition or complement fixation will reveal a greater than fourfold increase in titer.

D. *Maternal treatment*
1. Treatment is supportive with the use of analgesics and antipyretics.
2. The development of bacterial pneumonia requires specific antibiotic treatment.

E. *Neonatal clinical manifestations.* The neonate may develop typical exanthematous lesions. An increased incidence of congenital malformations is disputed.

F. *Neonatal diagnosis* is based on viral identification and serologic testing.

G. *Neonatal treatment.* No specific treatment is available.

VARICELLA (Chickenpox)

A. *General principles*
1. In utero infection may occur by transplacental passage of the virus.
2. Maternal infection that occurs within 7 to 10 days of delivery is associated with severe fetal infection that may result in neonatal death in one-third of cases.

B. *Maternal clinical manifestations*
1. A vesiculopapular rash occurs shortly after prodromal symptoms of fever and malaise.
2. Pneumonia is a common complication.

C. *Diagnosis*
1. Typical intranuclear inclusion bodies may be demonstrated in scrapings of the base of the vesicles.
2. Antibodies are detectable two to four weeks after infection.

D. *Maternal treatment*
   1. Treatment is generally supportive with the use of antihis-
      tamines to control pruritus and local cleansing to prevent
      secondary infection of open lesions.
   2. Pneumonia may lead to significant alveolar-capillary
      block, hypoxia, and death. Hospitalization and aggres-
      sive support are indicated.
E. *Neonatal clinical manifestations*
   1. Maternal infection early in pregnancy has been associated
      with numerous fetal anomalies including limb atrophy,
      cortical atrophy, and scarring of the skin. Convulsive
      disorders and paralysis in the neonate have been repor-
      ted.
   2. Infants born within 7 to 10 days of maternal infection will
      generally develop severe infection with significant mor-
      tality.
F. *Neonatal Treatment.* No generally satisfactory treatment is
   available, though the use of Zoster immune globulin may be
   of some benefit.

OTHER INFECTIOUS ILLNESSES

A. *Mumps.* An increased incidence of spontaneous abortion is
   associated with first-trimester infection. No association with
   congenital anomalies has been reported. Maternal treatment
   is supportive.
B. *Poliomyelitis.* This disease is rare in the United States due to
   widespread vaccination. The fetus may become infected,
   leading to paralysis and retarded growth. Maternal treatment is supportive, with ventilatory assistance often necessary.
C. *Bacterial infections and sexually transmitted diseases.* These
   topics are discussed in other chapters.

BIBLIOGRAPHY

Mandell GL, Douglas RG, Bennett JE (eds): Principles and Practice of Infectious Diseases. New York, John Wiley, 1979

Monif GRG (ed): Infectious Diseases in Obstetrics and Gynecology. Hagerstown, Md., Harper & Row, 1974

Remington JS, Klein J (eds): Infectious Diseases of the Fetus and Newborn Infant. Philadelphia, Saunders, 1976

Sever JL, Larsen JW, Grossman JH: Handbook of Perinatal Infections. Boston, Little, Brown, 1979

Section 11
Psychiatric Disease
Henry Lahmeyer, M.D.

PRACTICE PRINCIPLES

Few branches of medicine beside obstetrics and gynecology deal with so many issues associated with deep emotional responses — birth, pregnancy, abortion, sterilization, cancer, death, change of life, human sexuality — or in such intimate association. An appreciation of the psychiatric aspects of reproductive medicine is essential for the comprehensive and compassionate care of the patient.

PREGNANCY

A. *Introduction*

From a psychologic point of view, pregnancy generally follows the traditional trimester definition. Each trimester has a unique set of psychologic issues.

1. *Conception and the first trimester*

a) If pregnancy is planned, a good support system is available, and the mother is comfortable with the role of motherhood, this period will usually be accompanied only by increased sleep, eating, and lethargy.

b) *Hyperemesis gravidarum* has been ascribed psychologically to an attempt to expunge the pregnancy. Hormonal changes may also play a role. Certainly *anxiety* and *ambivalence* over mothering can contribute. Medically, the condition can become serious since electrolyte imbalance and weight loss may develop.

    (1) *Management.* The presence of this condition requires that the obstetrician meet with the patient and spouse to determine sources of *marital tension* and *financial* and *emotional stresses* currently and in the past for the expectant mother. A first occurence in a multigravida alerts the physician to psychologic stresses or biologic risk factors.

    (2) *Psychiatric referral* is usally indicated and treatment may involve counseling, hypnosis, or behavioral therapy.

2. *Second trimester*

  a) Usually this period is a relatively quiescent one psychologically. Distress during this period is therefore ominous. *Sleep* and *appetite disturbances, anxiety,* and *depression* now mean that the issues of the first trimester have not been resolved psychologically or that medically the pregnancy is not progressing properly.

  b) *Management.* Continued distress alerts one to the possibility of extreme *immaturity, depression,* or impending *psychosis. Preeclampsia* can present late in the second trimester and usually presents with *anxiety, irritability, sleep disturbance,* and *headache,* often before the classic symptoms of edema, proteinuria, and hypertension emerge. Psychiatric symptoms in the second trimester therefore require additional psychologic inventory and careful medical monitoring.

  c) *Psychotropic medications* are safer now than during the first trimester, but should be avoided if possible, since neurologic maturation is still an active process.

3. *Third trimester*
   a) *Physical and emotional discomfort* reemerge during this period. Increased girth leads to dyspnea, slowed mobility, poor sleep, and uneven appetite. Muscle aches, cramps, and peripheral edema are common. Changes in girth, hair color, and skin tone, all lead to distress about *body image. Sexual functioning* is difficult. As delivery nears, the mother's concern draws inward often to the exclusion of the father. He thus can become less available to comfort her mounting anxiety and anticipation.
   b) *Preeclampsia* can again present with *anxiety, headache,* and *irritability.*
   c) Other obstetric complications increase during this period increasing *regression* in the mother around the issues of fetal deformity, her own disfigurement, and loss of her own childhood with imminent motherhood. *Third trimester anxiety* is associated with fear of prolonged and precipitous labor, postpartum hemorrhage and fetal distress.
   d) *Management*
      (1) *Prenatal classes* are invaluable during this period to fulfill some of the function that a mother and extended family used to play. More frequent contact with the obstetrician occurs but may need to be further increased if anxiety escalates.
      (2) If anxiety does not improve, lorzaepam (Ativan), 1 to 2 mg (or other short half-life benzodiazepine) for anxiety or 2 to 5 mg p.r.n. for sleep, is now safe. Do not put the patient on a regular schedule of medication and try to discontinue lorazepam one to two days before labor. The *short half-life* benzodiazepine will minimize the risk of neonatal sedation.

B. *Abortion*
   1. Planned first-trimester abortions are associated with fewer psychologic sequelae than is childbirth, or stillbirth

later in pregnancy; late abortions with delivery of a viable fetus lead to more remorse and guilt in mother and obstetric staff.

2. Precounseling is desirable to:
   a) Help the patient make the best decision
   b) Encourage the patient to involve her support system of father and/or parents
   c) Identify patients with extreme anxiety or guilt about abortion so that follow-up counseling can be arranged
3. *Risk factors* associated with negative postabortion reactions include young age, unmarried status, certain religious faiths, and poor social supports.

C. *Fetal death*
   1. Significant *grief reaction* is almost universal after stillbirth or early infant death. Grief can lead to true depression, where guilt, and self-depreciation are prominent in a woman who was previously vulnerable to depression or was ambivalent about the child, or in a woman with some of the risk factors mentioned for abortion depression, particularly *poor support system.*
   2. *Management*
      (1) Facilitate the grief work by allowing her to talk about her feelings, her *fear* of future pregnancies, and her anger at fate and herself. The physician should be aware, however, that the *anger* that is so common during this period, will sometimes be directed toward him. It is important to understand that this anger usually is not personally directed at the physician. Acceptance of the upset is important; try not to react. If grief is prolonged for six weeks or more, or becomes worse, *depression* could be developing. The reason for the depression should be sought. If the reasons are vague or guilt and remorse are excessive, psychiatric referral is indicated. Antidepressants can be useful if a depressive syndrome has developed (Table 15–7).
      (2) Nursing and other staff often become depressed after fetal death, especially when legal issues complicate

TABLE 15–7. SYMPTOMS OF DEPRESSION

1. Insomnia
2. Anorexia and weight loss
3. Sadness and crying
4. Suicidal thoughts
5. Decreased interest in spouse, sex, child, and other previous interests
6. Low energy
7. Unreasonable guilt or remorse

the professional-patient relationship (e.g., in cases of weight criteria that requires a funeral, need for coroner's report, etc.).

D. *Prematurity*
1. Parents often have considerable fear, guilt, and worry. Mothers will usually be intimidated by the intensive care unit and hesitant to get involved in the infant's care. The *medical team* will often covertly discourage involvement as well.
2. *Management.* It is important to inform the parents about the possible causes of the infant's distress and the long-term prognosis, as the parents become receptive to this information. If the *infant* is at high risk, the parents should be told the risks and asked how much contact they would like to have with the infant. They may choose to have little contact until the danger is over in an intuitive attempt to minimize bonding until infant viability is assured. Parents of premature infants with better prognosis should be encouraged to have contact with the premature infant to enhance bonding and to help them overcome their natural reluctance to interfere with the professional staff.

E. *Psychosis and pregnancy*
   1. *Incidence.* From 0.1 to 0.25 percent. But in women with a history of previous psychosis during pregnancy, the incidence may be as high as 50 percent or higher.
   2. *Types of psychoses*
      a) Schizophrenia
         (1) *Incidence.* Common psychiatric problem in the public setting
         (2) *Clinical picture.* A chronic psychotic illness characterized by delusions, often auditory hallucinations and often the feeling that one's thoughts are being influenced or controlled by others. Some schizophrenics improve during pregnancy, but others deteriorate under the added stress.
         (3) *Management*
            (a) *Psychiatric involvement* is essential in order to assess the current psychiatric status, the need for psychotropics, and the ability of mother to care for the child.
            (b) *Social service* should be involved to help with assessing the support network and the desire of mother to keep the child and to find alternate caregivers if necessary.
            (c) *Psychiatric hospitalization* may be needed during pregnancy and often is recommended immediately postpartum if the mother is psychotic and unable to care for child. Psychiatric hospitalization of mother and child is optimal if the mother plans to keep the child. *Conjoint hospitalization* can help her with bonding and basic mothering skills.
         (4) *Psychotropic medication. Major tranquilizers* can be used safely. *Fetal effects* are not of concern until childbirth when *fetal tremors, restlessness* and *rigidity,* as well as respiratory distress, may occur. The drugs can be tapered 10 to 15 days

prior to anticipated labor. Use sufficient dosage to control psychotic symptoms but not fog the patient's thinking. Treatment should be done in conjunction with a psychiatrist.

- (a) *Anticholinergic side effects.* Dry mouth, blurred vision, urinary retention, constipation
- (b) *Extrapyramidal side effects.* Acute dystonia most common. This occurs early in treatment and can be corrected by lowering the dosage of the major tranquilizer or by adding benzodiazepine, 1 to 2 mg b.i.d. for 7 days before the dose is tapered.

b) *Manic-depressive (bipolar) psychoses*
  - (1) *Incidence.* More common than schizophrenia in private clinics.
  - (2) *Clinical picture.* A history of significant mood swings that significantly interfere with job or family and have required psychiatric hospitalization or led to suicide attempt. The past episodes involved both periods of depression and mania (Table 15–7).
  - (3) *Management.* Many of these patients will be on maintenance *lithium carbonate.* This should be suspended during the first trimester, or longer, if at all possible; reinstated during the middle phase; and discontinued near term to avoid some of the neonatal effects of *cyanosis, goiter, hypoglycemia, hypotonia,* and rarely *diabetes insipidus.* The risk for mania is high in the puerperium, so that lithium should again be reinstituted postpartum.

c) *Depression*
  - (1) *Incidence.* Depression is much more common in the puerperium than during pregnancy but occurs in those with a previous history of depression.
  - (2) *Management.* Try to avoid *tricyclic antidepressants*

in the *first trimester,* but teratogenic risk is very low.

(3) *Tricyclic neonatal effects.* Tachypnea, tachycardia, and hyperhidrosis that may last for up to a week after delivery. Try to discontinue tricyclics 10 to 15 days prior to delivery. They can be safely reinstated immediately postpartum even in lactating mothers.

LABOR AND DELIVERY
Extreme anxiety often occurs as a direct result of pain or a fear of mutilation or fetal distress.

1. *Management. Prenatal classes* and *a birthplan.* If she is well practiced and trusts those around her, the new mother will follow instructions during painful periods.

2. *Psychotropics.* If analgesics and psychologic support fail and anxiety becomes uncontrollable, haloperidol, 2 mg IM repeated every 30 minutes until anxiety is controlled, can be used. The baby will not be excessively sleepy but may develop tremor or dystonia for a day or two.

POSTPARTUM

A. *"Blues"*
  1. *Incidence.* From 20 to 70 percent.
  2. *Clinical presentation.* After a symptom-free period of one to three days, feelings of exhaustion, poor appetite, and "blues" are accompanied by a seemingly unexplainable tearfulness.
  3. *Management.* Most cases are self-limiting in three to seven days as exhaustion and pain from labor subside. Bonding to the child seems to account for the change. Family support in the form of assisting the patient with

the newborn and allowing her to obtain some sleep are important.

B. *Depression*

1. *Incidence.* From 5 to 15 percent of the general population; 50 percent if there is a previous bipolar history and 50 percent if there has been a previous postpartum depression

2. *Clinical presentation.* The "blues" progress instead of remitting. The full depressive syndrome can occur (Table 15–7). Interest in the infant fails to develop

3. *Risk factors*
   a) Previous history of depression or family history of depression
   b) Obstetric complications. Especially during labor and delivery, or third-trimester anxiety
   c) Poor social supports

4. *Management.* Same as for depression during pregnancy

C. *Psychoses*

1. *Incidence.* From 1 to 3/1000 births

2. *Clinical picture.* Most postpartum psychoses are predominantly affective, but depression mixed with confusion, delusions, and perplexity is common. Often this is coupled with delusions, extreme social withdrawal, failure to care for the infant or overt aggression towards the infant

3. *Management*
   a) *Psychiatric consultation* essential
   b) Search for possible *medical etiology*
      (1) Infections
      (2) Drug toxicity
      (3) Thromboembolic
      (4) Postanesthesia or spinal block
   c) *Psychiatric hospitalization* usually needed
   d) *Social service intervention* with family for:
      (1) Support and explanation
      (2) Arrangements for infant if conjoint hospitalization not possible

BIBLIOGRAPHY

Anath J: Side effects on fetus and infant of psychotropic drug use during pregnancy. Int Pharmacopsychiatry 11:246, 1976

Brown WA: Psychological Care During Pregnancy and the Postpartum Period. New York, Raven Press, 1979

Lahmeyer HW, Jackson C: Affective disorders and mental illness during the puerperium. In Val E, Gaviria M, Flaherty J (eds): Affective Disorders: Diagnosis and Treatment in Clinical Practice. Chicago, Year Book Medical Publishers, 1982

Protheroe C: Puerperal psychosis: a long term study 1927–1961. Br J Psychiatry 115:9, 1969

Section 12
Neurologic Disease
Jeffrey W. Ellis, M.D.

PRACTICE PRINCIPLES

During the course of pregnancy and the puerperium, the patient may develop a variety of neurologic symptoms that may be trivial or may represent serious underlying disease. All neurologic symptoms should be carefully evaluated by a thorough history and physical examination. Many neurologic conditions are self-limiting and will require no specific treatment. The evaluation and treatment of severe neurologic complications should not be attempted by the obstetrician and will require neurologic and medical consultation. Details of treatment and evaluation will not be discussed in this chapter but may be found in standard neurology and medicine texts.

NEUROLOGIC SYMPTOMS

Symptoms that may be encountered in the pregnant patient include headache, seizure, coma, effects of nerve palsy, and neurologic deficit. A consideration of the differential diagnosis will aid in an orderly evaluation and treatment sequence.

HEADACHE

Headache is the most common neurologic complaint of the pregnant woman

A. *Differential diagnosis.*
   1. Common etiologies
      a) Migraine
      b) Tension
      c) Sinusitis
      d) Ocular disturbance
      e) Cervical disease
      f) Otitis media
      g) Dental abscess or disease
      h) Trauma
      i) Hypertension (chronic hypertension, pregnancy-induced hypertension)
      j) Temporal arteritis
      k) Trigeminal neuralgia
   2. Headache associated with other neurologic symptoms may be due to:
      a) Mass lesion (seizure, focal neurologic deficit)
      b) Subarachnoid hemorrhage (meningeal irritation, altered consciousness, no gross localizing signs)
      c) Intracerebral hemorrhage (altered consciousness, focal neurologic deficit)
      d) Cerebral venous thrombosis (altered consciousness, seizure, focal neurologic deficit)
B. *Diagnosis.* In many cases, the cause of headache will be evident after history and physical examination. Careful neurologic examination is mandatory. Consultation should be obtained when the cause of headache cannot be determined or when associated neurologic signs and symptoms are present. Additional evaluation might include cerebrospinal fluid examination, electroencephalogram, computerized axial tomography, and angiography.
C. *Treatment.* Therapy when possible is aimed at treating the

cause of the headache. In cases where primary neurologic disease is suspected, therapy should be conducted by a neurologist.

SEIZURE

Seizure is the most common complex neurologic problem that confronts the obstetrician. In general, seizure disorders have little effect on pregnancy as long as appropriate anticonvulsant medications are maintained. In most cases, the seizure disorder was recognized prior to pregnancy with adequate therapy already initiated.

A. *Principles of drug management*
   1. Patients should be followed during pregnancy by both obstetrician and neurologist.
   2. Frequent assessment of drug levels is necessary, since diphenylhydantoin and phenobarbital are cleared more rapidly, leading to lower blood levels. Adjustment of dosage may be necessary.
   3. The teratogenic effects of anticonvulsant drugs must be considered.
   4. Trimethadione should never be used in pregnancy, because it has serious teratogenic effects.
   5. The neonate may develop deficiencies in vitamin K-dependent coagulation factors. The pediatric service should be notified of all patients who have been on anticonvulsant therapy.
B. *Clinical course.* The course of seizure disorders during pregnancy is variable and unpredictable. Approximately one-half of patients will have an increase in seizure activity; approximately one-half of patients will have no change in seizure activity; approximately 5 percent will have a decrease in seizure activity.
C. *Status epilepticus.* This disorder is characterized by the occurrence of two or more major seizures without an intervening return of consciousness. This poses a major

threat to both mother and fetus. Hypoxia is the most severe problem and may occur as a result of impaired ventilation during the seizure or as a result of aspiration, with resultant impaired ventilation. Death or severe central nervous system damage may occur. Therapy must be carried out rapidly.

1. *Management.* The objectives of management are to maintain adequate ventilation, prevent physical damage during violent seizure activity, and control seizure activity with medication.

   a) *Supportive therapy*

      (1) An adequate airway must be maintained. An oropharyngeal airway is usually sufficient. An endotracheal tube may be necessary if adequate ventilation cannot otherwise be maintained. In the absence of an airway, a padded tongue blade should be placed between the teeth.

      (2) The oropharynx should be thoroughly cleared using suction.

      (3) High-flow oxygen is administered.

      (4) A large-bore intravenous catheter is inserted and physiologic fluids are administered.

      (5) A nasogastric tube may be necessary to control persistent vomiting.

      (6) Arterial blood gases and electrolytes should be monitored frequently, with appropriate correction as necessary.

   b) *Drug therapy.* The objective of anticonvulsant drug therapy is to control seizure activity without producing untoward effects such as hypotension, respiratory depression, and cardiac arryhthmia. Vital signs must be monitored frequently during and after drug administration. The patient must not be left unattended during therapy.

      (1) *Diazepam.* This is a rapidly acting anticonvulsant associated with little hypotension and respiratory depression. Diazepam is administered in doses of

5 to 10 mg IV at a rate of no more than 5 mg/minute. If seizure activity has not stopped within 10 minutes, an additional 5 to 10 mg may be administered. Other drugs must be used if seizures are not controlled after the administration of 25 to 30 mg. Longer-acting anticonvulsants must be administered after seizure activity has been controlled.

(2) *Barbiturates.* Vital signs must be monitored closely because of the frequent association with hypotension and respiratory depression.

   (a) *Phenobarbital.* An initial dose of 150 mg is administered intravenously at a rate of 25 mg/minute. Additional doses of 25 to 50 mg may be given after 15 to 20 minutes, with a total dose not to exceed 400 mg.

   (b) *Amobarbital.* This is administered at a rate of 25 mg/minute until seizures are controlled or until a total dose of 250 mg is reached. An additional dose of 250 mg may be administered after 10 to 20 minutes if seizures are not controlled.

(3) *Diphenylhydantoin.* This drug may be given at a rate not to exceed 50 mg/minute to a total dose of 1000 mg if needed. Pulse, blood pressure, and ECG must be closely monitored during and after infusion because of associated hypotension and cardiac arryhthmia.

(4) *General anesthesia* may be necessary if seizure activity cannot be controlled within two hours or if an uncontrollable, life-threatening situation develops.

2. *Diagnosis.* During the course of treatment, a rapid evaluation of underlying causes should be undertaken. Specific treatment should then be initiated. Differential diagnosis includes: tumor, abscess, hematoma, aneurysm, meningitis, encephalitis, subarachnoid hemor-

rhage, hyponatremia, hypocalcemia, hypoglycemia, uremia, sudden withdrawal of anticonvulsant medication. Any seizure in a pregnant patient, especially the primigravida, should be assumed an eclamptic seizure until the diagnosis of preeclampsia/eclampsia is disproven.

COMA

This is an uncommon occurrence in pregnancy and demands rapid evaluation, support, and treatment.

A. *Differential diagnosis.* The following etiologies must be considered during the evaluation and treatment of coma:
  1. Intoxication (alcohol, drugs, toxic agents)
  2. Intracranial pathology (subarachnoid hemorrhage, intracranial hemorrhage, tumor, hematoma, concussion)
  3. Eclampsia
  4. Infection (meningitis, encephalitis, sepsis)
  5. Hypovolemia (hemorrhagic shock)
  6. Respiratory compromise (embolism, pulmonary insufficiency)
  7. Metabolic disturbance (electrolyte abnormality, hypoglycemia, acidosis, alkalosis, hepatic coma, renal failure, myxedema)
B. *Management.* Management should be conducted with consultation from the neurology and internal medicine staff. Initial management by the obstetric staff should include:
  1. Thorough history if possible
  2. Thorough and rapid physical examination
  3. Frequent determination of vital signs with cardiorespiratory support as needed
  4. Maintenance of an adequate airway
  5. Insertion of a large-bore IV catheter with maintenance of adequate blood pressure and tissue perfusion
  6. Rapid assessment of electrolytes, blood gases, hematocrit, blood urea nitrogen, and glucose.

NERVE PALSY

A variety of nerve palsies may occur during pregnancy; they are generally self-limiting.

A. *Carpal tunnel syndrome.* Symptoms of median nerve compression (numbness and tingling of the hands) are relatively common during pregnancy and generally occur to a mild degree. Significant sensory loss and weakness may occur in some cases. An increase in interstitial fluid during pregnancy may lead to compression of the median nerve within the carpal tunnel. Splinting of the hands or local injection of steroids may be necessary to control severe symptoms. This problem generally resolves after pregnancy. Surgical decompression of the nerve is rarely indicated.

B. *Bell's palsy.* Compression of the facial nerve is uncommon in pregnancy and may occur as a result of increased interstitial fluid. This problem resolves after pregnancy.

C. *Obstetric injury.* Peripheral nerve injury is relatively common and may occur as a result of normal vaginal delivery or operative delivery. Malpositioning of the legs during delivery may also lead to transient nerve injury. After delivery, the patient will experience pain along the distribution of the effected nerve. The most commonly involved nerves are the obturator, femoral, and common peroneal. Analgesics and physiotherapy are usually sufficient to control symptoms. Pain generally resolves within several days after injury.

D. *Meralgia paresthetica.* Compression of the lateral cutaneous nerve beneath the inguinal ligament may lead to pain and burning over the outer aspect of the thigh. This usually occurs during the third trimester and will resolve within weeks after delivery. Analgesics and avoidance of prolonged standing and walking will generally control symptoms. Injection of local anesthetics is rarely indicated.

SPECIFIC NEUROLOGIC DISEASES

A. *Myasthenia gravis.* Generally no increased difficulty is encountered during pregnancy as long as appropriate drug therapy is maintained. The course of the disease is variable: one-third of patients improve, one-third become more symptomatic, and one-third are unchanged. During labor, there may be decreased ability to bear down during the second stage, thus requiring forceps delivery. Transient symptoms of myasthenia gravis may occur in the newborn, with resolution occurring in four to six weeks.

B. *Paraplegia.* There are usually no specific complications during pregnancy except for recurrent urinary tract infection. Forceps delivery may be necessary because of decreased ability to bear down during the second stage of labor.

C. *Multiple sclerosis.* Pregnancy has no effect on the course of the disease and the newborn is unaffected.

D. *Guillain-Barré syndrome.* Respiratory insufficiency may develop during pregnancy, requiring hospitalization and support of ventilation. Forceps delivery is often required because of weakened abdominal muscles. The fetus is unaffected.

E. *Chorea gravidarum.* This uncommon condition is characterized by almost constant unintentional movements of the body, face, and extremities. The course is generally self-limiting. Severe cases may be controlled using chlorpromazine, 25 to 50 mg three times a day.

DRUG INTOXICATION

The obstetrician may be presented with a patient with signs and symptoms suggestive of drug intoxication. Rapid evaluation and treatment will often be necessary to prevent serious injury and complications. After initial assessment by the obstetric staff, medical and psychiatric consultation should be obtained.

A. *Narcotic intoxication*
   1. *Clinical findings*
      a) *Mild intoxication.* Euphoria, drowsiness, anxiety, mood swings, nausea, vomiting, apparent analgesia
      b) *Overdosage.* Respiratory depression, respiratory ar-

    rest, coma, vomiting, pulmonary edema, evidence of vasodilatation

    c) *Withdrawal.* Symptoms may be of variable intensity and include anxiety, perspiration, myalgia, anorexia, restlessness, increased blood pressure, pulse, and respiratory rate

2. *Differential diagnosis.* Intoxication from other drugs or toxic agents.

3. *Diagnosis.* Chemical identification of opiates in urine.

4. *Treatment*
    a) *Overdosage.* Hospitalization is required. Initial management is directed at maintaining adequate ventilation, preventing aspiration, and supporting the cardiovascular system. A narcotic antagonist such as naloxone 0.4 mg should be administered intravenously. This dose may be repeated every 5 to 10 minutes as necessary. Rapid improvement generally occurs if the offending drug was a narcotic. If no immediate improvement occurs, intoxication from other agents must be considered.

    b) *Withdrawal.* Methadone therapy should be conducted in consultation with the medical or psychiatric staff.

5. *Obstetric considerations*
    a) Narcotic addiction has been associated with intrauterine growth retardation and prematurity.
    b) Narcotic withdrawal will occur in the newborn, requiring aggressive management.
    c) During labor, analgesics and anesthetics must be used with caution.

B. *Depressant intoxication.* Commonly abused depressants include the barbiturates, sedative-hypnotics, and minor tranquilizers.

1. *Clinical findings*
    a) *Mild intoxication.* Euphoria, drowsiness, respiratory depression, ataxia, and impaired speech, memory and motor ability
    b) *Overdosage.* Severe respiratory depression, hypotension, coma, stupor

    c) *Withdrawal.* Symptoms may be of variable intensity and include anxiety, nausea, vomiting, tremors, muscular weakness, seizures, hallucination, delirium

2. *Differential diagnosis.* Intoxication from other drugs and toxic agents; organic disease such as diabetic acidosis, trauma, etc.

3. *Diagnosis.* Chemical identification of drug in the blood or urine

4. *Treatment*
    a) *Overdosage.* Hospitalization is required. Initial management is directed at maintaining adequate ventilation, preventing aspiration, and supporting the cardiovascular system. Gastric lavage may be attempted to remove drugs yet unabsorbed.
    b) *Withdrawal.* Management is best conducted in consultation with the medical or psychiatric staff. Medical detoxification should be combined with social and psychologic measures.

5. *Obstetric considerations*
    a) Certain drugs have been associated with congenital anomalies. Diazepam has been associated with cleft palate and cleft lip. Sporadic cases of nonspecific anomalies have been reported in association with meprobamate and chlordiazepoxide.
    b) All tranquilizers have been associated with withdrawal symptoms in the neonate.
    c) Barbiturates have been associated with the following neonatal problems: apnea, decreased responsiveness, bleeding, decreased sucking ability, increased neonatal drug metabolism.
    d) Depressants may potentiate the effects of narcotics and inhalation agents.

C. *Amphetamine intoxication*
  1. *Clinical findings*
    a) *Mild intoxication.* Hyperactivity, insomnia, anorexia
    b) *Overdosage.* Restlessness, tremor, confusion, rapid respiration, arrhythmia, hypotension or hypertension, nausea, vomiting, diarrhea, seizure, coma, psychosis

c) *Withdrawal.* Depression, prolonged sleep, hyperphagia
2. *Differential diagnosis.* Schizophrenia
3. *Diagnosis.* Chemical identification of the drug in blood or urine
4. *Treatment*
   a) *Overdosage.* Hospitalization is required. Supportive management is initiated. Acidification of urine increases amphetamine excretion. Gastric lavage should be attempted. Major tranquilizers should be administered to control agitation. There is no need to slowly taper amphetamine dosage, since there is no physiologic dependence.
   b) *Withdrawal.* In general, no specific treatment is required. Social and psychologic services should be offered.
5. *Obstetric considerations*
   a) Teratogenicity has not been determined, though biliary atresia and cleft deformities have been reported.
   b) Cardiorespiratory disturbances may be noted in the neonate.
   c) Anesthetic agents must be used with caution in the presence of cardiac arrhythmia and alterations in blood pressure.
D. *Alcohol intoxication*
   1. *Clinical findings*
      a) *Acute intoxication.* Tremor, confusion, ataxia, respiratory depression, stupor, coma
      b) *Withdrawal.* Wide range of manifestations from anxiety and restlessness to delirium tremens
   2. *Differential diagnosis.* It is important to differentiate an acute alcoholic spree from chronic alcoholism.
   3. *Diagnosis.* Ethyl alcohol may be identified in blood.
   4. *Treatment*
      a) *Acute intoxication.* Hospitalization may be necessary. Major tranquilizers such as haloperidol may be

needed to control acute agitation and hallucination. Airway maintenance and support of ventilation may be required.

b) *Withdrawal.* Delirium tremens may be associated with significant morbidity and mortality. Psychiatric and medical consultation will be necessary. Social and psychiatric services should be offered.

5. *Obstetric considerations*
   a) Multiple congenital anomalies (fetal alcohol syndrome) have been associated with maternal alcohol ingestion. No safe level of alcohol use has been determined.
   b) Neonatal depression generally does not occur. Hyperirritability, twitching, sweating, and fever may be present.

BIBLIOGRAPHY

Bjerkedal T, Bahna SL: The course and outcome of pregnancy in women with epilepsy. Acta Obstet Gynecol Scand 52:245, 1973

Donaldson JO: Neurology of Pregnancy. Philadelphia, Saunders, 1978

Fraser D, Turner J: Myasthenia gravis and pregnancy. Lancet 2:417, 1953

Gomberg B: Spontaneous subarachnoid hemorrhage in pregnancy not complicated by toxemia. Am J Obstet Gynecol 77:430, 1959

Hunt HB, et al.: Ruptured berry aneurysms and pregnancy. Obstet Gynecol 43:827, 1974

Lander CM, et al.: Plasma anticonvulsant concentrations during pregnancy. Neurology 27:128, 1977

Sweeney WJ: Pregnancy and multiple sclerosis. Am J Obstet Gynecol 66:124, 1953

Zegart KN, Schwarz RH: Chorea gravidarum. Obstet Gynecol 32:24, 1968

Section 13
Dermatologic Disease
Jeffrey W. Ellis, M.D.

PRACTICE PRINCIPLES
The pregnant woman is as susceptible to ordinary cutaneous diseases as is the nonpregnant woman. Several dermatologic changes are commonly associated with pregnancy and result from the endocrinologic changes of pregnancy. Four dermatologic diseases are unique to pregnancy, and one dermatologic disease is significantly associated with pregnancy.

DERMATOLOGIC CHANGES ASSOCIATED WITH NORMAL PREGNANCY

A. *Increased pigmentation.* An increase in pigmentation is common in pregnancy and occurs as a result of stimulation of melanocytes by estrogen and progesterone. A diffuse increase in pigmentation may be seen in the areola, nipples, axillae, umbilicus, linea alba, vulva, perineum, and thighs. *Chloasma gravidarum* (melasma) is hyperpigmentation of the face, which occurs primarily on the forehead and malar eminences. This may occur in varying degrees in 50 to 70 percent of pregnant women. In most cases, pigmentation fades after pregnancy and will not present a cosmetic problem. Chloasma associated with deep pigmentation may require treatment. Bleaching agents generally yield poor results. Some reports have claimed satisfactory depigmentation after pregnancy using a formulation of tretinoin, 0.1 percent; hydroquinone, 5.0 percent; and dexamethasone, 0.1 percent.

B. *Striae gravidarum.* Striae develop in approximately 90 percent of pregnant women and occur primarily on areas of excessive stretch such as the breasts, abdomen, and thighs. Histologically, striae are characterized by rupture and retraction of elastic fibers of the skin. Initially, striae appear pink and linear. They may widen as pregnancy progresses. After pregnancy, discoloration generally fades and the striae may then have a silver appearance. There is no known prevention for the development of striae.

C. *Vascular changes*

1. *Palmar erythema* develops in approximately 70 percent of white women and 30 percent of black women. The erythema may occur as a diffuse mottling of the skin or in sharply separated areas. In most cases, the erythema resolves completely after pregnancy.

2. *Vascular spiders* (spider angiomata, nevi aranei) develop in approximately 70 percent of white women and 10 percent of black women. The lesion appears as a small central papule with radiating telangiectatic vessels ranging in size between 2 and 10 mm. They appear most commonly on the upper extremities, trunk, and face. Vascular spiders generally appear during the first half of pregnancy and may subsequently increase in size and number. Most lesions disappear after delivery. If necessary, the lesions may be treated using either electrodesiccation or cautery.

D. *Changes in hair growth.* A moderate degree of hair loss for four to six months after pregnancy is termed *postpartum alopecia.* During pregnancy, more hairs are in an active growth phase than in a resting phase. After delivery, there is a conversion to an increased number of hairs in the resting phase. The number of hairs shedding per day may then increase to several times normal. After several months, there is generally complete regrowth of normal hair. There is no therapy to prevent hair loss or stimulate regrowth.

DERMATOLOGIC DISEASES UNIQUE TO PREGNANCY

A. *Herpes gestationis*
   1. *Type of lesion.* Macular erythema progresses to papules, vesicules, and bullae
   2. *Incidence.* 1/3000 to 4000 pregnancies
   3. *Onset.* Generally in the second and third trimesters
   4. *Location of lesions.* Mucous membranes, extremities, abdomen, buttocks
   5. *Symptoms.* Pruritis, fever, chills, discomfort from secondary infection
   6. *Clinical course.* The disease generally progresses through pregnancy. Secondary infection of the bullae may occur. Resolution of the lesions generally occurs after delivery. Recurrence in subsequent pregnancies is common. Lesions that arise late in pregnancy are likely to persist into the puerperium.
   7. *Laboratory findings.* Leukocytosis, eosinophilia, C_3 and IgG in the basement membrane zone of the skin demonstrated by immunofluorescent staining
   8. *Maternal-fetal complications*
      a) *Maternal.* Mild recurrences may occur during menses for 6 to 18 months after delivery.
      b) *Fetal.* A transient herpetiform eruption may occur in the neonate; however, this will clear in several weeks. Reports of neonatal mortality are inconclusive.
   9. *Differential diagnosis.* Erythema multiforme, bullous pemphigoid, dermatitis herpetiformis
   10. *Therapy.* *Corticosteroids* generally provide satisfactory results. Oral prednisone is administered initially in doses

of 20 to 40 mg/day. The dosage is then tapered to maintenance levels. Frequent cleansing and antibiotics may be necessary to control infection of open lesions.

B. *Prurigo gestationis*
1. *Type of lesion.* 1- to 2-mm papules
2. *Incidence.* 2 percent of pregnancies
3. *Onset.* Second half of pregnancy
4. *Location of lesions.* Upper trunk, extensor surface of extremities
5. *Symptoms.* Pruritis
6. *Clinical course.* The disease generally progresses through pregnancy. Resolution occurs after delivery. Recurrence in subsequent pregnancies is common.
7. *Laboratory findings.* None
8. *Maternal-fetal complications.* None
9. *Differential diagnosis.* Papular dermatitis of pregnancy, pruritus gravidarum
10. *Therapy.* Antipruritis (oral antihistamines) and topical corticosteroids are generally effective in controlling symptoms.

C. *Papular dermatitis of pregnancy*
1. *Type of lesion.* 3- to 5-mm erythematous papules
2. *Incidence.* 1 in 2000 pregnancies
3. *Onset.* At any time during pregnancy
4. *Location of lesions.* Generalized
5. *Symptoms.* Pruritis
6. *Clinical course.* The disease generally progresses throughout pregnancy. Resolution occurs after delivery. Recurrence in subsequent pregnancies is common.
7. *Laboratory findings.* Elevated urinary chorionic gonadotropin levels, decreased estrogen and cortisol
8. *Maternal-fetal complications*
   a) *Maternal.* None
   b) *Fetal.* Mortality is reported as 30 percent in untreated cases. Mortality is decreased when corticosteroid treatment is initiated.
9. *Differential diagnosis.* Herpes gestationis, dermatitis herpetiformis, infestations, drug reactions

   10. *Therapy.* Oral prednisone in doses of 40 to 200 mg/day is reported to control the disease and reduce fetal mortality.
D. *Pruritus gravidarum*
   1. *Type of lesion.* No primary lesion
   2. *Incidence.* 17 percent of pregnancies
   3. *Onset.* Third trimester
   4. *Location of symptoms.* May be generalized or localized to the abdomen
   5. *Symptoms.* Pruritus, anorexia, nausea, vomiting
   6. *Clinical course.* Resolution occurs after delivery. Recurrence in subsequent pregnancies is common
   7. *Laboratory findings.* Elevated bilirubin
   8. *Maternal-fetal complications*
      a) *Maternal.* None
      b) *Fetal.* Increased incidence of prematurity
   9. *Differential diagnosis.* Infestations, drug reactions
   10. *Therapy.* Antipruritics, cholestyramine

DERMATOLOGIC DISEASE ASSOCIATED WITH PREGNANCY

A. *Impetigo herpetiformis*
   1. *Type of lesion.* Small pustules
   2. *Incidence.* Rare
   3. *Onset.* Acute onset usually in the second half of pregnancy
   4. *Location of lesions.* Neck, axillae, extremities, inguinal areas, inner thighs, occasionally mucous membranes
   5. *Symptoms.* The patient may present severely ill with fever, nausea, vomiting, diarrhea, tetany, and convulsions. Pruritus and burning may occur over lesions.
   6. *Clinical course.* There is acute onset of erythematous macules that develop sterile pustules along the margins. New pustules form at the margins as the central lesion clears. The disease progresses throughout pregnancy with resolution generally occurring after delivery. Recurrence in subsequent pregnancies is rare.

7. *Laboratory findings*. Hypocalcemia and hyperphosphatemia have been reported in some cases
8. *Maternal-fetal complications*
   a) *Maternal*. Death may occur in cases with severe constitutional symptoms.
   b) *Fetal*. An increase in intrauterine demise has been reported.
9. *Differential diagnosis*. Pustular psoriasis, dermatitis herpetiformis, erythema multiforme
10. *Therapy*. Oral prednisone in doses of 20 to 60 mg/day has been effective in some cases. Underlying hypocalcemia should be corrected

BIBLIOGRAPHY

Bean WB, et al.: Vascular change of the skin in pregnancy. Surg Gynecol Obstet 88:739, 1949

Bushkell L, et al.: Herpes gestationis. Arch Dermatol 110:65, 1974

Kolodny RC: Herpes gestationis. Am J Obstet Gynecol 104:39, 1969

Liu DT: Striae gravidarum. Lancet 1:625, 1974

Rook A: Diseases of pregnancy. In Rook A, Wilkinson D, Ebling F (eds): Textbook of Dermatology. Oxford, UK, Blackwell Scientific, 1972

Sauer G, Geha BJ: Impetigo herpetiformis. Arch Dermatol 83:173, 1961

Schiff B, Kern AB: Study of postpartum alopecia. Arch Dermatol 87:609, 1963

Spangler AS, et al.: Papular dermatitis of pregnancy. JAMA 181:577, 1962

Section 14
Rheumatic Diseases
Milo B. Sampson, M.D.

PRACTICE PRINCIPLES

The etiology of the rheumatic diseases is unknown. However, autoimmune mechanisms may play a major role, since immune phenomena are prominent features of these diseases. Many of these diseases occur in women during the childbearing years and may affect the outcome of pregnancy. Rheumatoid arthritis and systemic lupus erythematosus are the most important of these diseases. Scleroderma, acute rheumatic fever, and gonococcal arthritis can also occur in pregnancy.

RHEUMATOID ARTHRITIS

A. Rheumatoid arthritis is a multisystem disease affecting connective tissue with joint inflammation as the major manifestation. The course is variable but tends to become chronic and leads to characteristic deformities and disability. When the disease is active, leukocytosis, elevated C-reactive protein, and a normocytic, hypochromic anemia are common. It usually occurs in the fourth decade and is three times as common in women as in men. A positive test for rheumatoid factor is found in 70 to 80 percent of cases.

B. *Diagnosis* is made when specific American Rheumatism Association criteria are present:
   1. Morning stiffness
   2. Pain, tenderness on motion in at least one joint
   3. Swelling in at least one joint for six weeks
   4. Swelling of another joint
   5. Symmetrical joint swelling
   6. Subcutaneous nodules
   7. Bony decalcification in involved joints
   8. Positive test for rheumatoid factor
   9. Poor mucin precipitation of synovial fluid
   10. Typical histologic changes in synovium
   11. Characteristic histologic changes in nodules
   12. *Seven* criteria are required for diagnosis of classical rheumatoid arthritis, *five* criteria for rheumatoid arthritis. Patients excluded from diagnosis include those with features characteristically associated with other collagen vascular diseases (e.g., lupus erythematosus and scleroderma), infectious diseases (e.g., tuberculosis), neurologic syndromes (such as shoulder-hand syndrome), the myelomas, leukemias, and agammaglobulinemias.

C. In general, *pregnancy has a beneficial effect on RA* that extends into the postpartum period, although symptoms may first present in pregnancy. Fertility is unaffected in rheumatoid arthritis, and therapeutic abortion is not indicated.

D. *Treatment*
   1. *Aspirin.* Still the safest and most useful of the anti-inflammatory agents.
   2. *Indomethacin.* Safety has not been established in pregnancy and may cause closing of the ductus arteriosus.
   3. *Phenylbutazone.* Should be avoided if possible, since there may be an embryotoxic effect.
   4. *Gold salts.* Although not contraindicated, these are best not used in pregnancy.
   5. *Systemic corticosteroids.* Many patients can be maintained on steroids; however, the hazards of these drugs are not diminished in pregnancy.

6. *Intra-articular steroids.* Useful when rheumatoid arthritis is active in one or two joints.
7. Immunosuppressive drugs should not be used in pregnancy if possible (see discussion of systemic lupus erythematosus).

SYSTEMIC LUPUS ERYTHEMATOSUS

A. *The outcome of pregnancy* complicated by systemic lupus erythematosus (SLE) depends on the severity and whether renal disease or hypertension is present. Congenital heart block in infants of mothers with SLE has been reported and is thought to be due to transplacental passage of LE factor.
B. SLE is a *multisystem disease* characterized by inflammation in many organ systems, development of antibodies to native DNA and other nuclear materials, and a wide variety of symptoms with remissions and exacerbations. The etiology of the disease is unknown, although host responses to immunologic events may be important.
C. *Diagnosis*
   1. Anemia, leukopenia, and slight thrombocytopenia may be present in SLE.
   2. The two most useful *tests* in diagnosis of SLE are measurement of IgG antibody directed against DNA histones (anti-ANA), and antibody directed against double-stranded DNA (anti-DNA). Low complement levels (C_3 and C_4) are found in all immune complex disease, including SLE, and fall when exacerbation occurs.
   3. *Initial symptoms* usually involve joints or skin; however, patients may present with depression or central nervous system symptoms. The American Rheumatism Association criteria to diagnose SLE (four of which are necessary for diagnosis) include:
      a) Facial erythema
      b) Discoid lupus
      c) Raynaud phenomenon
      d) Alopecia

    e) Photosensitivity
    f) Nasopharyngeal or oral ulceration
    g) Arthritis without deformity
    h) LE cells
    i) Chronic false-positive test for syphilis
    j) Profuse proteinuria
    k) Cellular casts
    l) Pleuritis or pericarditis
    m) Psychosis or convulsion
    n) Hemolytic anemia, leukopenia, or thrombocytopenia

4. *Effect of pregnancy on SLE*. There is a slight risk SLE will worsen during pregnancy. Patients in remission at conception will usually remain in remission. Patients with active disease will seldom go into remission. The disease may vary from pregnancy to pregnancy. Patients with significant cardiac or renal disease should not become pregnant. Falling complement levels may herald a poor pregnancy outcome, and treatment with steroids has been recommended.

5. *Effect of SLE on pregnancy*. Forty percent of patients will abort spontaneously. This figure is increased to 50 percent when renal disease is present. One third of infants will be premature and the stillbirth rate will be increased.

6. *Therapy in pregnancy*
    a) *Sunlight* will aggravate the disease and should be avoided.
    b) *Steroids* should be given with active disease and postpartum, since exacerbations usually occur in the first month postpartum (the initial onset of disease may be at this time). Therapeutic abortion may also cause exacerbations similar to those encountered in the postpartum period.
    c) *Immunosuppressives* used for diffuse glomerulonephritis include azothiaprine, cyclophosphamide, and cholorambucil.
    d) *LE cells found in the newborn* can cause a transient hemolytic anemia, leukopenia, or thrombocytopenia.

BIBLIOGRAPHY

American Arthritis Foundation: Primer on the Rheumatic Diseases.

Bear R: Pregnancy and lupus nephritis. Obstet Gynecol 47:715, 1976

Gifford R: Rheumatic diseases. In Burrow GN, Ferris TF: Medical Complications During Pregnancy. Philadelphia, Saunders, 1975 Chap 19

Zurier RB, Argyros TG, Urman JD, et al.: Systemic lupus erythematosus, management during pregnancy. Obstet Gynecol 51:178, 1977

16

Altered Fetal Growth

Ralph K. Tamura, M.D.
Rudy E. Sabbagha, M.D.

PRACTICE PRINCIPLES

Altered fetal growth, either too slow or too rapid, may be caused by several distinctly different fetal and maternal conditions. With the advent of sophisticated antenatal assessment tools and new therapeutic modalities, many of these problems will probably become manageable in the future.

INTRAUTERINE GROWTH RETARDATION (IUGR) OR SMALL FOR GESTATIONAL AGE FETUSES (SGA)

A. *Definition of IUGR*
   1. *Birth weight ≤ 10th percentile for a given gestational age* — determined by accurate menstrual dates or by fetal sonar crown-rump length (CRL) from 8 to 10 weeks' gestation or by biparietal diameter (BPD) from 14 to 26 weeks' gestation or by pediatric examination of the neonate.
   2. *Presence of fetal malnutrition* (FM) as evidenced by tissue

wasting, i.e., decrease in muscle mass, subcutaneous tissue, and fat. *Note:* In FM, birth weight may fall above the 10th percentile for dates.

3. By either definition, IUGR can occur in term as well as preterm and postterm pregnancies.

4. *IUGR is considered moderately severe if birth weight is ≤ 3rd percentile for dates and especially if it is also accompanied by reduction in body length.*

5. Other characteristics of IUGR

   a) *Duration of IUGR*

      (1) Early fetal growth occurs primarily by cell hyperplasia or cell division. This is followed by both progressive hyperplasia and hypertrophy. Finally, in the latter stage of pregnancy, growth occurs by cellular hypertrophy alone.

      (2) Consequently, *early onset of IUGR* is likely to affect cell division adversely, leading to irreversible diminution in organ size and possibly function. Factors associated with early IUGR include: heritable causes, immunologic abnormalities, fetal infections, chronic maternal diseases (e.g., cardiovascular, metabolic), poor maternal nutrition, multiple pregnancy, and irradiation.

      (3) By contrast, *delayed onset of growth retardation* (after organ cell number is completed) tends to result only in decreased cell size and is usually reversible. The most common etiology of the latter is uteroplacental insufficiency.

   b) *Symmetric versus asymmetric IUGR.* Antenatally, this differentiation is possible only if serial cephalic (BPD) and abdominal circumference (AC) measurements are obtained. In symmetric IUGR, the result may be of long duration. As a result, both BPD and AC are < 25th percentile. In asymmetric IUGR, the BPD is normal, but the AC is < 25th percentile.

B. *Perinatal risk*

1. Seven- to eightfold increase in perinatal mortality

2. Tenfold increase in perinatal mortality if birth weight falls below 2 standard deviations of the mean for gestational age

3. Long-term physical and neurologic sequelae in approximately one-third of cases

C. *Antenatal diagnosis of IUGR*

1. *Clinical methods.* Serial evaluation of fundal height and maternal weight gain allow diagnosis in only one-third of cases. Reasons for low yield are related to inaccurate assessment of gestational age and fetal weight by parameters such as menstrual dates and uterine fundal height.

2. *Serial cephalometry*

a) There are variable degrees of success in the antenatal diagnosis of IUGR by BPD with different rates of false-positive and false-negative results. Discrepancy in these results is due to:

(1) Nonuniformity in method of obtaining sonar BPDs

(2) Insufficient BPD data prior to 26 weeks of gestation or during the interval when the BPD is an accurate predictor of fetal age

(3) Evaluation of BPD growth in relation to a mean value derived from a heterogeneous population of fetuses rather than to the growth potential of each individual fetus as established from the first BPD value

(4) Similarity in the mean BPD growth rates for IUGR and normal fetuses over short intervals of two to four weeks

b) These discrepancies suggest that *cephalometry should not be used to make definitive diagnosis of IUGR; rather, serial BPDs should be used to identify fetuses at high risk for IUGR,* with the understanding that a certain proportion will be normal.

c) The sensitivity of cephalometry is about 50 percent (i.e., the proportion of undergrown neonates correctly predicted by a ≤ 25th percentile).

3. *Fetal abdominal circumference measurements (AC)*
   a) The fetal AC is more likely to predict IUGR, since the measurement reflects the size of the fetal liver and amount of subcutaneous tissue, both of which are small in SGA fetuses.
   b) AC measurements correctly detect IUGR in approximately 70 percent of cases in the third trimester of pregnancy.
4. *Head-to-abdomen circumference ratios (H/A).* In normal pregnancies, the H/A ratio is > 1.0 until 35 to 37 weeks of gestation. Following this interval, the AC increases rapidly and the H/A declines to < 1.0. Nonetheless, in approximately 70 percent of cases with asymmetric IUGR, the H/A ratio remains > 1.0 and at least > 2 standard deviations above the mean H/A value.
5. *Total intrauterine volume (TIUV)*
   a) The TIUV is obtained from multiple ultrasound measurements of the uterus (length × width × height × 0.5)
   b) The sensitivity of TIUV (proportion of undergrown fetsues with TIUV < 1 standard deviation) is about 50 percent.
   c) It should be noted that placental hypertrophy or polyhydramnios would invalidate TIUV for the detection of IUGR. In addition, dates should be objectively defined by fetal CRL or early BPD measurement for proper interpretation of TIUV.
6. *Assessment of individual fetal growth potential using both BPD and AC*
   a) *BPD measurements* are obtained in the intervals of 18 to 26 weeks and 30 to 33 weeks of pregnancy. Based on curves relating BPD to gestational age, the fetus is assigned a BPD growth percentile which:
      (1) Defines its gestational age to within ± 3 days by using the growth-adjusted sonar age method (GASA)
      (2) Establishes its potential cephalic growth for the remainder of the pregnancy

b) *AC measurements* are obtained at the 30 to 33 week interval or between 34 and 37 weeks of gestation, depending on the BPD percentile rank and/or presence of adverse clinical conditions. Based on curves relating AC to gestational age, the fetus is assigned a growth percentile for the AC. The AC percentile measurement serves primarily to estimate fetal body size.

c) Sonar measurements allow classification of each of the BPD and AC values into three possible growth patterns: large (> 75th percentile), small (< 25th percentile), and average (25th to 75th percentiles). *By relating the three BPD growth patterns to a specific AC percentile rank, nine fetal growth combinations are possible* (Fig. 16–1). Preliminary data indicate the following:

   (1) *Large for gestational age fetuses (LGA)* are likely to fall into growth patterns 1 and 4.

   (2) *Asymmetric IUGR fetuses* are likely to fall into

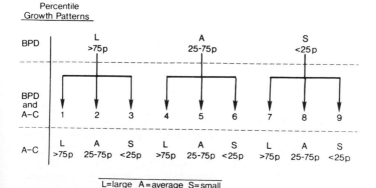

Figure 16–1. Nine fetal growth patterns noted by using both BPD and AC percentile (*p*).(From Tamura RK, Sabbagha RE: Am J Obstet Gynecol 138 No. 5:475–479, 1980.)

growth patterns 3 and 6. TIUV measurements may lend further credence to the diagnosis.

   (3) *Symmetric IUGR fetuses* are likely to fall into growth pattern 9. TIUV measurements may lend further credence to the diagnosis.

   (4) *Appropriate for gestational age fetuses (AGA)* are likely to fall into growth patterns 2, 5, 7, and 8.

  d) Preliminary results indicate that approximately 70 to 75 percent of IUGR fetuses would be detected by this method.

D. *Antenatal management of IUGR*

  1. Use of sonar BPD and AC at intervals of approximately three weeks to diagnose and to make prospective evaluations of the course of the individual fetus with suspected IUGR.

  2. Bioelectric testing. Nonstress tests (NSTs) weekly and oxytocin challenge tests (OCTs) when indicated.

  3. Biochemical testing (e.g., estriol) when indicated.

  4. Dynamic ultrasound modalities to assess fetal breathing movements, fetal movements, fetal tone, and qualitative amniotic fluid volume. These methods are investigational at present and together with the NST constitute the biophysical profile of the fetus.

  5. Assessment of pulmonary maturity by amniocentesis.

  6. The final decision for delivery of a pregnancy complicated by IUGR must be individualized on the basis of the available antepartum data.

E. *Neonatal complications*

  1. Asphyxia and associated meconium aspiration, pneumonia, and intracranial hemorrhage.

  2. Hypoglycemia (blood glucose values less than 30 to 40 mg/ml)

   a) Incidence: 29 to 67 percent

   b) Most frequently observed in preterm IUGR neonates and in the presence of hypoxia or hypothermia or both

   c) Etiology related to deficient reserves, high brain-to-liver ratio (resulting in glucose demands that outstrip

      rates of production), and delayed onset of gluconeogenesis
3. Transient neonatal hyperglycemia usually preceded by hypoglycemia
4. Hypocalcemia
5. Electrolyte disturbances
6. Polycythemia
7. Massive pulmonary hemorrhage

F. *Prognosis for growth and development*
1. Prognosis is difficult to assess because of the heterogeneity of IUGR fetuses, i.e., symmetric versus asymmetric.
2. With appropriate postnatal nutrition, there is evidence for "catch-up" growth in the first year of life.
3. In one prospective study, IUGR infants progressed to normal IQ. However, 25 percent of 96 full-term SGA infants had evidence of minimal cerebral dysfunction.

ACCELERATED FETAL GROWTH: MACROSOMIA

A. *Definitions*
1. Birth weights $\geq$ 4500 gm
2. Recent pediatric studies using skin-fold thickness measurements in the immediate neonatal period may serve to further delineate these LGA infants.

B. *Perinatal risk*
1. Three-fold increase in perinatal mortality.
2. Fetuses weighing more than 4000 gm are at risk for prolonged second stage of labor, midforceps delivery, shoulder dystocia, and immediate neonatal injury.
3. Severe neurologic disability in approximately 11 percent of infants.

C. *Antenatal diagnosis of accelerated fetal growth*
1. Macrosomia tends to occur with greater frequency in class A, B, and C diabetic gravidas.
2. Macrosomia is observed in a variety of conditions includ-

ing: fetuses of diabetic mothers, fetal insulinomas, nesidioblastosis, and Beckwith-Wiedman syndrome.

3. Recent studies utilizing ultrasound measurement of the BPD and AC (see section on IUGR above — assessment of fetal growth potential using both BPD and AC percentile measurements) appear promising for the detection of macrosomia. For example, for 23 infants of diabetic mothers (White's classes A to C), the BPD values for all fetuses fell in the normal range, whereas the AC values of 10 of the 23 fetuses were greater than 2 standard deviations above the mean. The birth weights and skin-fold thicknesses of the latter infants were significantly greater than for the others.

4. Because of the paucity of data, the accuracy of antenatal prediction of macrosomia cannot be determined at this time.

D. *Antenatal management of macrosomia*
   1. The antenatal management of macrosomia is essentially that for the management of the diabetic pregnancy.
   2. Ultrasound assessment of fetal weight may be of some assistance in determining the mode of delivery.

BIBLIOGRAPHY

Sabbagha RE: Biparietal diameter and gestational age. In Sabbagha RE (ed): Ultrasound Applied to Obstetrics and Gynecology. Hagerstown, Md, Harper & Row, 1980, pp 79–91

Sabbagha RE: Intrauterine growth retardation. In Sabbagha RE (ed): Ultrasound Applied to Obstetrics and Gynecology. Hagerstown, Md, Harper & Row, 1980, pp 103–110

Tamura RK, Sabbagha RE: Altered fetal growth. In Sciarra JJ, and Depp R (eds): Gynecology and Obstetrics, Vol 3: Maternal-Fetal Medicine. Hagerstown, Md, Harper & Row (in press)

17

Determination of Gestational Age and the Management of Postdatism

Bruce A. Work, Jr., M.D.

PRACTICE PRINCIPLES

Precise knowledge of age of the fetus is imperative for ideal obstetric management. Therefore, expert attention must be given to this important measurement. The clinically appropriate unit of measure is *weeks of gestation completed*.

DURATION OF HUMAN PREGNANCY

A. *Definition*
   1. *Clinical age:* 280 days or 40 weeks (9 calendar months or 10 lunar months) from last *normal* menstrual period (LNMP)
   2. *Ovulatory or fertilization age:* 266 days or 38 weeks from ovulation in 28-day ovarian cycle
B. *Calculation of duration of pregnancy or estimated date of confinement* (EDC)
   1. By use of a gestational age calendar, or calculator (Fig. 17–1).

461

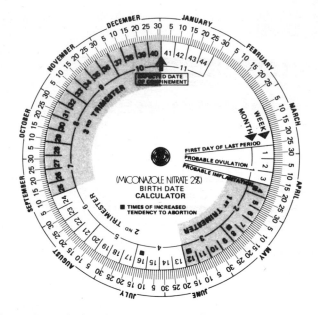

Figure 17–1. Gestational age calculator. For example, an LNMP of April 18 gives an EDC of January 21. (Used with permission from Ortho Pharmaceutical Corporation, Raritan, New Jersey.)

   2. By Naegele's rule: Subtract 3 from month of LNMP and add 7 to first day of LNMP. *Example:* LNMP September 13 gives EDC of June 20.

CLINICAL PARAMETERS

A. Evaluation of uterine size at first visit if patient seen before 12 to 16 weeks
B. Growth of uterus
   1. Fundus palpable over symphysis pubis at 12 to 14 weeks
   2. Fundus palpable at umbilicus at 20 weeks
   3. Average fundal height at 40 weeks 35 cm
   4. Graph of fundal heights per visit—most dynamic means

of visualizing relative age, as well as relative growth assessment (Fig. 17–2).

5. Quickening (maternal appreciation of fetal movement) is noted in the 17th week by the average multiparous patient and the 18th week by the average primiparous patient

6. Fetal heart tones by auscultation can be heard during the 20th week

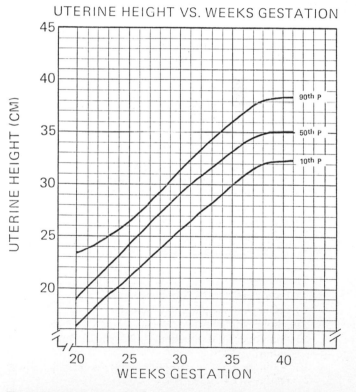

UTERINE HEIGHT VS. WEEKS GESTATION

Figure 17–2. Uterine growth curve chart. (Courtesy of the Department of Obstetrics and Gynecology, University of Illinois School of Medicine.)

    7. All factors are influenced by size of mother, size of baby, maternal conditions with possible effects on growth such as hypertension, and volume of amniotic fluid

C. Imaging techniques for assessment for gestational age
  1. X-ray examination
    a) Used before introduction of sonography
    b) Ossification centers
      (1) Distal femoral epiphysis at 36 weeks in 80 percent of fetuses
      (2) Proximal tibial epiphysis at 40 weeks in 70 to 75 percent of fetuses
    c) Degree of calcification of skull and long bones compared to mature bone, i.e., maternal pelvis, suggests duration as near 40 weeks
    d) Presence of fetal fat line in nondiabetic pregnancy suggest maturity and thus correlates with gestational age as approaching 40 weeks
  2. Ultrasound examination
    a) Measurement of early gestational sac: 2 cm at 6 weeks, 5 cm at 10 weeks
    b) Biparietal diameter: measured from 12 weeks to 33 weeks with good accuracy (Table 17–1)
    c) Intrauterine volumes (less used currently)
    d) Abdominal circumferences (Table 17–2)

D. Associated parameters *not* correlated with gestational age (how old?), but associated with *functional maturity* (does it work?) of different organ systems or status of *well-being* (is it sick?).
  1. Well-being
    a) Estrogens: total, estriol, estetrol
    b) Serum human placental lactogen
  2. Functional maturity
    a) Amniotic fluid creatinine (2.0 mg/dl indicative of maturity)
    b) Amniotic fluid spectrophotometric determinations at 650 μm (< 0.15)
    c) "Fetal fat cells": sebaceous material free or in cells in amniotic fluid

TABLE 17–1. NOMOGRAM FOR BIPARIETAL DIAMETER VERSUS GESTATIONAL AGE USING EDGE TO LEADING EDGE (YALE)*

cm	Weeks gestation	cm	Weeks gestation	cm	Weeks gestation
1.9	12.0	4.5	20.5	6.9	29.0
2.0	12.0	4.6	21.0	7.0	29.5
2.1	12.5	4.7	21.0	7.1	30.0
2.2	13.0	4.8	21.5	7.3	30.5
2.3	13.0	4.9	22.0	7.4	31.0
2.4	13.5	5.0	22.0	7.5	31.5
2.5	14.0	5.1	22.5	7.6	32.0
2.6	14.0	5.2	23.0	7.7	32.5
2.7	14.5	5.3	23.0	7.8	33.0
2.8	15.0	5.4	23.5	7.9	33.5
2.9	15.0	5.5	24.0	8.0	34.0
3.0	15.5	5.6	24.0	8.2	34.5
3.1	16.0	5.7	24.5	8.3	35.0
3.2	16.0	5.8	25.0	8.4	35.5
3.3	16.5	5.9	25.0	8.5	36.0
3.4	17.0	6.0	25.5	8.6	36.5 *mature*
3.5	17.0	6.1	26.0	8.8	37.0
3.6	17.5	6.2	26.0	8.9	37.5
3.7	18.0	6.3	26.5	9.0	38.0
3.8	18.5	6.4	27.0	9.1	38.5
4.0	19.0	6.5	27.0	9.2	39.0
4.2	19.5	6.6	27.5	9.3	39.5
4.3	20.0	6.7	28.0	9.4	40.0
4.4	20.0	6.8	28.5	9.6	40.5
				9.7	41.0

*Measurements on bistable grid.

d) Phospholipids and other measurements of surfactant activity. Surfactant lowers surface tension of alveoli and allows alveoli to expand. Phospholipid measurements reflect surfactant activity, since surfactant is 90 percent lipid and 10 percent protein: 90 percent of the lipids are phospholipids, the bulk being lecithin. Two acidic phospholipids phosphatidyl inositol (PI) and phosphatidyl glycerol (PG) are involved in

TABLE 17–2. ABDOMINAL CIRCUMFERENCE VERSUS ESTIMATED BIRTH WEIGHT

Abdominal circumference (cm)	Estimated birth weight centiles (kg) 5*		50	95*
21	0.78	(86.4)	0.90 1.04	(115.7)
22	0.90	(86.7)	1.03 1.19	(115.3)
23	1.03	(86.9)	1.18 1.36	(115.0)
24	1.17	(87.1)	1.34 1.54	(114.8)
25	1.32	(87.2)	1.51 1.73	(114.7)
26	1.47	(87.3)	1.69 1.94	(114.6)
27	1.64	(87.3)	1.88 2.15	(114.5)
28	1.81	(87.3)	2.09 2.38	(114.5)
29	1.99	(87.3)	2.28 2.61	(114.5)
30	2.17	(87.4)	2.49 2.85	(114.5)
31	2.35	(87.4)	2.69 3.08	(114.5)
32	2.53	(87.4)	2.90 3.32	(114.4)
33	2.71	(87.4)	3.10 3.55	(114.4)
34	2.88	(87.4)	3.29 3.76	(114.4)
35	3.03	(87.4)	3.47 3.97	(114.4)
36	3.18	(87.4)	3.64 4.16	(114.4)
37	3.31	(87.3)	3.79 4.33	(114.5)
38	3.42	(87.3)	3.92 4.49	(114.6)
39	3.51	(87.2)	4.02 4.61	(114.7)
40	3.57	(87.0)	4.10 4.72	(115.0)

*Figures in brackets represent the centile limit expressed as a percentage of the median birth weight.

metabolism of the AF phospholipids and surfactant. PI peaks at 35 to 36 weeks; PG increases after 36 weeks; and PG > PI at term

POSTDATISM AND POSTMATURITY

A. *Definitions*
   1. *Postdatism* is any pregnancy exceeding 42 weeks of gestation completed regardless of state of well-being.
   2. *Postmaturity* represents a dysmature state found in some

postdatism pregnancies and represents compromise of well-being.

  3. Clifford's stages

    a) *Stage I.* Infant has long nails and abundant hair; he or she is alert but has apprehensive facies and exhibits depletion of subcutaneous tissue. Mild respiratory distress syndrome (RDS) in 30 percent.

    b) *Stage II.* All the above plus meconium staining of skin and fetal membranes. Poor prognosis.

    c) *Stage III.* Yellow staining of skin and membranes. Severe RDS and often central nervous system damage.

B. *Occurrence*

  1. Approximately 80 percent of all pregnancies delivered between 37 and 42 weeks.

  2. Approximately 10 percent of pregnancies exceed 42 weeks' gestation and approximately 10 percent of these will manifest postmaturity or dysmaturity findings.

  3. Perinatal mortality from intrapartum fetal distress, meconium aspiration, and RDS:

    a) Lowest in 40 to 41-week group, doubles by 43 weeks, and trebles by 44 weeks.

    b) With evidence of toxemia, perinatal mortality doubles at 42 weeks, triples at 42½, and quadruples at 43.

C. *Etiology*

  1. Apparent postdatism may be the result of an error in dates or delayed ovulation, i.e., LNMP as remembered may be off by a month or may represent delayed ovulation in a given cycle, e.g., occurring on day 21 versus the average of day 14.

  2. Postmaturity appears to be due to failing placental function with subsequent compromise of fetus.

D. *Management*

  1. Antepartum

    a) Weeks 40 and 41

      (1) Reassess gestational age data.

      (2) Begin gestational age graph as device for summary of data (Fig. 17–3).

LEGEND:
+ EDC
● Fundal height
O Fetal heart tones first heard
△ Quickening:
   Primigravida = 19 weeks
   Multigravida = 17 weeks

❙ First exam
▼ Ultrasound
◇ X-ray
★ Positive UCG

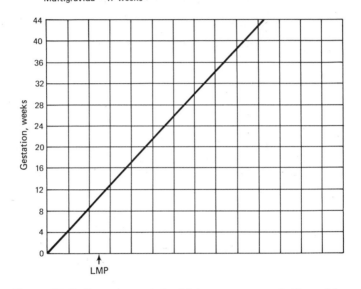

Figure 17–3. Dynamic graph for fetal age assessment. (From Johnson TR, Work BA Jr: Obstet Gynecol 54:115, 1979.)

      (3) In addition to weight and fundal height, measure girth and record.

      (4) Assess cervix as to favorability for induction (Bishop score, > 6 suggests suitability).

      (5) Proceed to *prompt* delivery with *evidence of toxemia or maternal age > 35 years.*

   b) Week 42

      (1) Measure serum estriol (E_{3s}) three times in week.

      (2) Perform NST two times in week, OCT if nonreactive.

      (3) Perform amniocentesis for lecithin/sphingomyelin ratio and presence of meconium in amniotic fluid.

      (4) Consider amnioscopy if equipped and experienced.

      (5) Proceed to prompt delivery if:

         (a) Favorable cervix

         (b) Large fetus (> 4000 gm)

         (c) Suspicious or positive OCT

         (d) Meconium in amniotic fluid

         (e) Evidence of toxemia

  c) Week 43

      (1) All of the above

      (2) In view of increased perinatal mortality, consider delivery of all cases regardless of other factors.

2. Intrapartum

  a) Continuously monitor FHR and uterine activity by direct mode.

  b) Avoid prolonged labor.

  c) Avoid difficult or traumatic vaginal delivery.

  d) Suction nares and nasopharynx as soon as head appears before delivery of shoulders if meconium present.

  e) Have neonatologist in attendance.

BIBLIOGRAPHY

Anderson GG: Postmaturity: A review. Obstet Gynecol Surv 27:65, 1972

Anderson HF, et al.: Gestational age assessment. Am J. Obstet Gynecol 139:173, 1981

Ballantyne JW: The problem of the postmature infant. J Obstet Gynecol Br Emp 2:521, 1902

Brown JCM: Postmaturity. Am J Obstet Gynecol 85:573, 1963

Clifford SH: Postmaturity — with placental dysfunctions. J Pediatr 44:1, 1954

Johnson TR, Work BA Jr: A dynamic graph for documentation of gestational age. Obstet Gynecol 54:115, 1979

Vorhere H: Placental insufficiency in relation to post term pregnancy and fetal postmaturity. Am J Obstet Gynecol 123:67, 1975

18

Fetal Monitoring and Fetal Distress

Jeffrey C. King, M.D.

PRACTICE PRINCIPLES

Since its introduction in the late 1960s, continuous electronic monitoring of the fetal heart rate (FHR) has become one of the mainstays of both antepartum and intrapartum fetal surveillance. Today, continuous electronic fetal monitoring (EFM) is used during labor in as many as 60 to 70 percent of pregnancies. The advantage of EFM is that it allows the physician to record the fetal response to recurrent stress, i.e., uterine contractions. While intrapartum EFM is considered mandatory for the high-risk population, its exact value in the management of low-risk patients remains questionable.

REGULATION OF FHR

Baseline FHR reflects the instantaneous product of accelerator (sympathetic) and decelerator (parasympathetic or vagal) signals to the fetal cardioregulatory center located in the midbrain. Since these signals exert their control in a push-pull fashion, the presence of normal FHR variability probably indicates that both inputs are functioning appropriately. The autonomic nerve pathways are established very early during fetal development. There is a slight slowing of FHR when followed serially from the first trimester to term. This confirms the experiments of Caldeyro-Barcia, which indicate an increasing vagal effect as gestational age advances. However, base-line FHR outside the normal range [120 to 160 beats per minute (bpm)] cannot be explained solely by prematurity.

Activation of the sympathetic nerve trunks results in acceleration of fetal heart rate and increase in force of cardiac contraction. While epinephrine, the sympathetic neurotransmitter, produces similar effects on the fetal heart, it causes vasoconstriction and fetal hypertension, which may result in reflex bradycardia.

REFLEXES AFFECTING FHR

Arterial blood pressure is primarily regulated by the baroreceptor reflex. Fetal hypertension increases the activity of these receptors located in the aortic arch and carotid sinuses. Stimulation results in increased parasympathetic activity and decreased sympathetic activity. The overall effect is deceleration with arterial hypertension, acceleration with hypotension.

A fall in the P_{O_2} of arterial blood acts as the primary stimulus to the carotid and aortic chemoreceptors. In addition, changes in pH and P_{CO_2} may also result in activation. Stimulation of these chemoreceptors results in peripheral vasoconstriction, with unpredictable changes in FHR. Martin has shown that acute hypoxia produces slowing of FHR and increased variability.

INSTRUMENTATION OF FHR MONITORING

An electronic fetal monitor obtains, processes, and records signals from both mother and fetus. The fetal signal is obtained by either an electrode or a transducer. It is then converted to an electrical signal within the monitor and amplified; a "heart signal" results. The interval between successive signals is measured and an instantaneous FHR determined. Most modern monitors have the capacity to electrically filter the signal in order to remove extraneous noise and enhance its clarity. This "logic" rejects rate changes of 30 bpm or more between successive beats or an absolute rate greater than 240 bpm. If this data is received, it is rejected and not recorded. While this may be helpful to "clean up" an external monitor tracing, it may prevent identification of fetal cardiac arrhythmias during direct monitoring of labor.

A. *Indirect*

1. *Phonocardiography.* Valvular motion may be used to define the time interval between cardiac cycles precisely. An extremely sensitive microphone has been developed to "listen" to those frequencies associated with heart sounds. However, during labor, the noise of uterine contractions, bowel sounds, maternal vessels, and maternal movement may interfere with the ability to detect the fetal signal, thereby making this technique unacceptable. Phonocardiography may be unsuccessful in producing an acceptable tracing when obesity or polyhydramniosis complicates the pregnancy.

2. *Abdominal ECG.* The present technology allows separation of the fetal and maternal ECG signal. Logic circuitry is very important in separating these signals to determine the interval between successive fetal cardiac events. While this technique may be successful (25 to 50 percent) during the antepartum period when the uterus is quiescent, it is useless during labor due to extraneous muscular and maternal activity.

3. *Doppler ultrasound.* The principle of Doppler-shift ultrasonography is the most common noninvasive method for determining fetal heart rate. The ultrasound beam is reflected off various tissue interfaces back to the transducer. Since there is continuous reflection during both systole and diastole, the monitor uses a logic circuit to extrapolate the FHR and reject "illogical" information. Since it is impossible to keep the beam directed at a particular point of fetal intracardiac anatomy, the exact rate cannot be determined. Therefore, beat-to-beat

variability (BBV) cannot be interpreted using this indirect method.

B. *Direct*

1. By attaching a bipolar spiral electrode to the fetal presenting part a fetal electrocardiogram (FECG) is obtained. The interval between each fetal R wave is recognized by the monitor and an exact FHR is determined. *It is essential that the obstetrician be aware that the FECG provides an indication of the electrical activity of the fetal heart and does not necessarily represent mechanical cardiac activity.*

2. Since the exact fetal heart rate is displayed by the monitor, fetal beat-to-beat variability is reliably represented. Obviously, since the electrode is attached to the fetus directly, the fetal membranes must be ruptured. Care must be taken when the electrode is attached to the presenting part. When the fetal head is flexed, cranial suture lines and fontanels must be avoided. If the head is extended, facial structures (eyes, nose, mouth) can be injured by application of the electrode. With breech presentations, the genitalia must be avoided, and the electrode should be attached only to the fetal buttocks. Serious complications, most commonly infections, occur as a result of electrode placement in about 1 of 700 to 1000 attachments.

MEASUREMENT OF UTERINE ACTIVITY

Indirect

Indirect measurement is used when fetal membranes have not yet ruptured or the cervix is closed. An external tocodynamometer is used to record uterine activity. A change in shape and hardness of the uterus moves a plunger within the tocotransducer, resulting in a deflection on the monitor tracing. It is important to remember that *external monitoring only documents movement and the exact strength of contraction cannot be inferred.* Base-line tone and peak amplitude of uterine contractions cannot be measured. The tocodynamometer is attached to the maternal abdomen by elastic belts, and the location of the transducer should be adjusted every hour to prevent skin irritation.

Direct

Measurement of actual intrauterine pressure can be recorded by inserting a small fluid-filled catheter into the amniotic space. This catheter may be inserted transabdominally or, more commonly, transcervically via an introducer. Transcervical insertion requires that the membranes be ruptured. Care must be taken during insertion to prevent the complications of lower uterine segment perforation by the introducer. Multiple studies have examined the relationship between intrauterine pressure catheters and infection. It appears that there is no direct relationship. However, aseptic techniques should be used during insertion.

FETAL MONITOR INTERPRETATION

Each fetal monitor tracing should be interpreted using a routine systematic approach. The obstetrician then is sure of "looking" at all aspects of the tracing. Base-line fetal heart rate, variability, periodic changes, and uterine activity must be determined (Fig. 18–1).

A. *Baseline*. Baseline refers to the FHR occurring between periodic changes. Sympathetic stimulation increases baseline, while parasympathetic activity causes a slowing of FHR. The *normal baseline ranges* between 120 and 160 bmp. Rates greater than 160 bpm (*fetal tachycardia*) may be due to maternal fever, hyperthyroidism, hypoxia, anemia, or tachyarrhythmias. *Fetal bradycardia* (rates below 120 bpm) can result from congenital heart defects, heart block, or hypoxia (Fig. 18–2).

B. *Variability*. When FHR is obtained by a direct electrode, the monitor can determine instantaneous FHR, which results in accurate BBV. *Short-term variability* refers to the change of FHR from one beat to another. The normal short-term BBV

476

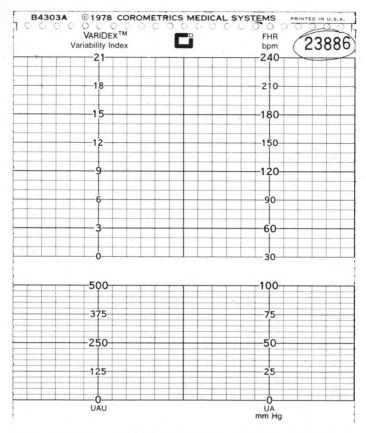

Figure 18–1. Standard fetal monitor paper with FHR values between 30 and 240 bpm. Uterine activity is displayed from 0 to 100 mm Hg. Varidex and UAU are developments of Corometrics Medical Systems to provide the clinician with added information about fetal status. It is standard that the paper speed be run at 3 cm/minute. All examples in this chapter are at that paper speed.

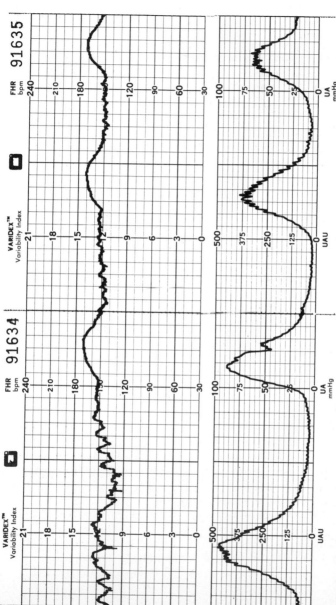

Figure 18–2. External tocodynamometer and direct scalp electrode tracings showing normal FHR baseline with good variability. Smooth accelerations are evident, occurring with each contraction. The clinician should be aware that this type of acceleration may represent early umbilical vein occlusion that can progress to variable decelerations.

ranges between 5 and 10 bpm. *Long-term variability* is the general undulation or waviness of the FHR tracing, occurring with a frequency of 3 to 5 cycles/minute. Variability seems to be a reflection of an intact or normal cardioregulatory center and cardiac responsiveness. Most investigators agree that normal variability is predictive of normal fetal pH. The significance of increased or decreased variability remains questionable. Increased variability may be associated with fetal movement but is often seen early in the development of late decelerations. Certain medications (narcotics or $MgSO_4$, for example) and fetal "sleep" can produce decreased variability, but fetal acidosis/hypoxia is its most common cause (Figs. 18–3, 18–4).

C. *Periodic changes.* Short-term alterations of FHR, either accelerations or decelerations, associated with fetal movement, stimulation, or uterine contractions are periodic changes. *Accelerations* are generally considered to be a sign of good fetal well-being. They indicate the ability of the fetus to respond to a sympathetic discharge. Conversely, *decelerations* of fetal heart rate are always abnormal and may reflect poor fetal health (Fig. 18–5).

D. *Uterine contractions. Normal baseline uterine tone* is between 5 and 12 mm Hg. Values above 15 to 20 mm Hg are defined as *hypertonous*. Studies have shown that when intraamniotic pressure rises above 30 mm Hg, intervillous space perfusion ceases and maternal perception of uterine contractions begins. During normal labor, the strength of contractions varies from an average of 30 mm Hg in early labor to 50 mm Hg in late first stage and 80 to 120 mm Hg during second stage. Generally, contractions last 60 seconds during normal labor.

Types of Decelerations

A. *Early decelerations*
   1. Early decelerations are uniformly U-shaped decelerations of both slow onset and return to baseline. They

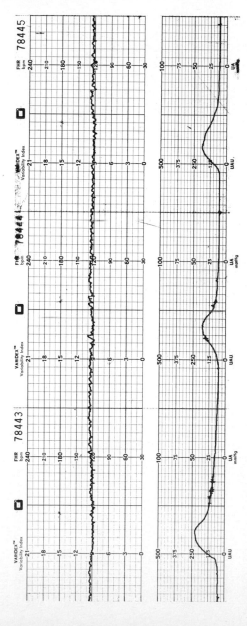

Figure 18–3. Intrauterine pressure catheter and scalp electrode tracings showing normal uterine tone and normal baseline FHR. The long-term variability is decreased but the short-term variability appears to be normal.

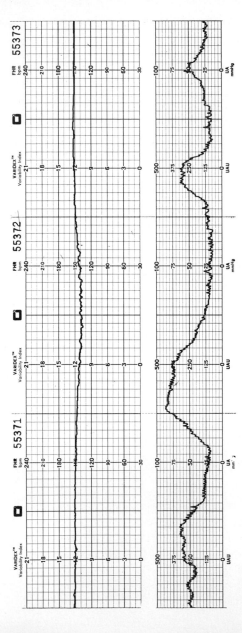

Figure 18–4. External uterine tocodynamometer and direct fetal scalp electrode tracings showing absent short- and long-term variability with a suggestion of a late deceleration due to prolonged uterine hypertonus. Fetal scalp blood sampling is suggested for further evaluation of this type of tracing.

begin early in the contraction cycle, have their nadir at the peak of the contraction, and return to baseline prior to completion of the contraction. The extent of FHR descent generally parallels the strength of uterine contraction.

2. Rarely does the FHR fall below 100 bpm. It appears that *head compression* and increased intracranial pressure cause cardiac slowing through a vagal reflex; therefore, it may be blocked by atropine. Early decelerations are a reassuring heart rate pattern and felt to be innocuous. Since they are not associated with fetal hypoxia, acidosis, or low Apgar scores, no treatment is necessary (Fig. 18–6).

B. *Late decelerations*

1. This type of deceleration is similar in shape and uniformity to early decelerations, but the timing is delayed relative to the contraction. The onset of deceleration is 30 seconds or more after the onset of the contraction, and the FHR returns to baseline significantly after the contraction has ended. Late decelerations are rarely more than 10 to 20 bpm below baseline. It is generally believed that hypoxia due to *uteroplacental insufficiency* results in either direct myocardial suppression or a chemoreceptor reflex. This type of deceleration is *always pathologic if repetitive.*

2. *Uteroplacental insufficiency* is treated by discontinuing oxytocics, expanding maternal volume, left uterine displacement, and oxygen. Persistence of late decelerations mandates further investigation, i.e., fetal scalp blood sampling. The development of fetal tachycardia and absent variability indicates fetal distress, and delivery should be accomplished immediately (Fig. 18–7).

C. *Variable decelerations*

1. The most frequently observed FHR deceleration pattern during labor is variable decelerations. It is variable in configuration, duration, intensity, and timing relative to

482

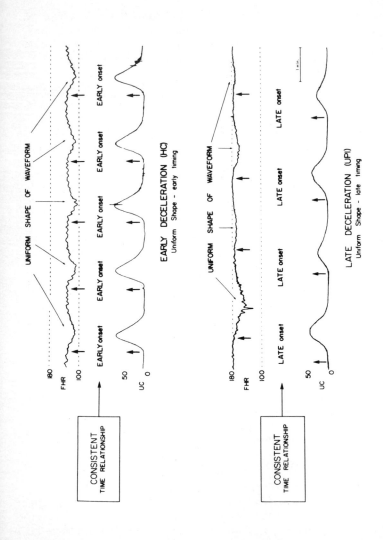

CONSISTENT TIME RELATIONSHIP

UNIFORM SHAPE OF WAVEFORM

180
FHR
100

EARLY onset   EARLY onset   EARLY onset   EARLY onset   EARLY onset   EARLY onset

50
UC 0

EARLY DECELERATION (HC)
Uniform Shape - early timing

CONSISTENT TIME RELATIONSHIP

UNIFORM SHAPE OF WAVEFORM

180
FHR
100

LATE onset   LATE onset   LATE onset   LATE onset   LATE onset

50
UC 0

1 min.

LATE DECELERATION (UPI)
Uniform Shape - late timing

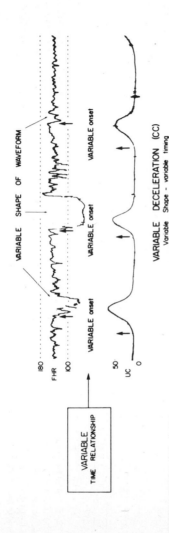

Figure 18–5. Fetal heart rate decelerations in relation to the time of onset of uterine contractions. (From Hon: An Atlas of Fetal Heart Rate Patterns. New Haven, Harty Press, 1968.)

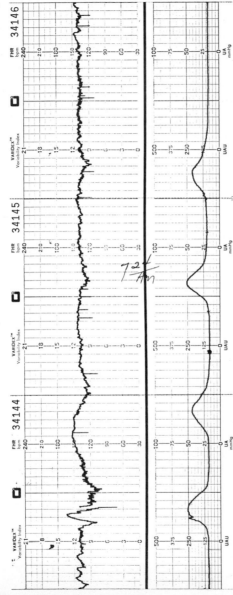

Figure 18–6. Intrauterine pressure catheter tracings showing a borderline increased uterine tonus; however, values such as this can be obtained if the transducer is not properly leveled with regard to the maternal xiphoid. The direct electrode reveals a combined pattern of FHR decelerations. The first deceleration is an obvious variable. At 34144, a late deceleration can be seen, which is followed by what appears to be an early deceleration. Following 34145, a fetal deceleration occurs that assumes the onset timing and shape of a late deceleration, but there is return to baseline by the end of the contraction.

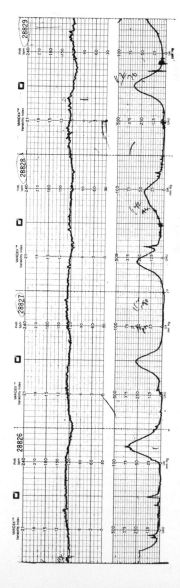

Figure 18–7. Recurrent late decelerations shown on scalp electrode with intrauterine pressure catheter tracings. Fetal scalp blood sampling was performed, revealing a pH of 7.22, but because of the persistence of this abnormal pattern, an emergency cesarean section was performed. The neonate had a central pH at birth of 7.20.

485

uterine contractions. They appear to result from *compression of the umbilical cord,* and their resultant fetal insult will vary with the duration and degree of compression.

2. Accelerations may precede or follow the deceleration. It is felt that they represent a compensatory fetal response to umbilical vein obstruction.

3. Kubli has graded variable decelerations as:
   a) *Mild.* Duration less than 30 seconds regardless of level or FHR greater than 80 bpm regardless of duration.
   b) *Moderate.* FHR less than 80 bpm regardless of duration.
   c) *Severe.* Less than 70 bpm for greater than 60 seconds.

4. The clinician should make every attempt to alter maternal position in order to relieve the cord compression. If there are persistent moderate to severe variable decelerations associated with tachycardia or loss of variability, scalp blood sampling is necessary (Fig. 18–8).

D. *Arrhythmia.* Arrhythmias occur in about 5% of all monitor tracings. Usually, they do not represent fetal hypoxia. Fortunately, most cases of arrhythmia resolve spontaneously following delivery. When complete fetal heart block occurs, evidence of maternal autoimmune disease may be found. The fetus must be closely watched for the development of congestive failure if tachyarrhythmias develop. Multiple reports have suggested maternal treatment with digoxin or propranolol is effective in controlling fetal tachyarrhythmias (Figs. 18–9 to 18–11).

E. *Second-stage patterns.* Late in the second stage of labor, severe and prolonged decelerations of the FHR may occur from any combination of cord compression, placental insufficiency, or head compression. Generally, these patterns are benign but can result in fetal acidosis. Other monitors of fetal condition are necessary, such as scalp blood sampling. If BBV disappears, the fetus must be suspected of deterioration.

487

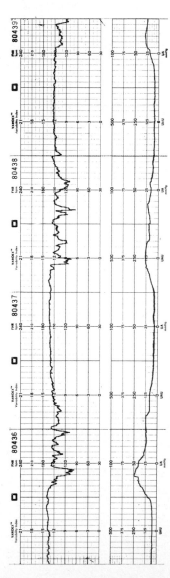

Figure 18–8. External uterine tocodynamometer and direct electrode tracings showing classic variable decelerations. Alterations of maternal position resulted in a normal FHR within 10 minutes.

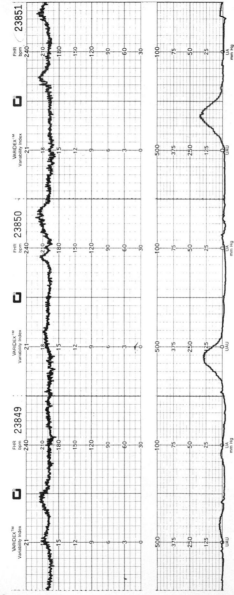

Figure 18–9. External monitoring of a patient at 38 weeks gestation who was found to have an elevated FHR at a routine prenatal visit. Maternal fever, amnionitis, and hyperthyroidism were ruled out. Ultrasonography showed that the fetal atria and ventricles were contracting synchronously, and evidence of congestive heart failure (fetal) was absent. The neonate was found to have paroxysmal atrial tachycardia that responded to digoxin.

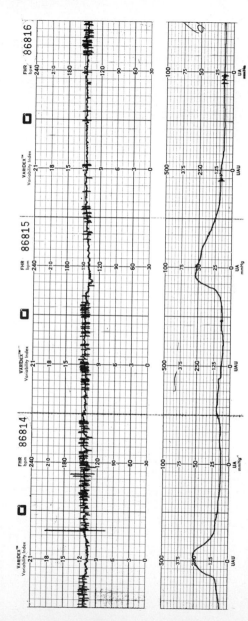

Figure 18–10. Direct scalp electrode tracing reveals a fetal arrhythmia that proved to be unifocal premature ventricular contractions. This abnormality resolved within 48 hours of delivery.

489

490

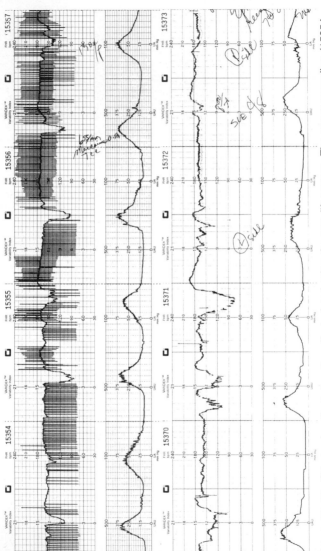

Figure 18–11. This tracing illustrates the effect of activating the pen lift system. The upper recording (15354–15357) shows evidence of multifocal premature ventricular contractions with the pen lift out and variable decelerations. The lower recording (15370–15373) shows variable decelerations after the tracing has been "cleaned up" with the pen lift in.

FETAL SCALP BLOOD SAMPLING

A. *Physiology*
1. It appears that the interpretation of FHR patterns with fetal scalp blood sampling increases the accuracy of the predictability for fetal well-being or fetal distress. Fetal acidosis results from decreased oxygen availability to fetal tissue, causing a change from aerobic to anaerobic glycolysis. This leads to an accumulation of carbon dioxide, hydrogen ions, and lactate.
2. After the formation of lactate in the presence of excess hydrogen ions, there is a reaction with bicarbonate to cause a reduction in hydrogen ions (buffer effect) and liberation of carbon dioxide. This carbon dioxide can then be exchanged across the placenta and eliminated by the mother. However, when cord compression or uteroplacental insufficiency occurs, there is accumulation of carbon dioxide and hydrogen ions in the fetus. Therefore, determination of pH will show the extent of fetal impairment of these metabolic pathways.

B. *Technic.* Fetal blood may be obtained by inserting a vaginal obturator against the fetal presenting part when the cervix is more than 3 cm dilated and membranes are ruptured. An incision (1 to 2 mm in depth) is made, and the sample is collected in long glass or nylon capillary tubes. It has been shown that up to 10 percent contamination with air does not significantly alter pH values. Since fetal infection is an ever-present concern, aseptic technique is necessary. Hemostasis must be assured following blood sampling by holding pressure against the wound through two contraction cycles.

C. *Interpretation.* A scalp blood pH between 7.25 and 7.40 is consistent with normal fetal oxygenation. Values between 7.20 and 7.25 should be repeated in 20 to 30 minutes to determine the trend. If the pH is less than 7.20, fetal acidosis is suspected, and delivery should be accomplished. Values less than 7.10 are associated with neonatal depression in 90 percent of cases.

Experimental Techniques

Multiple centers have explored the use of pH electrodes to provide continuous pH values. However, there have been many problems with electrode safety and reliability. Therefore, this remains a research tool.

Additionally, the use of continuous transcutaneous PO_2 monitors applied to the fetal presenting part during labor is currently being explored. While some understanding of the relationship between FHR patterns and continuous fetal PO_2 measurement has been determined, the exact significance of this remains to be elucidated.

ANTEPARTUM TESTING

A. *Nonstress Test (NST)*
   1. The rationale of the NST as an effective modality for assessment of fetal well-being is based on the association of FHR accelerations with fetal movement and an intact central nervous system controlling FHR.
   2. It is felt that the fetal rest-activity cycle varies from 40 to 90 minutes; therefore, *appropriate duration of monitoring is essential* when fetal movements do not occur spontaneously.
   3. NST is indicated in the surveillance of all high-risk pregnancy conditions. There are no known contraindications to its use.
   4. *If two FHR accelerations of 15 bpm lasting 15 seconds associated with fetal movement occur during a 20-minute monitoring interval, the test is* **reactive**. *A* **nonreactive** *pattern is one where there are no accelerations of less than 15 bpm lasting less than 15 seconds. When a nonreactive test is obtained, a contraction stress test should be performed to further evaluate fetal status.*
   5. A reactive test is found in almost 90 percent of patients and has been shown to be a reliable indicator of fetal health. A false reactive test (fetal death within one week) occurs in less than 1 percent of patients (Fig. 18–12).

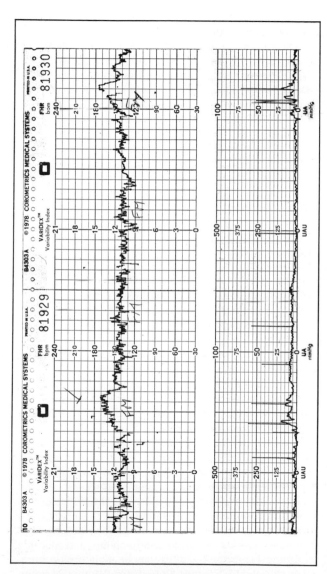

Figure 18–12. External monitoring for NST showing angular accelerations of FHR associated with fetal movements. This represents a reactive test.

B. *Contraction Stress Test (CST)*
1. Since fetal well-being is dependent on the blood flow through the intervillous space, the concept of controlled "stress" was developed to assess fetal status. When uteroplacental insufficiency develops, the fetus may be in a chronic state of compensated distress. Interruption of placental blood flow by uterine contraction should indentify these fetuses at risk for intrauterine demise.
2. *Indications for CST* include all conditions where uteroplacental insufficiency is suspected, such as, diabetes, postdatism, hypertension, intrauterine growth retardation, previous stillbirth, and hemoglobinopathies. Contraindications to CST are those patients at risk of uterine rupture or preterm labor, such as multiple gestation, preterm rupture of membranes, incompetent cervix, or any patient with a contraindication to the occurrence of labor itself.
3. The test should be performed in the labor suite or in close proximity. A dilute infusion of pitocin is begun after a 15-minute baseline FHR is obtained. *A **negative test** shows no late decelerations anywhere on the tracing and there is a minimum of three contractions lasting longer than 40 seconds in 10 minutes. A **positive test** result involves persistent late decelerations in the absence of uterine hyperstimulation.* If contractions are occurring, spontaneously or pitocin-induced, at a rate less than three every 10 minutes with late decelerations, further uterine stimulation should not be undertaken (Fig. 18–13).
4. When late decelerations occur intermittently, but not persistently, the tracing should be interpreted as *suspicious* and inconclusive. Many believe that this result indicates fetal stress and marginal fetal reserve. Further evaluation is mandatory and must take into consideration maternal condition and gestational age. Fetal condition can be evaluated by observation of fetal activity (kick count), breathing, amniotic fluid volume, and placental morphology. While the fetus may be monitored continuously, a repeat CST must be performed within 24 hours.

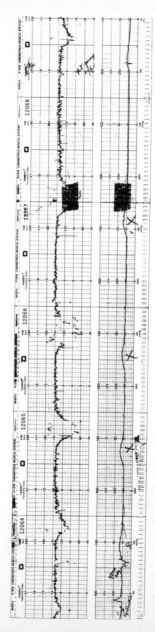

Figure 18–13. Full external monitoring of a patient at 30 weeks' gestation with severe pregnancy-induced hypertension. The tracing shows severe late decelerations occurring with every mild uterine contraction. This patient underwent emergency cesarean section under general anesthesia. The neonate weighed 1050 gm and, in spite of intermittent abdominal distention (possible necrotizing enterocolitis), did well. No respiratory assistance was necessary during the neonatal period.

495

ANTEPARTUM FHR TESTING MANAGEMENT SCHEME

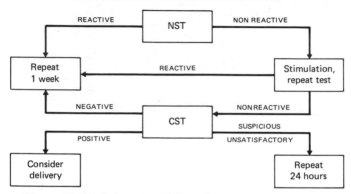

Figure 18–14. Antepartum FHR testing management scheme.

If uterine contractions are of inadequate duration or frequency, or FHR is of a quality that cannot be interpreted, the test is *unsatisfactory*. Continuing attempts should be made to obtain a satisfactory tracing; if not possible, repeat testing should be done within 24 hours.

5. A *negative test* is found in 85 to 90 percent of patients and is a reliable indicator of fetal health. A *false-negative* (fetal death within one week) occurs in less than 1 percent of patients. When a *positive test* is obtained, careful consideration of delivery is indicated. While maternal estriol values may be helpful, sampling of amniotic fluid to detect fetal lung maturity should be done to aid in deciding the optimal timing of delivery. It must be remembered that 25 to 50 percent of patients with a positive CST will tolerate labor without evidence of fetal distress (false-positive). Therefore, cesarean section is not always indicated when a positive CST is found (Fig. 18–14).

BIBLIOGRAPHY

Cibils L: Electronic Fetal-Maternal Monitoring Antepartum/Intrapartum. Boston, PSG Publishing, 1981

Freeman R, Garite T: Fetal Heart Rate Monitoring. Baltimore, Williams & Wilkins, 1981

Gratacos J, Paul R: Antepartum fetal heart rate monitoring: Nonstress test versus contraction stress test. Clin Perinatol 7:387, 1980

Lauersen N, Hochberg H: Clinical Perinatal Biochemical Monitoring. Baltimore, Williams & Wilkins, 1981

Parer J (ed): Fetal monitoring. Semin Perinatol 2:113, 1978

Quilligan EJ (ed): Update on fetal monitoring. Clin Obstet Gynecol 6:207, 1979

Rosen M (ed): Bioelectric methods of fetal assessment. Clin Obstet Gynecol 22:545, 1979

Willcourt R, Queenan J: Fetal scalp blood sampling and transcutaneous Po_2. Clin Perinatol 8:87, 1981

19

Abnormalities of Labor and Delivery

Jeffrey W. Ellis, M.D.
Edward F. Lis, M.D.

PRACTICE PRINCIPLES

In normal labor, uterine contractions lead to progressive cervical effacement and dilatation. The fetus descends through the pelvis in a sequence that results in vaginal delivery. Abnormalities of either the first or second stage of labor are characterized by lack of appropriate cervical dilatation and descent. Abnormalities of labor and delivery may be caused by ineffective uterine contractions (powers), by excessive fetal size or malpresentation (passenger), or by abnormal structure of the birth canal (passage).

ABNORMAL LABOR

Abnormal labor (dysfunctional labor) occurs when there is any variation in the normal pattern of cervical dilatation or descent of the presenting part. Curvimetric analysis of the labor should be used as a guide and should allow rapid assessment of abnormal labor patterns (Fig. 19–1). Numerous terms have been used to describe the abnormalities of labor. *In its simplest terms, labor may (1) progress normally, (2) progress too fast (precipitous labor), (3) progress too slowly (prolonged or protracted labor), or (4) may not progress (arrested labor).*

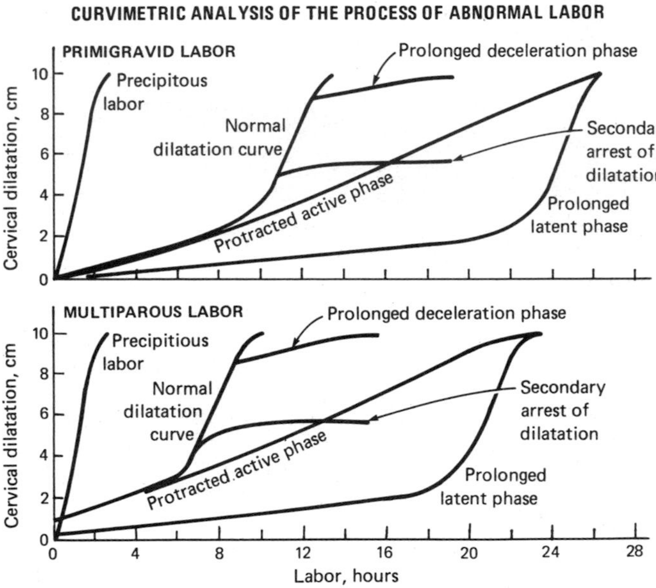

Figure 19–1. Curvimetric analysis of the progress of abnormal labor.

Precipitous Labor

A. *Definition*. Labor lasting three hours or less. The maximum slope of dilatation is 5 cm/hour or more.
B. *Etiology*. Forceful uterine contractions in the presence of minimal resistance to descent.
C. *Complications*. In most cases, there is no harm to the mother or fetus. The following complications may occur
   1. Maternal lacerations (cervix, vagina, perineum) from an unattended delivery
   2. Fetal hypoxia from frequent strong contractions
   3. Cerebral trauma resulting from rapid, unattended delivery

    4. Uterine rupture
    5. Amniotic fluid embolism
D. *Management*
    1. When recognized, immediate preparations should be made for delivery.
    2. Tocolytic agents may be administered to decrease the frequency and intensity of contractions. Often, there is little time to administer medications.

Prolonged Labor

A. *Prolonged latent phase*
    1. *Definition*
        a) Primigravida. Latent phase duration of 20 hours or more
        b) Multigravida. Latent phase duration of 14 hours or more
    2. *Etiology*
        a) False labor
        b) Firm, long, closed cervix at the beginning of labor
        c) Excessive sedation
        d) Regional anesthesia given too early
        e) Uterine dysfunction
        f) Fetopelvic disproportion is *not* associated with prolonged latent phase
    3. *Management.* For appropriate management, it is necessary to determine if the patient is actually in labor.
        a) *Sedation.* The administration of 10 to 15 mg morphine IM or 200 mg secobarbital IM will generally cause the patient to sleep for two to four hours. If the patient was in false labor, contractions generally do not resume after the patient awakens. If true labor had been present, effective contractions often occur after the patient awakens.
        b) *Oxytocin stimulation.* If uterine contractions continue after sedation and further progress is not made, oxytocin stimulation is indicated. Many authorities

believe that amniotomy alone at this stage will be ineffective in stimulating effective contractions, and may expose the patient to chorioamnionitis if labor is prolonged.

B. *Prolonged active phase*
1. *Definition*
   a) Primigravida. Dilatation of the cervix at less than 1.2 cm/hour in the active phase
   b) Multigravida. Dilatation of the cervix at less than 1.5 cm/hour in the active phase
2. *Etiology*
   a) Fetopelvic disproportion
   b) Malpresentation
   c) Excessive sedation
   d) Regional anesthesia given too early
   e) Rigid cervix
   f) Premature rupture of the membranes
   g) Uterine overdistention due to hydramnios or multiple gestation
3. *Management*
   a) When a prolonged active phase pattern is identified, the physician should begin a systematic evaluation of the uterine contractions, fetus, and pelvis. The frequency, duration, and intensity of the uterine contractions should be assessed, with the placement of an intrauterine pressure catheter as indicated. The fetal lie, presentation, and attitude are evaluated using both abdominal and vaginal palpation. Ultrasonography or x-ray films of the maternal abdomen may be necessary to detect congenital anomaly, malpresentation, and macrosomia. Clinical pelvimetry should be performed by an experienced examiner to detect pelvic contraction, pelvic deformity, and obstructing soft tissue masses. The use of x-ray pelvimetry in evaluating abnormal labors is controversial, but may be necessary if the physician is inexperienced in manual pelvimetry or wishes to confirm his findings.

b) In most cases, labor will progress without further intervention. Having previously evaluated all aspects of the labor, the physician will be prepared to act accordingly if an arrest pattern develops.

c) In the absence of fetopelvic disproportion, some authorities will administer oxytocin.

C. *Prolonged descent pattern*

1. *Definition*

   a) Primigravida. Descent of 1 cm/hour or less

   b) Multigravida. Descent of 2 cm/hour or less

2. *Etiology.* Similar to the etiologies of prolonged active phase.

3. *Management*

   a) Management is similar to that of prolonged active phase.

   b) Midforceps procedures are to be avoided, since maternal and fetal morbidity are significantly increased in the presence of high fetal station and malpresentation.

   c) In many cases, labor will progress to uneventful delivery. The physician should nevertheless be prepared for the possibility of an arrest disorder.

Arrested Labor

Four distinct arrest disorders have been identified that are related in etiology, response to therapy, and prognosis. Because of the common etiology, these disorders often occur in combination. Arrest disorders are associated with increased maternal and fetal morbidity due to the frequent need for operative delivery and the potential for fetal cerebral trauma.

A. *Definitions*

1. *Secondary arrest of dilatation.* Cessation of cervical dilatation for two hours or more in the active phase

2. *Prolonged deceleration phase.* Primigravidas: deceleration phase duration of three hours or more; multigravidas: deceleration phase duration of one hour or more

3. *Arrest of descent.* Cessation of progressive descent for one hour or more after the beginning of the descent process

4. *Failure of descent.* Lack of descent during the deceleration phase and second stage

B. *Etiology*
1. Fetopelvic disproportion — 50 percent of cases
2. Malpresentation
3. Regional anesthesia
4. Excessive sedation

C. *Management*
1. In all cases of arrested labor, preparations should be made for the possibility of cesarean section and should include all necessary preoperative blood studies and the availability of two units of typed and crossmatched blood.

2. The physician should undertake a thorough and systematic evaluation of the uterine contractions, fetus, and pelvis.

3. If fetopelvic disproportion is detected, a cesarean section should be performed.

4. If no fetopelvic disproportion has been detected and uterine contractions are suboptimal as diagnosed by evaluation of frequency, duration, and intensity, amniotomy should be performed and oxytocin stimulation initiated. The prognosis for vaginal delivery is good if the postarrest slope of dilatation and descent exceeds the prearrest pattern. If appropriate dilatation and descent do not occur after two hours of adequate uterine contractions, cesarean section should be performed.

5. If no fetopelvic disproportion has been detected and the patient has experienced adequate uterine contractions for two hours, no further stimulation of contractions should be attempted, and a cesarean section should be performed.

6. Forceps delivery is indicated if all of the criteria for safe forceps delivery have been met and if forceps delivery will occur with minimum traction from a low station. In

cases of high fetal station and malpresentation, cesarean section is the appropriate treatment for arrest disorders.

UTERINE DYSFUNCTION AS A CAUSE OF ABNORMAL LABOR

Abnormalities of uterine contractions may be associated with disorders in all stages of labor. Uterine dysfunction may be classified as either hypertonic or hypotonic.

A. *Hypertonic uterine dysfunction.* This form of uterine dysfunction generally occurs during the latent phase of labor and is characterized by pain that is out of proportion to the intensity of the uterine contraction and out of proportion to the progress of cervical effacement and dilatation. Uterine contractions are uncoordinated and lack fundal dominance, and are not effective in effacing and dilating the cervix. Fetal distress in early labor has been associated with hypertonic dysfunction.

1. *Diagnosis.* Hypertonic dysfunction should be suspected during evaluation of prolonged latent phase. Palpation of the uterus will reveal mild contractions out of proportion to the amount of pain experienced by the patient.

2. *Management*

a) *Sedation* should be administered in the form of 10 to 15 mg morphine or 200 mg secobarbital. This will often allow two to four hours of sleep, with normal uterine contractions often occurring after the patient awakens.

b) The administration of *low doses of oxytocin* has been suggested by some authorities, but this form of treatment has not been widely recognized.

c) *Cesarean section* will be necessary if fetal distress develops or if the hypertonic pattern continues despite sedation.

B. *Hypotonic uterine dysfunction.* This form of uterine dysfunction generally occurs during the active phase of labor and is characterized by relatively painless, mild contractions of short duration. In contrast to hypertonic dysfunction, the uterine contractions of hypotonic dysfunction are coordinated and exhibit fundal dominance with a normal gradient. Cervical effacement and dilatation will generally be slow. Hypotonic dysfunction has been associated with obstructed labors and is often seen in association with overdistention of the uterus caused by hydramnios, multiple gestation, and macrosomia.

1. *Diagnosis.* Hypotonic dysfunction should be suspected during the evaluation of prolonged or arrested labor. The uterus will often be easily indentable at the height of the contraction. The use of the intrauterine pressure catheter will generally reveal contractions developing less than 30 mm Hg of pressure.

2. *Management.* If fetopelvic disproportion has been ruled out, oxytocin stimulation should be initiated. Guidelines for the use of oxytocin in the stimulation of labor are similar to its use for induction of labor.

FETAL FACTORS AS A CAUSE OF ABNORMAL LABOR

Fetal factors associated with abnormal labor include excessive size, abnormal development, and malpresentation.

A. *Excessive size.* Excessive fetal size (macrosomia) is generally defined as a fetal weight in excess of 4000 gm. Five percent of pregnancies are associated with a fetal weight of greater than 4000 gm and 0.5 percent of pregnancies are associated with a fetal weight of greater than 4500 gm. Macrosomia has been related to the following factors: heredity, maternal diabetes mellitus, excessive maternal weight gain, prolonged pregnancy, multiparity, congenital anomalies.

1. *Diagnosis.* Macrosomia should be suspected when excessive uterine size is detected or when the patient has a history of a previous macrosomic infant. Ultrasound examination will generally confirm the diagnosis; how-

ever, ultrasound may be relatively inaccurate in estimating the weight of a large infant.

2. *Complications.* The major complications of macrosomia include arrested labor due to cephalopelvic disproportion, shoulder dystocia, traumatic operative delivery, and entrapment of the fetal head in breech presentation.

3. *Management*

   a) *Breech presentation.* Most authorities advise cesarean section for delivery of a fetus in breech presentation weighing in excess of 3800 gm. The major danger in vaginal delivery is entrapment of the aftercoming head.

   b) *Cephalic presentation.* Management is controversial. Some authorities will perform a cesarean section in all cases of infants weighing in excess of 4000 gm, citing the hazards of shoulder dystocia and traumatic operative vaginal delivery. Others advocate expectant management with a trial of labor. Cesarean section is performed if arrested labor occurs.

B. *Abnormal development*

   1. *Anomalies of the head and neck*

      a) *Hydrocephalus.* Hydrocephalus should be suspected in the following clinical situations:

      - In all cases of breech presentation
      - When a large fetal head is palpated during abdominal examination
      - When vaginal examination reveals large fontanelles and widely spaced sutures
      - In a primigravida when engagement does not occur before the onset of labor
      - In all cases of failure of engagement of the fetal head during the active phase of labor

      (1) *Diagnosis.* Hydrocephalus may be confirmed by either ultrasound or radiographic examination of the abdomen.

      (2) *Management.* The pediatric and neurosurgical

services should be notified when hydrocephalus is diagnosed. The management of the delivery will depend on the size of the head and the presence of other anomalies such as meningomyelocele. Transvaginal decompression of the head with drainage of cerebrospinal fluid may significantly decrease the head size and allow vaginal delivery. Alternately, the fetal head may be decompressed transabdominally. In each case, a 16- or 18-gauge spinal needle is inserted into the fetal skull using aseptic technique. In cases of associated meningomyelocele or other open neural tube defects, cesarean section should be performed, since the thin-walled neural sac may rupture during vaginal delivery, leading to meningitis.

b) *Anomalies of the neck.* A variety of anomalies may cause massive enlargement of the fetal neck, including congenital goiter, lymphocele, and tumors. Abnormal extension of the fetal head may develop leading to face or brow presentation.

(1) *Diagnosis.* Ultrasonography or an amniogram will confirm the diagnosis. An abdominal x-ray film may reveal abnormal extension of the head.

(2) *Management.* Cesarean section is often necessary because of the development of arrest of labor due to malpresentation or absolute fetopelvic disproportion. Vaginal delivery may occur if the fetus is small.

2. *Anomalies of the trunk.* Major anomalies of the trunk should be suspected in cases of transverse lie, arrested labor, and shoulder dystocia. The following anomalies of the trunk may occur: teratoma, hepatic tumor, cystic disease of the kidneys, ascites, fetal hydrops with anasarca, distended bladder, and conjoined twins.

a) *Diagnosis.* Large trunk anomalies may be diagnosed by either ultrasonography, roentgenography, or amniography.

b) *Management.* Many anomalies of the trunk are not detected until after partial delivery of the fetus with failure to complete delivery. Destructive procedures may be necessary to complete delivery. Transabdominal aspiration of obstructing cystic structures may decompress the trunk and allow the completion of delivery. Cesarean section should be performed if a massive obstructing anomaly is detected before delivery.

C. *Malpresentation.* Abnormalities of presentation are a common cause of abnormal labor. Diagnosis and management are discussed in the following chapter.

PELVIC ABNORMALITIES AS A CAUSE OF ABNORMAL LABOR

A. *Contracted pelvis.* Shortening of one or more of the critical internal diameters of the pelvis may impede or prevent delivery. Obstruction may develop at the inlet, midpelvis, or outlet. Pelvic measurements are important only in relation to the size of the infant, since a small infant may easily deliver through a contracted pelvis.

1. *Etiology.* Alterations in pelvic dimensions and structure are associated with the following factors:
   a) Congenital anomaly
   b) Malnutrition (rickets, osteomalacia)
   c) Injury (fracture and misalignment)
   d) Tumors
   e) Disorders of the spine, hips, and lower extremities (lumbar kyphoscoliosis, shortening of an extremity)

2. *Diagnosis.* Pelvic contraction may be diagnosed by either manual pelvimetry or x-ray pelvimetry. The following factors should alert the physician to the possibility of pelvic contraction:
   a) History of difficult forceps procedures
   b) History of dysfunctional labor

    c) Short maternal stature (less than 5 feet)
    d) History of pelvic fracture
    e) Physical examination revealing disorders of the spine, hips, or lower extremities

3. *Complications*
    a) Malpresentation
    b) Uterine dysfunction
    c) Uterine rupture
    d) Fistula formation from pressure necrosis
    e) Cord prolapse
    f) Fetal cerebral trauma

4. *Classification*
    a) *Generally contracted pelvis.* This is the most common pelvic deformity found in the United States and is generally associated with women of short stature. The pelvis is contracted proportionately in all diameters with somewhat greater contraction in the anterior-posterior (AP) diameters.
    b) *Inlet contraction.* An inlet contraction exists when the AP diameter is less than 10 cm or the transverse diameter less than 12 cm. Spontaneous delivery with a contracted inlet depends on the size, position, and attitude of the fetus, the malleability of the fetal head, and the adequacy of uterine contractions. Inlet contraction should be suspected in all cases of malpresentation and failure of the presenting part to engage.
    c) *Midpelvic contraction.* Contraction of the midpelvis is more common than inlet contraction. Midpelvic contraction exists when the AP diameter is less than 11.5 cm or the transverse diameter is less than 9.5 cm. The following characteristics are commonly associated with a contracted midpelvis: converging side walls, prominent ischial spines, flat sacrum, and narrow sacrosciatic notch.
    d) *Outlet contraction.* Isolated outlet contraction is rare, and it is usually associated with midpelvic contraction. Outlet contraction exists when the bituberous diameter is less than 8 cm.

B. *Soft tissue abnormalities.* The following conditions have been associated with abnormal labor:
   1. *Rigid cervix* resulting from cauterization, conization, or cerclage
   2. *Pelvic tumors* interfering with engagement and descent: myomata, ovarian masses, vaginal masses
   3. Extreme distention of the bladder or rectum

ADDITIONAL COMPLICATIONS OF LABOR AND DELIVERY

The complications described below may occur during abnormal labor and are often related to abnormalities of the fetus or abnormalities of the pelvis.

A. *Uterine rupture.* Rupture of the uterus is an obstetric emergency and is one of the leading causes of maternal death.
   1. *Definition*
      a) *Incomplete rupture.* The uterine laceration is separated from the peritoneal cavity by visceral peritoneum.
      b) *Complete rupture.* The uterine laceration communicates with the peritoneal cavity, with all or part of the fetus extruded into the peritoneal cavity.
      c) *Dehiscence versus rupture of a cesarean section incision.* Traditionally, the separation of a previous cesarean section scar may be either a rupture or a dehiscence. The characteristics of each are described below.

	Dehiscence	**Rupture**
Fetal membranes	Intact	Ruptured
Visceral peritoneum	Intact	Ruptured
Fetus	Remains in uterus	Partially or completely extruded

	Dehiscence	**Rupture**
Bleeding	None to minimal	Moderate to massive
Scar involvement	Usually partial separation	May involve entire scar with extension
Development	Gradual	Rapid

2. *Etiology.* The following classification of the etiologies of uterine rupture has been proposed by Pritchard and MacDonald (*Williams Obstetrics,* 16th ed.).
   a) Uterine injury *before* current pregnancy
      (1) Surgery involving myometrium
         (a) Cesarean section or hysterotomy
         (b) Repaired previous uterine rupture
         (c) Myomectomy incision close to or through endometrium
         (d) Deep cornual resection to remove interstitial oviduct
         (e) Excision of uterine septum
      (2) Coincidental trauma to uterus
         (a) Instrumented abortion
         (b) Sharp or blunt trauma
         (c) Silent rupture during previous pregnancy
   b) Uterine injury *during* current pregnancy
      (1) Before delivery
         (a) Persistent, intense, spontaneous contractions
         (b) Oxytocin or prostaglandin administration (hypertonic uterine contractions)
         (c) Hypertonic solution injected intraamniotically
         (d) Perforation by monitor catheter
         (e) External trauma, sharp or blunt
         (f) Marked uterine overdistention (twins, hydramnios, macrosomic fetus)
      (2) During delivery
         (a) Internal podalic version

          (b) Difficult forceps delivery

          (c) Breech extraction

          (d) Fetal anomaly overdistending lower uterine segment

          (e) Vigorous fundal pressure

          (f) Difficult manual removal of placenta

    c) Uterine defects not necesarily related to trauma

       (1) Congenital. Pregnancy in an incompletely developed uterus or uterine horn

       (2) Acquired

          (1) Placenta increta or percreta

          (b) Invasive mole or choriocarcinoma

          (c) Adenomyosis

          (d) Sacculation of adherent retroverted uterus

3. *Symptoms.* The patient will complain of severe abdominal pain prior to rupture. Pain during rupture may be described as "tearing." Abdominal pain may resolve for a short time after rupture. Labor pain usually ceases abruptly.

4. *Diagnosis*

    a) Physical signs. Uterine tenderness, easily palpable fetal parts, vaginal bleeding, shock

    b) Diagnostic studies. Falling hematocrit, abdominal x-ray revealing abnormal fetal position or free intraperitoneal air, ultrasound showing fetus partially or totally outside the uterus

    c) Labor monitoring. Cessation of uterine contractions, cessation of fetal heart rate, or evidence of late decelerations or fetal bradycardia

5. *Management.* Rapid recognition and treatment of uterine rupture is mandatory to prevent maternal mortality and to preserve reproductive capability, if possible.

    a) Two large-bore intravenous catheters are inserted and physiologic solutions are infused at a rate that maintains adequate tissue perfusion.

    b) An indwelling urinary catheter is inserted, and if time permits, a central venous pressure line is inserted to aid in fluid management.

    c) Four to six units of whole blood are typed and crossmatched. Type-specific blood is administered only if there is severe volume depletion.

    d) The abdomen is opened through a midline incision to give maximum exposure.

    e) Upon entry into the abdomen, the location and severity of the rupture are rapidly assessed.

    f) In cases of minor dehiscence or a small rupture not associated with major tissue damage, repair of the defect may be attempted. Two or three layers of closure will be necesary.

    g) In cases of major tissue damage or when the rupture has lead to expanding hematomas in the broad ligament, hysterectomy may be required.

    h) Hypogastric artery ligation will generally decrease bleeding substantially, thus allowing more time to make an adequate assessment of the extent of the rupture and perform hysterectomy if necessary.

B. *Prolapse of the umbilical cord*

  1. Types of cord prolapse

    a) *Cord (funic) presentation.* The cord lies below the presenting part and the membranes are intact.

    b) *Cord prolapse.* The cord lies below the presenting part and the membranes are ruptured. The cord may then prolapse into the vagina or out through the introitus.

    c) *Occult cord prolapse.* The cord lies alongside the presenting part and is generally not palpable on vaginal examination.

  2. *Incidence.* Overt prolapse of the cord is found in 0.3 to 0.6 percent of labors.

  3. *Danger to fetus.* After cord prolapse, compression of the cord between the presenting part and the walls of the pelvis may significantly interfere with blood flow to the fetus. Severe hypoxia may result, leading to irreversible organ damage and death. In cases of occult cord prolapse, intermittent compression of the cord will occur during uterine contractions, leading to impaired fetal

circulation. Variable decelerations of the fetal heart rate or prolonged periods of bradycardia will be noted.

4. *Etiology.* Prolapse of the cord is associated with factors that interfere with the normal adaptation of the presenting part to the pelvic inlet. If the presenting part does not form an adequate seal at the inlet, the cord may pass through a defect. Cord prolapse is often associated with a long cord or a cord attached to a low-lying placenta.

The following are associated with cord prolapse:

a) *Abnormal presentation.* Transverse lie, breech, face, brow, compound presentations. Cord prolapse will occur in approximately 10 percent of transverse lies and 3 percent of breech presentations.

b) *Cephalopelvic disproportion*

c) *Multiple pregnancy*

d) *Prematurity*

e) *Hydramnios*

f) *Rupture of membranes with a high presenting part*

g) *Iatrogenic.* Artifical rupture of membranes with an unengaged presenting part.

5. *Diagnosis.* The key to early diagnosis and treatment is suspicion. In patients who are at high risk for cord prolapse (See Etiology), frequent vaginal examinations will be necessary to detect a cord presentation. After spontaneous rupture of membranes, an immediate vaginal examination is mandatory to detect cord prolapse. Overt or occult prolapse should be suspected in all cases of recurrent fetal heart rate deceleration or prolonged bradycardia.

a) *Occult cord prolapse.* Palpation through the cervix may reveal a pulsatile, cordlike structure alongside the presenting part. Often the cord is not palpable, and occult prolapse is merely suspected on the basis of variable deceleration of the fetal heart rate.

b) *Cord presentation.* The pulsating cord is felt through the membranes. This must be differentiated from vasa previa and pulsations from vaginal vessels.

c) *Cord prolapse.* The cord is palpable in the vagina or is visible outside of the introitus.

6. *Management.* A prolapse of the cord is an obstetric emergency. Management decisions and treatment must proceed quickly. Management ultimately depends on the status of the fetus and the extent of cervical dilatation.

a) In the following situations, no further therapy is indicated, and the labor is allowed to continue: dead fetus, fetal anomaly incompatible with survival, extreme prematurity incompatible with survival.

b) In all other cases, immediate preparations for delivery should be made. The mother is placed in a deep Trendelenburg or knee-chest position, and the presenting part is pushed out of the pelvis by a vaginal hand. These manuevers may reduce the pressure on the cord and should be continued until delivery is effected. High concentrations of oxygen are administered to the mother by mask. No attempts should be made to reposition the cord up into the uterus since this usually fails.

c) If the cervix is completely dilated and the presenting part is engaged, a vaginal delivery may be performed. If the fetus is in a cephalic presentation with a position and attitude suitable for vaginal delivery, a midforceps or vacuum extraction may be performed. When a difficult or time-consuming forceps rotation is expected, an immediate cesarean section should be performed. In a breech presentation suitable for vaginal delivery, total breech extraction may be performed. Version and extraction are indicated only if fetal death is imminent.

d) If the cervix is incompletely dilated or if the presenting part is unengaged, an immediate cesarean section should be performed.

e) Immediately prior to cesarean section, the presence of the fetal heart beat should be determined using either a Doppler device or stethoscope. Fetal cardiac activity may continue after pulsations in the cord stop.

7. *Prognosis.* In general, perinatal mortality increases as the time between cord prolapse and delivery increases. Perinatal mortality uncorrected for fetal anomaly and severe prematurity is 20 to 30 percent. The ultimate prognosis for the infant is related to the duration and extent of cord compression, fetal maturity and the extent of trauma associated with delivery. Maternal morbidity is increased due to complications of emergency operative delivery.

C. *Persistent occiput posterior positions.* A persistent occiput posterior position may be associated with prolongation of the second stage of labor.

1. *Incidence.* This position persists in approximately 5 percent of labors.

2. *Etiology.* Factors that prevent or delay anterior rotation of the occiput are associated with persistent posterior positions.

   a) The narrow forepelvis of the anthropoid and android pelvis favors engagement and descent in the posterior position.

   b) A narrow midpelvis usually associated with converging side walls may prevent or delay normal internal rotation.

3. *Diagnosis.* Vaginal examination will reveal the larger anterior fontanelle in the anterior segment of the pelvis and the smaller posterior fontanelle in the posterior segment of the pelvis. Extensive caput succedaneum is often associated with posterior positions and may obscure cranial landmarks.

4. *Mechanism of labor.* As descent progresses in the posterior position, internal rotation will occur at the midpelvis. In 90 percent of cases, the occiput will rotate to an anterior position. If the midpelvis is narrow, a posterior position will persist. The second stage of labor is then slightly prolonged. The head is initially born by flexion as the forehead, vertex, and occiput successively pass over the perineum. As the head falls back, the facial structures successively pass beneath the symphysis.

5. *Management*
   a) Since spontaneous rotation to an occiput anterior position generally occurs, expectant management is indicated as long as labor is progressing normally.
   b) Failure of rotation to the anterior position may be caused by inadequate uterine contractions, a narrow midpelvis, or slight deflexion of the head.
   c) If the occiput posterior position persists in the second stage of labor, spontaneous delivery in the posterior position may occur, especially in multiparas.
   d) An arrest of descent and rotation may occur during the second stage. Manual rotation of the head to an anterior position may be attempted. If rotation cannot be effected, forceps delivery is indicated. Manual pelvimetry is performed to evaluate the adequacy of the midpelvis. If the midpelvis is adequate, forceps rotation to an occiput anterior position may be performed by an experienced operator. Reapplication of the forceps to the new occiput anterior position will enable completion of delivery (Scanzoni maneuver). If the midpelvis is narrow or if the operator is not experienced in the midpelvic rotation, a forceps delivery in the occiput posterior position is performed.
   e) Cesarean section is uncommonly indicated but will be necessary in cases of a failed forceps procedure or if significant midpelvic contraction exists.
   f) If the fetus is delivered in the occiput posterior position, large head diameters will distend the vulva and perineum, frequently causing extension of the episiotomy. Many authors favor a mediolateral episiotomy in these cases.
   g) Extensive molding and caput succedaneum may give a false impression of engagement when the biparietal diameter actually lies above the inlet. An unintentional high forceps procedure may be performed if this is not recognized.

D. *Persistent occiput transverse positions.* Arrest of descent and rotation leading to a persistent occiput transverse position is a common cause of prolongation of the second stage of labor.

1. *Etiology.* Factors that prevent or delay normal internal rotation are associated with persistent transverse positions.

   a) *Pelvic variations:* android, platypelloid
   b) *Cephalopelvic disproportion*
   c) *Hypotonic uterine contractions*
   d) *Conduction anesthesia*

2. *Diagnosis.* Vaginal examination will reveal the sagittal suture in the transverse diameter of the pelvis. The lowest point of the head is at or below the level of the ischial spines.

3. *Management*

   a) If hypotonic uterine contractions are present, stimulation of labor with oxytocin is indicated.
   b) If there is no further descent and rotation despite adequate uterine contractions, manual pelvimetry should be performed to assess the adequacy of the pelvis. If cephalopelvic disproportion is suspected, a cesarean section should be performed.
   c) If cephalopelvic disproportion is not suspected, a forceps delivery may be performed. Prior to application of the forceps, manual rotation of the head to an occiput anterior position should be attempted. Detailed descriptions of forceps procedures for persistent occiput transverse positions may be found in the references listed.
   d) A cesarean section should be performed if a forceps procedure fails or if a difficult forceps procedure is anticipated.

E. *Shoulder dystocia.* A shoulder dystocia exists when the head has delivered and the shoulders cannot be delivered by the usual maneuvers. The posterior shoulder normally enters the pelvis; however, the anterior shoulder arrests above the symphysis pubis. Rarely, both shoulders arrest above the pelvic inlet.

1. *Incidence.* A shoulder dystocia occurs in 0.15 percent to 0.60 percent of deliveries. When the fetus is greater than 4000 gm, the incidence of shoulder dystocia is 1.7 percent.

2. *Etiology.* If the bisacromial diameter of the fetus is large relative to the AP and oblique diameters of the pelvic inlet, a shoulder dystocia may result. This is usually associated with a large fetus passing through an inlet of normal size. Shoulder dystocia may also occur when a normal-sized infant passes through a contracted inlet.

3. *Dangers to the fetus*
   a) Fetal cardiac function is severely compromised as the chest is compressed after delivery of the head. As venous drainage from the brain is delayed, stagnant hypoxia and hemorrhage may result. If delivery is further delayed, irreversable brain damage and fetal death may occur.
   b) Excessive traction applied to the head during delivery may lead to cord injuries and brachial plexus injuries. Clavicular fracture may lead to pneumothorax and subclavian vessel injury.

4. *Management.* If a shoulder dystocia develops, the following maneuvers are carried out rapidly:
   a) The nasopharynx and mouth of the infant are suctioned to ensure a clear airway.
   b) A hand is inserted into the vagina to detect anomalies of the neck or thorax that may prevent delivery.
   c) A large episiotomy is made or the previous episiotomy is extended.
   d) Firm suprapubic pressure is applied by an assistant as traction is applied to the head.
   e) If this maneuver fails, a hand is inserted into the vagina and the shoulders are rotated to an oblique diameter. Fundal and suprapubic pressure is applied by an assistant as traction is applied to the head.

f) If the shoulders cannot be delivered by the above maneuvers, the posterior shoulder is delivered by passing a hand beneath the posterior shoulder and sweeping the posterior arm across the chest. The hand is then grasped and the arm is pulled out through the vagina. The anterior shoulder is delivered by a combination of suprapubic pressure and traction on the head.

g) Since clavicular fracture is common during attempts at delivering the posterior shoulder, some authors advise first attempting the Woods screw maneuver. Fundal pressure is applied by an assistant. If the head is in the left occiput transverse position, two fingers are placed over the anterior aspect of the posterior shoulder. The shoulder is then rotated 180 degrees counterclockwise past the 12 o'clock position. The posterior shoulder is then delivered under the pubic arch. The shoulder that is now posterior is rotated clockwise 180 degrees and is delivered under the pubic arch.

h) If all other maneuvers fail, a clavicle may be intentionally fractured.

i) Complete failure to deliver the shoulders may be due to fetal anomaly (anasarca, neoplasm, conjoined twins) or cervical constriction ring.

BIBLIOGRAPHY

Abnormal Labor

Friedman EA: Dysfunctional labor. III. Secondary arrest of dilatation in the nullipara. Obstet Gynecol 19:576, 1962

Friedman EA: Failure to progress in labor: evaluation and management. Contemp Obstet Gynecol 4:41, 1974

Friedman EA: Labor: Clinical Evaluation and Management. New York, Appleton-Century-Crofts, 1978

Friedman EA, Sachtleben MR: Dysfunctional labor. V. Therapeutic trial of oxytocin in secondary arrest. Obstet Gynecol 21:13, 1963

Friedman EA, Sachtleben MR: Dysfunctional labor. I. Prolonged latent phase in the nullipara. Obstet Gynecol 17:135, 1961

Schifrin BS: The case against pelvimetry. Contemp Obstet Gynecol 4:77, 1974

Umbilical Cord Prolapse
Savage EW, et al.: Prolapse of the umbilical cord. Obstet Gynecol 35:502, 1970

Persistent Occiput Posterior
Phillips RD, Freeman M: The management of persistent occiput posterior position. Obstet Gynecol 43:171, 1974

Shoulder Dystocia
Benedetti TJ, Gabbe SG: Shoulder dystocia. Obstet Gynecol 52:526, 1978

20

Abnormalities of Presentation

Jeffrey W. Ellis, M.D.

PRACTICE PRINCIPLES

Abnormalities of presentation commonly lead to complications during labor and delivery. A thorough understanding of the mechanisms of labor and causes of abnormal presentation is mandatory for successful management. Abnormalities of presentation may complicate 5 to 6 percent of pregnancies at term.

Breech Presentation

The management of breech presentation is one of the most controversial areas in modern obstetrics. Numerous factors exist that may significantly increase fetal and maternal morbidity. When adjusted for complicating maternal and fetal factors, the intrinsic fetal risk in a vaginal delivery is approximately three times greater than with cephalic presentation.

A. *Incidence.* Breech presentation exists in approximately 25 percent of pregnancies at 28 weeks' gestation and progressively declines to an incidence of *3 to 4 percent at term.*
B. *Predisposing causes.* Breech presentation is associated with a variety of fetal and maternal anatomic conditions that

prevent normal adaptation of the fetal head to the pelvic
inlet:
1. Hydrocephalus, anencephaly
2. Polyhydramnios
3. Low-lying placenta or placenta previa
4. Uterine anomaly, e.g. acquired (myomata) or congenital
   (uterine septum)
5. Prematurity
6. Multiple gestation
7. Contracted pelvis

C. *Types and incidence*
   1. *Frank breech* (70 percent). Lower extremities flexed at
      the hips and extended at the knees resulting in the feet
      lying near the head
   2. *Complete breech* (5 percent). Knees and thighs flexed
   3. *Footling breech* (25 percent). One or both hips extended
      with one or both feet as the presenting part

D. *Diagnosis*
   1. *Abdominal examination.* The soft breech is palpable at
      the pelvic inlet and the firm, round head is palpable at the
      fundus.
   2. *Vaginal examination.* The buttocks and possibly one or
      both lower extremities are palpable. The anus and
      genitalia may be felt.
   3. *Ultrasonography.* Will confirm breech presentation and
      aid in identification of congenital anomalies.
   4. *Abdominal radiographs.* Useful in determining the type
      of breech presentation and will identify any deflexion of
      the head.

E. *Perinatal morbidity and mortality.* Breech presentation is
   associated with significantly increased perinatal morbidity
   and mortality as compared to a fetus of similar gestational
   age in a cephalic presentation. The principle causes of
   increased perinatal morbidity and mortality include:
   1. Low birth weight: incidence 20 to 30 percent (cephalic, 7
      to 10 percent)
   2. Congenital anomalies: incidence > 6 percent (cephalic, 2
      percent)

3. Birth hypoxia
4. Birth injury
F. *Hazards of vaginal delivery*
  1. *Cord prolapse*
     a) Complete breech: incidence, 4 percent
     b) Footling breach: incidence, 15 percent
  2. *Traction injuries.* Hip dislocation, brachial plexus injury from hyperextension of the fetal arms, cervical spine transection.
  3. *Compression injuries.* Laceration of the liver, spleen, or kidneys.
  4. *Cord compression.* Begins during the second stage of labor; prolonged compression may lead to sustained hypoxia.
  5. *Entrapment of the fetal head.* May result from delivery of the body through an incompletely dilated cervix or from delivery of a fetus with a hyperextended head. This occurs most commonly in delivery of a macrosomic fetus (large head) or a premature or growth-retarded fetus (head larger than trunk).
  6. *Intracranial hemorrhage.* May result from prolonged hypoxia or cerebral injury.
G. *Antepartum management.* Diagnosis of breech presentation prior to the onset of labor aids the obstetric team in formulating appropriate management.
  1. *Careful abdominal and vaginal palpation* should be performed during prenatal visits to determine presentation. If a breech presentation is suspected, ultrasound studies should be performed to confirm the diagnosis and detect congenital anomalies. Careful clinical pelvimetry should be performed to detect pelvic contraction or soft tissue masses.
  2. *External cephalic version* is a maneuver that attempts to convert a breech presentation or transverse lie into a cephalic presentation. This procedure is performed without anesthesia, so that excessive force is not exerted. It is performed before the onset of labor, generally between 32 and 36 weeks of gestation. The use of this procedure is

controversial. Many authorities feel that the risks of the procedure exceed the possible benefits, especially in view of the fact that a significant number of breech presentations will spontaneously convert to a cephalic presentation.

a) *Contraindications*
   (1) Previous cesarean section or uterine scar
   (2) Multiple gestation
   (3) Placenta previa
   (4) Low engagement of the presenting part
   (5) Marked fetopelvic disproportion
   (6) Known or suspected uterine anomaly
   (7) Oligohydramnios
   (8) Severe congenital anomaly of the fetus
   (9) Active labor
b) *Complications*
   (1) Placental abruption
   (2) Umbilical cord accident
   (3) Rupture of membranes
   (4) Uterine rupture
   (5) Fetal spinal cord injury
c) *Technique*
   (1) Perform an abdominal ultrasound to determine amount of amniotic fluid, presence of congenital anomaly, and location of placenta.
   (2) Using gentle abdominal pressure, with the aid of an assistant if necessary, the breech is deflected toward the fundus and the head toward the pelvis.
   (3) Fetal heart tones should be evaluated throughout the procedure.
   (4) This procedure should be performed only by physicians experienced in the technic and at a facility where rapid operative delivery may be performed if fetal distress develops.

3. *Patient education.* The patient should be instructed to report to the hospital immediately at the onset of labor or if membranes rupture.

H. *Intrapartum management.* Immediately on admission to the hospital, the following procedures and determinations should be performed:

1. Pelvic examination is performed to confirm breech presentation, to determine the variety of breech, to check for umbilical cord prolapse, and to assess cervical effacement, dilatation, and station.
2. Determine gestational age.
3. Determine the size of the fetus, using ultrasound if available.
4. Perform x-ray pelvimetry.
5. Obtain a flat A-P x-ray of the maternal abdomen to assess any deflexion of the fetal head, to determine the variety of breech, and to detect any congenital anomalies such as hydrocephalus.
6. Type and crossmatch two units of whole blood in case operative delivery becomes necessary.
7. Initiate continuous electronic monitoring of the uterine contractions and fetal heart rate.
8. Formulate a specific management plan and determine the appropriate route of delivery.

I. *Route of delivery.* The management of delivery of the fetus in breech presentation is controversial. The risks of vaginal delivery must be weighed against the risks to the mother of undergoing a cesarean section. Though some authorities advocate cesarean section for all breech deliveries, a critical analysis of the literature reveals that vaginal delivery is a safe route of delivery if the entire clinical setting is carefully analyzed and a specific management plan followed. The management of breech presentation must therefore be individualized.

1. *Indications for cesarean section.* In the following situations, most authorities agree that cesarean section should be performed without a trial of labor:
   a) Fetal distress
   b) Footling breech or complete breech
   c) Dysfunctional labor (especially failure of descent)

    d) Hyperextension of the fetal head
    e) Contracted pelvis or pelvic deformity
    f) Fetal weight greater than 3500 gm

2. *Optimum criteria for vaginal delivery*

    a) *Normal pelvic diameters and architecture.* Since a normal-sized but unmolded head may become entrapped, the pelvis must be at least of normal size — and preferably larger. The pelvic type should optimally be gynecoid. Many authorities consider a platypelloid or an android pelvis to be an indication for cesarean section. The critical pelvic diameters and pelvic type should be determined by x-ray pelvimetry. Optimum pelvic diameters are:

	Inlet	Midpelvis	Outlet
Anteroposterior	>11 cm	>11.5 cm	>11.5 cm
Transverse	>12 cm	>10 cm	>10 cm
Sacrum	Hollow, with no anterior inclination		

    b) *Frank breech presentation.* Since the breech nearly completely fills the pelvic inlet, the incidence of cord prolapse is reduced. The extended legs associated with the frank breech add to the trunk diameter, causing the trunk to deliver through a more completely dilated cervix.

    c) *No evidence of fetal head hyperextension.* The narrowest head diameters present with a completely flexed head. If extension of the head occurs, larger diameters are presented at the pelvic inlet. Extreme extension of the fetal head (greater than 90 degrees) has been associated with a high incidence of spinal cord injury. The degree of extension is determined by calculating the angle between the cervical vertebrae and the upward extension of the main axis of the thoracic vertebrae.

d) *Normal progress of labor.* The rate of dilatation and descent should be similar to that of a cephalic presentation. *Careful curvimetric analysis of the progress of labor is mandatory.*

e) *No evidence of abnormal fetal heart rate*

f) *Fetal weight between 2500 and 3500 gm.* The incidence of entrapped fetal head is increased in small and large fetuses.

g) *Obstetrician experienced in breech delivery*

3. *Special situations*

a) *Primigravida breech.* The management of the primigravida breech is especially controversial. Though some advocate routine cesarean section, many authorities feel that a safe vaginal delivery may be anticipated if optimum criteria for vaginal delivery are met.

b) *Premature or growth-retarded fetus.* Delivery of the small fetus may be hazardous for two reasons. The head of the premature or asymmetrically growth-retarded fetus is relatively larger than the trunk as compared to the normal term fetus, where the reverse is true. This may lead to entrapment of the head at delivery. Second, the incompletely developed cranium of the premature fetus is more susceptible to intracranial injuries as a result of the compression-decompression phenomena. For these reasons, some authorities advocate cesarean section, whereas others feel that a safe vaginal delivery may be anticipated if the optimum criteria for vaginal delivery are met.

c) *Induction of labor.* Induction of labor for whatever reason is generally considered contraindicated with breech presentation. Cesarean section should be performed if immediate delivery is necessary.

d) *Stimulation of labor.* Dysfunctional labor is generally considered an indication for cesarean section. Some authorities will cautiously administer oxytocin in cases of primary uterine dysfunction but not in cases of secondary dysfunction.

J. *Technic of cesarean section.* In general, the uterine incision must be large enough to allow for atraumatic delivery of the fetus. Most authorities agree that a *low segment vertical incision* is the procedure of choice, since it may be easily extended if a larger incision is needed to ensure atraumatic delivery.

K. *Technics of vaginal delivery. It must be emphasized that vaginal delivery of a breech presentation should only be attempted by physicians who are experienced in all aspects of the procedure.*

1. Delivery room team
   a) Obstetrician and assistant
   b) Anesthesiologist
   c) Pediatrician
   d) Complete nursing team

2. Methods of breech delivery
   a) *Spontaneous breech delivery.* The entire infant is expelled by natural forces of labor without any manipulation by the obstetrician. This form of delivery is uncommon in term infants.
   b) *Total breech extraction.* The entire body of the fetus is extracted by the obstetrician using both traction and manipulation. This technique is seldom used except in cases of imminent fetal death or in cases of delivery of a second twin that is either breech or in a transverse lie.
   c) *Partial breech extraction.* The fetus delivers spontaneously to the umbilicus and the remainder of the body is delivered by traction and manipulation.

3. *Technic of total breech extraction*
   a) General or regional anesthesia is administered.
   b) The patient is placed in the lithotomy position.
   c) The bladder is emptied by catheterization.
   d) The hand of the operator is inserted into the uterine cavity.

e) Both ankles of the fetus are grasped and brought down into the vagina.

f) If difficulty is experienced in grasping both ankles, one foot should be brought into the vagina, and then the second foot immediately grasped.

g) Gentle traction is applied until both feet appear at the vulva.

h) Downward traction is applied until the calves and thighs appear.

i) As the breech distends the vulva, upward traction is applied until the hips are delivered.

j) At this point, the infant is delivered according to the technic of partial breech extraction.

4. *Technic of partial breech extraction.* At this point, the fetus has delivered spontaneously to the level of the umbilicus.

a) An assistant applies fundal pressure to prevent extension of the head.

b) The thumbs of the operator are placed over the sacrum and the fingers are placed over the hips.

c) An episiotomy is performed by the assistant (mediolateral preferred).

d) When the umbilical cord appears, it is advanced to prevent excessive traction.

e) Downward traction is applied until the costal margins and scapulae are visible.

f) Slight rotation of the fetus will bring the shoulders into the anterior-posterior diameter of the outlet.

g) Continued downward traction is applied until the axilla of the anterior arm is visible.

h) Upward traction is applied until the posterior axilla is visible.

i) Clockwise rotation of the trunk will then allow spontaneous delivery of one arm; counterclockwise rotation will spontaneously deliver the other arm.

j) If the rotation technic for delivery of the arms fails, the arms should be gently grasped and delivered. The posterior arm is delivered first. Upward traction is applied to the fetus, and two fingers are passed over the humerus of the posterior arm until the elbow is contacted. The arm is then swept into the vagina and through the vulva.

k) Downward traction is applied to the fetus and the anterior arm is delivered in a similar fashion.

l) The body is placed over the palm and forearm of the operator as two fingers of that hand are placed over the maxilla of the fetus (Mauriceau maneuver). The other hand is placed over the fetal back.

m) Downward traction is applied until the suboccipital area of the head appears beneath the symphysis.

n) Upward traction is then applied as the head is held in flexion by slight traction applied over the maxilla.

o) The head is slowly delivered.

p) Some authorities advise the routine use of Piper forceps for delivery of the aftercoming head; others advise their use only if difficulty is encountered in delivery.

5. *Anesthesia for delivery*

a) In most cases of partial breech extraction, pudendal block or epidural anesthesia is adequate. Epidural anesthesia is preferred by many authorities, since it provides excellent anesthesia and reduces the maternal urge to bear down, thus reducing the incidence of delivery of the trunk through a partially dilated cervix.

b) During total breech extraction, a general anesthetic may be required to provide uterine relaxation.

c) Some obstetricians prefer the induction of general anesthesia during delivery of the head to ensure perineal relaxation.

TRANSVERSE AND OBLIQUE LIE

A transverse or oblique lie exists when an angle is formed between the long axis of the fetus and the long axis of the mother. If a right angle is formed, the fetus is in a transverse lie; if an acute angle is formed, the fetus is in an oblique lie. The presenting part is often a shoulder or the back. Prior to labor and rupture of membranes, the fetus may change frequently between a transverse and oblique lie.

A. *Incidence.* Transverse lie is found in approximately *0.3 percent of labors.* It is more common in multiparas.

B. *Etiology.* Transverse lie is associated with factors that either distort the normal shape of the uterine cavity or interfere with normal engagement of the presenting part.

1. *Variations in placental implantation.* Any implantation that shortens the longitudinal length of the uterine cavity may cause the fetus to accommodate to a transverse or oblique diameter. This includes placenta previa, lower-segment implantation, and fundal implantation.

2. *Uterine anomalies.* Congenital anomalies involving fusion defects (arcuate uterus, bicornuate uterus) may increase the width of the uterine cavity. Lower-segment or cervical myomata may interfere with engagement and descent.

3. *Pelvic anomalies.* A contracted pelvic inlet may interfere with engagement and descent. This is the most common cause of transverse lie in primigravidas.

4. *Pendulous abdomen.* General relaxation of the abdominal wall, often associated with multiparity, may cause forward and lateral movement of the uterus, thus interfering with normal engagement and descent.

5. *Fetal anomalies.* Abdominal or thoracic enlargements may distort the normal long axis of the fetus.

6. *Prematurity.* A small fetus is freely moveable in the uterine cavity and will often assume a transverse lie prior to its eventual accommodation along the longitudinal axis of the maternal abdomen.

7. *Hydramnios.* Overdistention of the uterine cavity will allow free movement of the fetus. The width of the uterine cavity may be increased.

8. *Multiple pregnancy*. Multiple fetuses will cause distortion of the normal longitudinal length of the uterine cavity. The pelvis may be occupied by the presenting part of one fetus, preventing engagement of the other fetus. Hydramnios will further increase the width of the uterine cavity.

9. *Dead fetus*. Softening of the fetus skeleton and connective structures may cause the fetus to assume an exaggerated degree of flexion.

C. *Mechanism of labor*. Spontaneous conversion of a transverse lie to a longitudinal lie may occur during the early stages of labor. If the fetus remains in a transverse lie, spontaneous delivery will not occur unless the fetus is very small or macerated. As labor progresses, the shoulder is forced into the pelvis, and further descent stops as the shoulder is arrested at the pelvic inlet. Commonly, an arm will prolapse into the vagina. Continued uterine contractions will lead to progressive thinning of the lower uterine segment until uterine rupture occurs.

D. *Dangers to mother and fetus*
   1. Prolapse of the umbilical cord and its attendant complications will frequently occur.
   2. Tetanic uterine contractions during late stages of labor will lead to compromised placental circulation, fetal hypoxia, and eventually fetal death.
   3. Extreme flexion of the fetal trunk may severely compromise circulation.
   4. Uterine rupture and intrauterine death will occur in cases of neglected transverse lie.

E. *Diagnosis and management*
   1. A careful abdominal examination to determine fetal lie is performed during every prenatal visit.
   2. Transverse lie is suspected when the abdomen appears wide and asymmetrical. Fundal height measurement will reveal the uterus to be smaller than would be expected for the period of gestation.
   3. Abdominal palpation will reveal the fetus to lie along the transverse axis of the maternal abdomen. The fetal head

will be palpable in one lower abdominal quadrant and the breech in the other.

4. Before a vaginal examination is performed, an ultrasound examination of the pelvis should be obtained to rule out placenta previa.

5. If placenta previa is excluded, a vaginal examination may be performed. Often no fetal structures are palpable. If the fetus is low in the abdomen, an arm, shoulder, or rib cage may be palpable.

6. A thorough manual examination of the pelvis should be performed to detect pelvic contraction or soft-tissue masses.

7. X-ray pelvimetry is performed if pelvic contraction is suspected. An ultrasound examination of the fetus or amniography may be performed to detect fetal anomaly.

8. If there is no contraindication to vaginal delivery, external cephalic version may be performed. After successful version, the presenting part should be held in the pelvis for approximately 10 minutes to allow uterine accommodation. This procedure may be repeated as often as necessary.

9. If a transverse or oblique lie persists after 34 weeks of gestation, the patient should be hospitalized, since spontaneous conversion to a longitudinal lie is unlikely. The patient should be observed closely for the onset of labor or spontaneous rupture of membranes.

10. Cesarean section should be performed if a transverse lie persists and the fetus is mature. Perinatal and maternal morbidity increases significantly after the onset of labor or rupture of membranes.

F. *Method of delivery*

1. *Fetus less than 800 gm.* If the fetus is extremely premature and not expected to survive, version and extraction may be performed after complete cervical dilatation. Spontaneous delivery may occasionally occur.

2. *Fetus greater than 800 gm.* All gestations that may be expected to survive should be delivered by cesarean section. Most authorities advocate the lower-segment

vertical incision, since the incision may be extended towards the fundus if difficulty is encountered during delivery.

3. *Internal podalic version* with a viable infant is not recommended, since it is often associated with unacceptable fetal and maternal morbidity.

4. *Intrauterine fetal demise.* Fetal death will often occur as a result of impaction or cord prolapse.

   a) If the cervix is completely dilated, internal podalic version and extraction may be performed under general anesthesia. This procedure may lead to uterine rupture if the lower segment is extremely thin.

   b) If the cervix is incompletely dilated, external cephalic version may be performed.

   c) Cesarean section should be performed if the above maneuvers fail.

   d) Destructive procedures are not recommended, since they often lead to serious maternal soft-tissue injury.

   e) Cesarean hysterectomy is indicated in cases of neglected transverse lie associated with uterine rupture or severe intrauterine infection.

FACE PRESENTATION

In a face presentation, there is extreme extension of the fetal head causing the occiput to nearly contact the back. The face becomes the presenting part. The presentation is cephalic and the attitude is complete extension.

A. *Incidence.* A face presentation is found in *0.2 to 0.3 percent of labors.* It is more common in multiparas.

B. *Etiology.* A face presentation may occur whenever there is a condition that either favors extension of the head or prevents flexion of the head. In approximately 30 percent of cases, no cause can be found.

   1. *Cephalopelvic disproportion.* The following factors may interfere with descent and lead to extension of the fetal head: inlet contraction, inlet deformity, soft-tissue mass, large fetal head.

2. *Pendulous abdomen,* often associated with multiparity, may lead to abnormal forward and lateral movement of the fetus and result in extension of the head.
3. *Conditions that favor increased fetal mobility.* In the following conditions the fetal head may remain freely moveable within the pelvis: hydramnios, a small infant in a normal-sized pelvis (premature), a normal-sized infant in a large pelvis.
4. *Low-lying placenta or placenta previa.* The placenta distorts the lower uterine segment, preventing normal accommodation of the head in the pelvis.
5. *Tumors of the neck or multiple loops of umbilical cord* may prevent normal flexion.
6. *Cervical muscle shortening or spasm* may prevent normal flexion.
7. *Congenital absence of cranial structures.* Anencephalic fetuses usually present as a face.

C. *Diagnosis*
1. *Abdominal examination.* The characteristic finding is the presence of the cephalic prominence on the same side as the fetal back.
2. *Vaginal examination.* Facial parts are easily palpated. The fontanelles and sutures are not palpable. The soft, irregular face may be confused with a breech. An ultrasound or x-ray examination may be necessary to confirm the diagnosis.

D. *Mechanism of labor.* The face presentation generally does not exist before the onset of labor. Complete extension usually occurs during descent. With complete extension, the submentobregmatic diameter of 9.5 cm presents. The biparietal diameter does not pass through the pelvic inlet until the chin has nearly reached the perineum.
1. *Mentum anterior.* Descent and rotation occur as with vertex presentations, with the chin (mentum) as the leading part. After internal rotation, the chin passes under the pubic arch. The chin pivots at the symphysis and the head delivers by flexion. The remainder of the mechanism is similar to the vertex presentation.

2. *Mentum posterior.* Marked molding usually occurs as the head passes through the inlet. After internal rotation, the chin is directed posteriorly into the hollow of the sacrum. In approximately two-thirds of cases, the chin will rotate to an anterior position when it reaches the pelvic floor. If the chin remains in a posterior position, further progress of labor is impossible, since the neck is shorter than the length of the sacrum.

E. *Management*

1. X-ray pelvimetry is indicated in cases of face presentation because of its common association with cephalopelvic disproportion. Ultrasound may be used to confirm anencephaly, a large fetal head, or anomalies of the neck.

2. *In mentum anterior positions,* spontaneous delivery or low-forceps delivery may be anticipated. Arrest of labor with a mentum anterior position should be treated by cesarean section rather than oxytocin stimulation because of the likelihood of cephalopelvic disproportion and associated birth trauma.

3. *In mentum posterior positions,* spontaneous rotation to a mentum anterior position will occur in two-thirds of cases. Rotation will often not occur until the face begins to distend the perineum. If a posterior position persists, cesarean section should be performed.

4. The following procedures are no longer accepted in modern practice: version-extraction, manual conversion of the face to a vertex presentation, manual or forceps rotation of a persistent mentum posterior to an anterior position. These procedures have been associated with unacceptable fetal and maternal morbidity.

BROW PRESENTATION

In a brow presentation, the head occupies an attitude midway between full extension and full flexion. The presenting part is the area between the orbital ridges and the anterior fontanelle. The brow is considered a transitional position during descent, since most brow presentations will convert to a vertex presentation by complete flexion or to a face presentation by complete extension.

A. *Incidence.* A persistent brow presentation is found in *0.1 percent of labors.*

B. *Etiology.* Brow presentations are generally associated with the same factors found in face presentations.

C. *Diagnosis*
   1. *Abdominal examination.* The cephalic prominence is palpable on the same side as the fetal back.
   2. *Vaginal examination.* The following structures are palpable: anterior fontanelle, frontal sutures, orbital ridges, nasal ridge. The mouth and chin are not palpable.

D. *Mechanism of labor.* The mechanism of labor will vary with the size of the infant. In a term infant, the largest diameter of the head (occipitomental, 13.5 cm) will present at the pelvic inlet. Engagement will occur only if there is extensive molding or if further extension or flexion occurs. If the brow presentation persists, descent will be slow. If the brow rotates anteriorly, the head is initially born by flexion, with the brow, bregma, and occiput successively passing over the perineum. Extension of the head will then occur with the mouth and chin passing under the pubic arch.

E. *Management*
   1. Spontaneous conversion of a brow presentation to a face or vertex presentation occurs in most cases; therefore, expectant management is indicated.
   2. If the infant is small or the pelvis large, spontaneous delivery may be anticipated.
   3. An arrest of labor should be treated by cesarean section rather than oxytocin stimulation because of the likelihood of cephalopelvic disproportion and associated birth trauma.
   4. Manual conversion of a brow to a face or vertex presentation is not recommended.

COMPOUND PRESENTATION

A compound presentation exists when an extremity prolapses alongside the presenting part and both enter the pelvis simultaneously. The most common compound presentation involves a hand prolapsed alongside the head.

A. *Incidence.* Compound presentation is found in *about 0.1 percent of labors*. It is more common in multiparas.

B. *Etiology.* Compound presentations usually occur in association with factors that interfere with normal occlusion of the pelvic inlet by the presenting part: pelvic contraction, pelvic deformity, hydrocephalus, hydramnios, prematurity, multiple gestation.

C. *Diagnosis.* Vaginal examination will reveal an extremity alongside the head or breech.

D. *Mechanism of labor.* In most cases, labor progresses normally according to the usual mechanism of the presenting part. Since engaging diameters are increased, labor may be prolonged due to delayed descent.

E. *Management*

1. In most cases, labor should be allowed to progress without interference. A normal vaginal delivery may be anticipated.

2. If a prolapsed extremity appears to interfere with descent, attempts should be made to replace the extremity above the presenting part. Cesarean section will be necessary if attempts at repositioning fail and there is a subsequent arrest of descent.

3. Forceps may be used for delivery if indicated. Care is taken not to include the extremity within the forceps, since serious compression injury may occur.

4. *Umbilical cord prolapse occurs in 15 to 20 percent of compound presentations.* Continuous electronic monitoring and frequent vaginal examinations will be necessary to detect cord prolapse.

BIBLIOGRAPHY

Breech Presentation

Ballas S, et al.: Deflextion of the fetal head in breech presentation: incidence, management, and outcome. Obstet Gynecol 52:653, 1978

Braun F, et al.: Breech presentation as an indicator of fetal abnormality. J Pediatr 86:419, 1975

Brenner W, et al.: The characteristics and perils of breech presentation. Am J Obstet Gynecol 118:700, 1974

Collea JV, et al.: The randomized management of term frank breech presentation: vaginal delivery versus cesarean section. Am J Obstet Gynecol 131:186, 1978

DeCrespigny L, Pepperell R: Perinatal mortality and morbidity in breech presentation. Obstet Gynecol 53:141, 1979

Duenhoelter JH, et al.: A paired controlled study of vaginal and abdominal delivery of the low birth weight breech fetus. Obstet Gynecol 54:310, 1979

Goldenberg RL, Nelson KG: The premature breech. Am J Obstet Gynecol 127:240, 1977

Kauppila O, et al.: Management of the low birth weight breech delivery: should cesarean section be routine? Obstet Gynecol 57:289, 1981

Neilson DR: Management of the large breech infant. Am J Obstet Gynecol 107:345, 1970

O'Leary JA: Vaginal delivery of the term breech. Obstet Gynecol 53:341, 1979

Piper E, Bachman C: The prevention of fetal injuries in breech delivery. JAMA 92:217, 1929

Ranney B: The gentle art of external cephalic version. Am J Obstet Gynecol 116:239, 1973

Todd D, Steer C: Term Breech: review of 1006 term breech deliveries. Obstet Gynecol 22: 583, 1963

Woods JR: Effects of low-birth-weight breech delivery on neonatal mortality. Obstet Gynecol 53:735, 1979

Zatuchni GI, Andros GJ: Prognostic index for vaginal delivery in breech presentation at term. Am J Obstet Gynecol 93:237, 1965

Transverse Lie
Sherline DM: Transverse and oblique lie. In Sciarra J (ed): Gynecology and Obstetrics, Vol. 2, New York, Harper & Row, 1978, Chap. 78

Face Presentation
Benedetti TJ, et al.: Face presentation at term. Obstet Gynecol 55:199, 1980

Duff P: Diagnosis and management of face presentation. Obstet Gynecol 84:1881, 1962

Brow Presentation
Jacobson L, Johnson C: Brow and face presentation. Am J Obstet Gynecol 84: 1881, 1962

Magid B, Gillespie C: Face and brow presentation. Obstet Gynecol 9:450, 1957

21

Premature Labor
Jeffrey W. Ellis, M.D.

PRACTICE PRINCIPLES
Prematurity is the major cause of perinatal mortality. Physiologic lung immaturity and sepsis (and its sequelae) are usually the underlying causative factors leading to infant death. Prematurity may also be associated with long-term sequelae of motor and intellectual handicaps. Eight to ten percent of births in the United States occur before 36 weeks' gestation.

DEFINITION OF PREMATURE LABOR
Premature labor is strictly defined as regular uterine contractions producing progressive cervical changes occurring between the 20th and 36th weeks of gestation.

1. In clinical practice, the physician will often not wait for cervical changes before initiating therapy. This is because the further cervical dilatation and effacement advance, the less successful are attempts at pharmacologic inhibition of labor.
2. Many centers have adopted the following "contraction frequency criteria" for diagnosing premature labor: 60 minutes of contractions occuring at least every 10 minutes with a 30-second duration.

ASSOCIATED FACTORS IN PREMATURE LABOR
In the majority of cases, no predisposing factors are identified. Factors known to be *associated* with premature labor include:

1. History of premature labor (25 percent risk of recurrence)
2. Multiple gestation
3. Polyhydramnios
4. Uterine anomalies (congenital, acquired: myomata)
5. Placental abruption, placenta previa
6. Trauma. Blunt or penetrating injury to the abdomen
7. Incompetent cervix
8. Maternal fever
9. Premature rupture of membranes
10. Untreated hyperthyroidism, hyperparathyroidism, or hyperadrenocorticism
11. Orgasm
12. Severe maternal systemic disease such as severe preeclampsia, diabetes, and chronic renal disease
13. Maternal infection, especially urinary tract infection (pyelonephritis)
14. Low socioeconomic status

During routine prenatal visits, it is mandatory to identify patients with any of these risk factors for premature labor. These patients should generally be followed on a weekly basis and counseled to immediately report any uterine contractions or other prodromes of labor. Pelvic examinations should be performed weekly, preferably by the same physician, to detect any early changes in cervical dilatation and effacement.

SELECTION OF PATIENTS FOR INHIBITION OF LABOR

A. *Determine if the patient is in labor.* Use either contraction criteria or note cervical changes.
B. *Determine the gestational age of the fetus.* With most

patients, the determination of a preterm gestation can be made on the basis of accurate dating established during previous prenatal visits. When accurate dating is unavailable, the physician is initially faced with an infant whose gestational age can be determined by size estimation alone. The fetus may be either small for gestational age and physiologically mature, appropriate for gestational age, or large for gestational age and physiologically immature. If doubt exists as to the maturity of the fetus, labor should be stopped and maturity studies undertaken.

C. *Determine cervical changes.* Labor is most successfully inhibited when it is in the latent phase, that is at a cervical dilatation less than 4 cm. Inhibition at greater degrees of dilatation has been attempted but is usually unsuccessful.

D. *Absolute contraindications.* In the following situations, the risks to the mother and fetus outweigh the benefits of prolonging the pregnancy:
    1. Severe preeclampsia/eclampsia
    2. Placental abruption
    3. Chorioamnionitis
    4. Dead fetus
    5. Fetal anomaly incompatible with life
    6. Fetal distress as evidenced by falling urinary estriol determinations, positive oxytocin challenge tests, etc.
    7. Severe maternal disease requiring delivery
    8. Mature fetus

E. *Relative contraindications.* In the following situations, premature labor may be inhibited only if neither the fetus nor the mother would be placed in jeopardy if the pregnancy is allowed to continue. If the clinical condition deteriorates during therapy, labor-inhibiting drugs must be stopped.
    1. Chronic hypertension
    2. Chronic renal disease
    3. Heart disease
    4. Diabetes mellitus
    5. Erythroblastosis fetalis
    6. Intrauterine growth retardation

F. *Additional indications.*

1. A patient with a previous cesarean section may have premature labor inhibited as long as abdominal examination and symptoms do not suggest uterine incision separation.

2. Though controversial, patients with premature rupture of membranes between the 28th and 32nd weeks of gestation may have labor inhibited for 48 hours to allow acceleration of biochemical lung maturation. Labor-inhibiting agents must be discontinued if signs of chorioamnionitis develop.

3. Bleeding as a result of placenta previa is usually aggravated by uterine contractions. If bleeding is minimal, no fetal distress is noted, and the fetus is premature, labor may be inhibited (but this is controversial). Corticosteroids may then be given to accelerate lung maturity (also controversial).

4. Labor-inhibiting drugs have been administered prophylactically to patients with multiple gestations beginning at 28 to 32 weeks of pregnancy. This use is presently investigational.

5. Uterine contractions are common after cervical cerclage. Labor-inhibiting drugs may be administered for 48 to 72 hours after the procedure. Some physicians give labor-inhibiting drugs to cerclage patients until documented fetal maturity.

6. Fetal heart rate decelerations suggesting fetal distress generally occur in relation to uterine contractions. Several authorities have advocated stopping uterine contractions while the patient is being prepared for operative delivery, although this is controversial.

TREATMENT: TOCOLYTIC DRUGS

Pharmacologic agents currently used in the inhibition of premature labor are divided into two categories depending on their site of action:

1. Drugs which repress substances which stimulate uterine contractions.
2. Drugs which directly inhibit myometrial contraction.

The choice of drugs is made on the basis of the patient's history and current physical condition. Though β-mimetic drugs are currently considered the most effective agents, certain conditions will necessitate the use of other drugs. Each drug will have specific advantages, disadvantages, and contraindications. In view of potentially serious side effects, these drugs should be administered only by physicians thoroughly familiar with their use and in a hospital equipped to monitor the mother and fetus closely. The dosage of any of these drugs involves a compromise between uterine response and unwanted effects.

The drugs described below are currently used in the United States for inhibition of preterm labor. Ritodrine is the only drug that has been approved by the Food and Drug Administration to carry the indication for use in inhibiting labor.

A. *Inhibitors of oxytocin and prostaglandin*
   1. *Prostaglandin inhibitors.* Aspirin, indomethacin, and naproxen are seldom used today because of the existence of more effective drugs.
      a) *Effectiveness.* Few clinical trials
      b) *Mechanism*
         (1) Prevention of prostaglandin synthesis
         (2) Possible blockade of prostaglandin
      c) *Administration.* Oral and rectal
      d) *Contraindications.* History of gastrointestinal bleeding or ulcer disease
      e) *Disadvantages*
         (1) Poor gastrointestinal toleration
         (2) Theoretical possibility of premature closure of the ductus arteriosis in the fetus
   2. *Ethanol*
      a) *Effectiveness.* 75 percent

b) *Mechanism*
   (1) Probably by direct blockade of oxytocin release from the posterior pituitary
   (2) Possibly by direct suppression of the myometrium
c) *Administration*
   (1) An intravenous infusion of 9.5 percent solution of ethanol in D_5/W is administered at a rate of 7.5 ml/kg of body weight per hour for 2 hours.
   (2) The rate is then decreased to 1.5 ml/kg/hour for 10 hours.
   (3) If contractions resume after the treatment period, a loading dose may be repeated as 10 percent of the initial loading dose for every hour that the ethanol infusion has stopped. If more than 10 hours have elapsed, the original loading dose should be readministered. Maintenance doses remain the same.
d) *Patient monitoring.* Maternal vital signs must be carefully monitored with specific reference to respiratory rate. The patient must be watched closely to prevent aspiration or physical injury if intoxication occurs. The patient must never be left unattended. Some authorities have advised periodic determinations of blood alcohol levels to detect toxic levels.
e) *Contraindications*
   (1) Severe liver disease
   (2) Alcoholism (active or inactive)
   (3) Drug addiction
   (4) Psychiatric disease where intoxication would render the patient unmanageable
f) *Disadvantages*
   (1) Maternal nausea, vomiting, aspiration, headache, anxiety, respiratory depression.
   (2) Continuous oral administration for maintenance therapy is often unacceptable to the patient and may cause fetal alcohol syndrome.

(3) Combination with narcotic analgesics and sedatives may cause severe respiratory depression.

(4) Maternal hypoglycemia may develop complicating diabetic management.

(5) Severe neonatal depression may result if delivery occurs during or shortly after the treatment period.

(6) Must carefully monitor serum sodium levels, as hyponatremia secondary to fluid load plus diuresis and subsequent hypovolemia and seizure are major risks.

B. *Direct inhibitors of myometrial contraction*
 1. *Magnesium sulfate*
   a) *Effectiveness.* 50 to 75 percent.
   b) *Mechanism.* Probably by uncoupling of the excitation-contraction response at the cellular level by displacing calcium.
   c) *Administration*
     (1) A 4-gm intravenous bolus given over 15 minutes.
     (2) This is followed by an infusion of 2gm/hour by pump via "piggyback" infusion system. Never infuse $MgSO_4$ directly.
     (3) After contractions have stopped, the infusion is reduced to 1 gm/hour.
     (4) The infusion is discontinued after 24 hours if the patient is acontractile.
   d) *Patient monitoring.* Maternal vital signs must be carefully monitored with specific reference to respiratory rate. Hourly urinary output must be monitored, since magnesium is excreted in the urine and low urinary output may lead to dangerously high serum levels. Some authorities advise periodic determinations of serum magnesium levels.
   e) *Contraindications*
     (1) Severe renal disease that impairs magnesium excretion.
     (2) Any degree of maternal heart block.

  f) *Advantages.* May be used in patients who have contraindications to the use of β-mimetic drugs.

  g) *Disadvantages*

    (1) No effective oral maintenance form.

    (2) Frequent clinical and laboratory assessment is needed to prevent magnesium toxicity.

    (3) Narcotics and barbiturates may potentiate maternal respiratory depression.

    (4) Infants born during or shortly after therapy may have respiratory depression and decreased muscle tone.

2. β-*Mimetic drugs:* isoxsuprine, terbutaline, ritodrine

  a) *Effectiveness.* 75 to 95 percent

  b) *Mechanism.* Stimulation of β-receptors on the myometrium causes muscle relaxation, possibly by affecting the potassium and sodium ion flux across the cell membrane.

  c) *Patient monitoring.* Cardiovascular effects are common and are generally related to dosage and the degree of maternal hydration. Maternal vital signs must be monitored every 15 minutes. Maternal tachycardia and a slight reduction in blood pressure are common. Severe hypotension may occur especially if there is hypovolemia. The fetal heart rate must be continuously monitored. During protracted therapy, maternal glucose and potassium levels should be evaluated.

  d) *Contraindications*

    (1) Cardiac disease that may be adversely affected by tachycardia or sudden hypotension

    (2) Maternal intravascular volume depletion

    (3) Uncontrolled hyperthyroidism

  e) *Disadvantages*

    (1) Maternal tachycardia and hypotension are common especially if there is intravascular volume depletion.

    (2) Maternal blood glucose levels will be increased

due to glycogenolysis. Frequent evaluations of blood glucose will be necessary in diabetic patients.

(3) Due to maternal hyperglycemia, the infant may become hypoglycemic after delivery due to increased fetal insulin secretion.

(4) Maternal potassium levels may be decreased with protracted therapy.

(5) Maternal pulmonary edema may occur in the presence of volume overload. Pulmonary edema has also been reported with concomitant administration of corticosteroids. Meticulous records of fluid intake and output must be kept.

(6) *Potentiation of drug effect* may occur with administration of anesthetic agents and other sympathomimetic amines.

(7) *Adverse reactions* are common and include palpitation, tremor, nausea, vomiting, headache, chest pain and tightness, and cardiac arrhythmia. These effects are related to the β-mimetic activity of the drugs.

f) *General principles of administration*

(1) The eventual dosage of the β-mimetic drug represents a balance between the uterine response and unwanted side effects.

(2) In view of the potentially serious adverse effects of β-mimetic drugs, their use should be supervised by physicians thoroughly familiar with the pharmacology, indications, contraindications, and adverse effects of these drugs.

(3) A secure indwelling intravenous line should be established using either a 16- or 18-gauge catheter.

(4) The patient should be adequately hydrated before and during drug administration.

(5) To promote uterine perfusion, the patient should remain in the left lateral position.

(6) The β-mimetic drug should always be administered in a dilute solution using a mechanical infusion pump.

(7) A "two-bottle" technique of infusion should be used. In the primary intravenous line, the patient should receive a solution of either D5/NS or D5/LR in the event that rapid volume expansion is necessary. The fluid containing the β-mimetic drug is connected to the main intravenous line using a Y-connector. This technique will ensure that the patient does not receive large quantities of the drug if the intravenous line is inadvertently allowed to run at a high rate.

(8) The patient must be attended constantly while the drug is administered.

g) *Drug administration.* The following β-mimetic drugs are currently used in the United States for the inhibition of premature labor. Ritodrine appears to have the fewest associated side effects.

(1) *Isoxsuprine (Vasodilan)*

(a) Prepare an IV solution of isoxsuprine: placing 30 mg of drug in 250 ml normal saline.

(b) Begin infusion using an infusion pump, giving a loading dose of 0.2 to 1.0 mg/minute for 10 to 15 minutes.

(c) Maintenance dose (IV): 0.1 to 0.3 mg/minute for 24 hours.

(d) If uterine activity is effectively inhibited, oral maintenance then may be begun: 10 to 20 mg p.o. every four to six hours.

(e) The same precautions apply to isoxsuprine as do to terbutaline.

(2) *Terbutaline*

(a) 0.25 mg IV bolus

(b) Prepare an IV solution of 5 mg terbutaline in 95 ml of 5 percent dextrose in water. The dilution will then be 50 μg/ml.

(c) Begin the IV infusion at 10 μg/minute using a mechanical infusion pump.

(d) Increase the infusion by 5 μg every 10 minutes until uterine contractions stop or until significant side effects occur.

(e) The usual therapeutic range is 10 to 80 μg/minute.

(f) After uterine activity has been suppressed for four hours, stop the infusion and begin subcutaneous administration of terbutaline 0.25 mg every four hours.

(g) Continue subcutaneous administration for 24 hours, then give 2.5 mg orally every four hours.

(h) Any patient who resumes uterine activity while on either subcutaneous or oral terbutaline should be restarted on the IV infusion. The initial IV bolus should be repeated.

(i) Reduce or discontinue the dosage if the patient has *tachycardia* greater than 120/minute; *fetal tachycardia* greater than 180/minute; *hypotension* to the point of decreased vital organ perfusion (usually a mean arterial pressure of less than 70 mm Hg).

(j) Discontinue the infusion if uterine contractions do not stop after two hours of maximum dosage.

(3) *Ritodrine (Yutopar)*

(a) Prepare an IV solution of 150 mg ritodrine in 500 ml of fluid. The dilution will then be 0.3 mg/ml. The diluting solution may be either D5/W, normal saline, or Ringer's solution.

(b) Begin the infusion at 0.1 mg/minute using a mechanical infusion pump.

(c) Increase the infusion by 0.05 mg/min every 10 minutes until uterine contractions stop or until significant side-effects occur.

(d) The usual therapeutic range is 0.15 to 0.35 mg/min.

(e) Discontinue the infusion if uterine contractions persist at the maximum dose.

(f) The infusion should be continued for 12 hours after uterine contractions have stopped.

(g) Thirty minutes before discontinuing the intravenous dosage, oral ritodrine is administered. The initial oral dosage is 10 mg. every two hours for the first 24 hours. The dosage is then changed to 10 mg or 20 mg every 4 to 6 hours depending upon uterine activity.

(h) Oral dosage is maintained as long as it is necessary to prolong pregnancy.

(i) The maximum daily dosage of ritodrine is 120 mg. in 24 hours.

(j) If uterine contractions recur on oral therapy, the intravenous regimen may be restarted.

Outpatient Management

The patient should remain hospitalized for at least 48 hours after uterine contractions have stopped. She may then be discharged from the hospital with the following instructions:

1. Oral medications must be taken according to a strict schedule.

2. Relative inactivity should be maintained and strenuous physical activity avoided.

3. Sexual intercourse and masturbation are prohibited.

4. The patient should be evaluated as an outpatient at least once a week for the remainder of the pregnancy.

5. Any evidence of renewed uterine activity should be reported promptly.

BIBLIOGRAPHY

Barden TP, et al.: Ritodrine hydrochloride; A betamimetic agent for use in preterm labor. Obstet Gynecol 56:1, 1980 (39 references)

Caritis SN, et al.: Pharmacologic inhibition of preterm labor. Am J Obstet Gynecol 133:557, 1979

Creasy RK, et al.: System for predicting spontaneous preterm birth. Obstet Gynecol 55:692, 1980

Csapo AL, Hereczeg J: Arrest of premature labor by isoxsuprine. Am J Obstet Gynecol 129:482, 1977

Petrie RH: Stopping premature labor with magnesium sulfate. Contemp Obstet Gynecol 11:187, 1978

Spearing G: Alcohol, indomethacin, and salbutamol: A comparative trial of their use in preterm labor. Obstet Gynecol 53:171, 1979

Wallace RL, et al.: Inhibiting of premature labor by terbutaline. Obstet Gynecol 51:387, 1978

22

Premature Rupture of Membranes

Jeffrey W. Ellis, M.D.

PRACTICE PRINCIPLES

Premature rupture of membranes is a common obstetric complication. Management is aimed at preventing neonatal and maternal infection while maximizing the infant's chances for survival. Management must be appropriate to the individual case.

- *Definition.* Premature rupture of the membranes (PROM) is the rupture of the amniotic sac before the onset of labor.
- *Incidence.* PROM occurs in 3 to 14 percent of pregnancies. The incidence increases with advancing gestational age. Twenty percent of cases of PROM occur before 36 weeks of gestation.

CLINICAL SIGNIFICANCE

A. *Onset of labor.* The latent period is defined as the interval between rupture of membranes and the onset of labor.
   1. Near term, approximately 80 percent of patients with PROM will begin labor within 24 hours; in 95 percent, within 72 hours.

2. Before 36 weeks of gestation, labor begins within 24 hours in 35 to 50 percent of patients. Seventy percent of patients will begin labor within 48 hours. Ten percent of patients will have a latent period greater than 14 days.

B. *Maternal complications.* Intrauterine infection (chorioamnionitis), sepsis, disseminated intravascular coagulation

C. *Fetal complications.* Premature delivery, sepsis, prolapse of cord or fetal part, increased incidence of operative delivery due to abnormal presentation (usually breech)

ETIOLOGY

The etiology of PROM is unknown in the majority of cases. PROM has been associated with amniocentesis, abdominal trauma, incompetent cervix, hydramnios, abnormal lie, placenta previa, viral and bacterial intrauterine infection, and ascorbic acid deficiency.

MANAGEMENT

The management of PROM is one of the most controversial areas in modern obstetrics, varying considerably among institutions based on individual experiences and regional preferences. Large-scale, prospective studies will be necessary to define optimum management.

A. *General principles. There is no single correct plan of management for all patients with PROM.* General management principles are outlined below, and should be followed in sequence.

1. *Confirm the presence of ruptured membranes.*

2. Determine approximate cervical dilatation and effacement *by speculum examination only*. The information obtained from a manual vaginal examination will normally not alter management and may introduce bacteria into the amniotic cavity.

3. Evaluate the patient for the presence of chorioamnionitis.

4. If chorioamnionitis is suspected, the fetus should be delivered regardless of gestational age.

5. If chorioamnionitis is not suspected, determine the gestational age of the fetus.

6. Further management will depend on gestational age assessment.

7. If necessary, transfer the patient to a medical center that has appropriate diagnostic facilities and a neonatal intensive care unit.

B. *Diagnosis.* Various techniques are commonly used to detect the presence of amniotic fluid in the vagina.

1. *Speculum examination of the vagina and cervix* may reveal free flow of fluid from the cervical os. A pool of amniotic fluid may be noted in the posterior fornix. Gentle fundal pressure may be applied if necessary to demonstrate free flow.

2. *Gross examination* of the fluid may reveal fetal hair, vernix caseosa, or meconium.

3. *pH testing* of the vaginal fluid using *nitrazine paper* will reveal a strongly alkaline pH if amniotic fluid is present (pH 7.0 to 7.5). The nitrazine paper will turn *dark blue to black*. Normal vaginal secretions have a pH of 4.5 to 5.5, and the nitrazine paper remains yellow. Additional fluids that may be found in the vagina may give false readings.

   a. *Urine.* Alkaline or acid
   b. *Blood.* Alkaline
   c. *Cervical secretions.* Alkaline
   d. *Antiseptic solutions.* Alkaline

4. *A fernlike pattern* will be noted if amniotic fluid is allowed to dry on a slide and is then examined under a microscope. This crystalization pattern is due to high concentrations of NaCl and protein. No other vaginal fluid will show a fernlike pattern.

5. *Nile blue stain,* when mixed in equal portions with amniotic fluid, may reveal orange-colored fetal fat cells of

sebaceous gland origin. These cells are present in significant quantity only in gestations greater than 36 weeks.

6. If no amniotic fluid can be identified using these techniques and if the diagnosis of PROM is *strongly* suspected, the following techniques may be used:

a) The patient should remain at rest in the supine position for one hour, thus allowing amniotic fluid to accumulate in the vagina. The speculum exam is then repeated.

b) *Ballotment* of the presenting part may release fluid into the vagina from behind the presenting part. There is a risk of umbilical cord prolapse with this procedure.

c) *Evans Blue dye* or other nontoxic dyes may be injected into the amniotic cavity. Gauze or cotton inserted into the vagina will be stained by the dye if membranes are ruptured.

d) *Ultrasound examination* of the uterus may reveal decreased amniotic fluid volume if significant fluid loss has occurred. This is a highly suggestive, but not a confirmatory, sign.

EVALUATION AND MANAGEMENT OF CHORIOAMNIONITIS

A. *Signs and symptoms*
  1. *Maternal.* Fever, tachycardia, uterine tenderness and irritability, purulent cervical discharge
  2. *Fetal.* Tachycardia, possible decreased beat-to-beat variability, and late decelerations during labor
B. *Laboratory studies*
  1. *Complete blood count.* Leukocytosis with a left shift is usually present with chorioamnionitis.
  2. *Cultures.* Aerobic and anaerobic cultures should be obtained from the endocervix. A Gram stain should also be performed.

3. *Amniocentesis.* In cases where chorioamnionitis is suspected but signs and symptoms do not establish the diagnosis, amniocentesis may be performed. A white blood cell count, Gram stain, and aerobic-anaerobic cultures should be performed on the fluid. The presence of white blood cells and bacteria is suggestive of intrauterine infection. (Several authorities feel that intrauterine infection can be proven only if more than 10^2 colonies of bacteria per milliliter of fluid are demonstrated on culture.)

C. If *intrauterine infection* is suspected, the following management plan should be followed:

1. If delivery will occur within one to two hours and the mother is not severely ill, antibiotics should be withheld until after the umbilical cord is clamped. This will allow the pediatrician to obtain pure cultures from the infant without the interference of antibiotics.

2. If delivery will be delayed beyond two hours, broad-spectrum (aerobic and anaerobic coverage) antibiotics should be administered parenterally to the mother.

3. Most authorities agree that either *ampicillin* or *cephalosporin* is the appropriate antibiotic in most cases. If the patient is severely ill or allergic to penicillin, appropriate parenteral doses of gentamicin and clindamycin should be administered.

4. Antibiotic regimens may be altered according to subsequent bacterial identification and drug sensitivities.

5. In general, delivery should occur within approximately eight hours from the development of chorioamnionitis. The route of delivery is determined by general obstetric factors such as gestational age and lie of the fetus, presence of cephalopelvic disproportion, and the presence of a uterine scar. If there is no initial indication for cesarean section, induction of labor with oxytocin should be started. Cesarean section will be necessary if delivery does not occur within eight hours. Continuous electronic monitoring is mandatory because of the increased incidence of fetal distress.

   6. A cord blood culture and Gram stain should be obtained at delivery.

D. *Determination of gestational age.* The following observations and studies should be used to determine maturity of the fetus:

   1. Review of prenatal records and previous fetal ultrasound studies if performed.

   2. Measurement of fundal height.

   3. Measurement of the fetal biparietal diameter by ultrasound.

   4. Amniocentesis with determination of lecithin-sphingomyelin ratio (L/S ratio) and phosphatidyl glycerol and creatinine levels. (Because of the reduction of the amniotic fluid volume, amniocentesis should be performed only with the aid of ultrasonography, obtaining fluid from the largest available pocket.)

   5. Collection of vaginal amniotic fluid and determination of L/S ratio and the presence of phosphatidyl glycerol. Since contamination by other vaginal fluids may falsely increase the L/S ratio, the findings of an L/S ratio greater than 2:1 does not always confirm maturity. An L/S ratio of less than 2:1 probably indicates an immature fetus. Many authorities believe that the shake test is a more accurate method for determining the quantity of surfactant, as it measures a physical property of the fluid and not a chemical property that may be altered by contamination.

E. *Management according to gestational age.* The most significant factors leading to perinatal mortality and morbidity are the consequences of prematurity and infection. Most authorities believe that the greatest hazard to the fetus before 33 weeks of gestation is prematurity. Based on this premise, the following guidelines for management have been proposed (provided there is no evidence of intrauterine infection):

   1. *Fetus with L/S ratio greater than 2:1.* The fetus should be delivered without prolonging the latent period.

   2. *Gestational age greater than 36 weeks.* The fetus should be delivered without prolonging the latent period.

3. *Gestational age between the beginning of the 33rd week through the end of the 36th week.* Delivery should be performed after a latent period of 12 to 24 hours from the time of membrane rupture to promote fetal lung maturation.

4. *Gestational age from the beginning of the 27th week of gestation through the 32nd week.* Delivery should be delayed until the end of the 32nd week.

5. *Gestational age less than 27 weeks.* Considerable controversy exists regarding management of PROM at less than 27 weeks of gestation. Many authorities feel that delivery should be delayed until the end of the 32nd week if possible. Others argue for "emptying the uterus." Each case must be decided on its own merits after fully discussing the results and benefits with the patient.

F. *Principles of conservative management.* If delivery is to be delayed, the management plan outlined below should be followed:

1. The patient should maintain bed rest until leakage of fluid stops.

2. Vital signs and fetal heart rate should be determined every four hours.

3. A CBC with white blood cell differential should be obtained every 12 to 36 hours as clinically indicated.

4. If chorioamnionitis is suspected, the fetus should be delivered.

5. If there is no evidence of chorioamnionitis after several days of hospitalization, the patient may be discharged from the hospital with the following instructions:

   a) The patient should take her oral temperature every four to six hours.

   b) Sexual intercourse, douching, and the use of vaginal tampons are prohibited.

   c) The patient should report to the hospital immediately if fever or a purulent vaginal drainage develops, or if labor begins.

   d) The patient should be examined in the office once a week. A CBC should be obtained at each visit.

G. *Management controversies.* The following issues are controversial and await the results of large-scale, prospective studies. Physicians should continue to consult the current literature in the field for new data. Management in individual institutions will depend on prevailing regional views and individual experience.

1. *Prophylactic antibiotics.* Most authorities currently feel that prophylactic antibiotics should not be administered to patients with PROM. Some studies have shown a decreased incidence of puerperal endometritis after the use of prophylactic antibiotics. However, no studies have shown a reduction in neonatal sepsis.

2. *Benefits of ruptured membranes in preventing RDS.* A review of the current literature (Table 22–1) reveals studies that both advocate and refute the benefits of prolonged rupture of membranes in accelerating fetal lung maturation and thus decreasing the incidence and severity of respiratory distress syndrome (RDS).

3. *Tocolytic agents.* Several authors have advocated the use of tocolytic agents to inhibit labor in patients with PROM who have no evidence of chorioamnionitis. It has been further suggested that tocolytic agents should be used only after amniotic fluid has been obtained by amniocentesis and no bacterial growth is found on cultures.

4. *Steroid acceleration of lung maturity.* Although some studies have suggested a decreased incidence of RDS after the administration of standard dosages of betamethasone, there has not been widespread acceptance of this form of management. Recent studies have suggested possible neurologic deficits in infants exposed to corticosteroids in utero.

5. *Surveillance and treatment of vaginal and cervical infections.* Many centers routinely obtain cultures for group B β-hemolytic streptococcus and *Neisseria gonococcus* at the time of initial evaluation of the patient with PROM. Treatment of positive cultures has ranged from immediate delivery under specific antibiotic coverage to

TABLE 22–1. REVIEW OF THE LITERATURE ON THE EFFECTS OF *PROM* ON THE INCIDENCE OF RDS

Studies Suggesting Benefit	Studies Suggesting No Benefit
Alden: Pediatrics 50:40, 1972	Bada: Pediatric Res 10:420, 1976
Bauer: Pediatrics 53:7, 1974	Barrada: Am J Obstet Gynecol 129:25, 1977
Berkowitz: Am J Obstet Gynecol 124:712, 1976	Dimmick: Obstet Gynecol 47:56, 1976
Chiswick: Lancet 1:1060, 1973	Jones: N Engl J Med 292:1253, 1975
Gluck: Am J Obstet Gynecol 115:539, 1973	Liggins: Mod Perinatal Med 1974
Miller: Am J Obstet Gynecol 132:1, 1978	Quirk: Am J Obstet Gynecol 134:768, 1979
Obladen: Am J Obstet Gynecol 135:1079, 1979	Schreiber: Am J Obstet Gynecol 136:92, 1980

expectant management with antibiotics administered only at the time of delivery.

BIBLIOGRAPHY

Abe T: The detection of the rupture of fetal membranes with the nitrazine indicator. Am J Obstet Gynecol 39:400, 1940

Atlay RD, Sutherst JR: Premature rupture of the fetal membranes confirmed by intra-amniotic injection of dye (Evans Blue T-1824). Am J Obstet Gynecol 108:993, 1970

Averette HE, et al.: Cytodiagnosis of ruptured fetal membranes. Am J Obstet Gynecol 87:226, 1963

Berkowitz RL: Premature rupture of membranes: a review and treatment plan. Comtemp Obstet Gynecol 10:35, 1977

Bobbitt JR, Ledger WJ: Amniotic fluid analysis—Its role in maternal and neonatal infection. Obstet Gynecol 51:56, 1978

Garite TJ, et al.: The use of amniocentesis in patients with premature rupture of membranes. Obstet Gynecol 54:226, 1979

Mead PB, Clapp JF: The use of betamethasone and timed delivery in the management of premature rupture of the membranes in the preterm pregnancy. J Reprod Med 19(1):3, 1977

23

Multiple Gestation
Jeffrey W. Ellis, M.D.

PRACTICE PRINCIPLES
Multiple gestations are associated with significantly increased maternal and perinatal morbidity. Careful antepartum management is necessary for the early diagnosis and treatment of maternal complications. Optimal intrapartum management remains controversial, with a greater tendency towards cesarean section.

A. *Incidence*
  1. *Spontaneous*
     a) Twins: 1/88 pregnancies
     b) Triplets: $1/88^2$ pregnancies (1/7744)
     c) Quadruplets: $1/88^3$ pregnancies (1/681,472)
  2. Significantly increased with the use of drugs stimulating ovulation, e.g., menotropins (Perganol)
B. *Predisposing factors*
  1. Increased age
  2. Multiparity
  3. Familial history of multiple gestation on maternal side
  4. Induced ovulation
C. *Varieties*
  1. *One-third*: single ovum (monozygotic) — "identical twins"

2. *Two-thirds*: two or more ova (polyzygotic) — "fraternal twins"

D. *Placenta and membrane types*
    1. One-third of single-ovum twins: two placentas (fused or unfused), two chorions (fused), two amnions
    2. Two-thirds of single-ovum twins: one placenta, one chorion, two amnions
    3. Rare in single-ovum twins: one placenta, one chorion, one amnion
    4. Double-ovum twins: two placentas (fused or unfused), two amnions, two chorions

ANTEPARTUM CARE

A. *Suspect* multiple gestation:
    1. When the uterus grows rapidly and out of proportion to calculated gestational age
    2. In patients with unexplained weight gain after the 20th week of pregnancy
    3. In patients who have received drugs for induction of ovulation
    4. In patients with a significant family history of multiple gestation

B. *Diagnosis*
    1. Suggested by hearing two separate areas of distinct fetal heart tones differing by at least 10 beats per minute
    2. Suggested by palpation of multiple extremities or two heads
    3. Multiple gestation will consistently be confirmed by *ultrasonography* or abdominal radiograph after 16 weeks of gestation

C. *Maternal complications.* Increased incidence of:
    1. Preeclampsia
    2. Anemia
    3. Premature rupture of membranes
    4. Premature labor

    5. Polyhydramnios

    6. Hyperemesis gravidarum

D. *Fetal complications.* Increased incidence of:

    1. Intrauterine growth retardation

    2. Congenital anomalies

    3. "Fetal transfusion syndrome" from common placental circulations

    4. The complications of premature delivery

E. *Antepartum management*

    1. As a result of the numerous maternal complications associated with multiple gestation, the patient should be followed on a weekly basis beginning at 25 weeks' gestation.

    2. *Adequate dietary intake* should be stressed with dietary consultation as needed.

    3. *Oral iron supplementation* is necessary for all patients, since a twin gestation will increase the iron requirement of the pregnancy nearly 100 percent. *Complete blood counts* should be performed every four weeks.

    4. The patient should be monitored carefully for the development of signs of preeclampsia, which may occur earlier in pregnancy than with singleton gestations.

    5. *Serial ultrasound* measurements of the fetal biparietal diameters and trunk diameters are necessary to detect intrauterine growth retardation and congenital anomalies.

    6. Though controversial, several recent studies indicate that *decreased maternal activity* with *frequent bed rest* beginning at approximately 30 weeks' gestation leads to increased fetal weight and a decreased incidence of premature labor.

       a) Hospitalization may be necessary to accomplish this goal.

       b) The prophylactic use of oral β-*mimetic drugs* is currently being investigated as a means of decreasing the incidence of premature labor. Their use in actual premature labor is indicated.

7. The patient should be counseled to report to the hospital immediately at the onset of labor or if membrane rupture occurs.

8. The standard tests of fetal well-being are difficult to interpret with multiple gestation. Because of the difficulty in monitoring each fetal heart rate, the nonstress test and oxytocin challenge test may effectively assess only one fetus. Urinary estriol levels may be within the normal range even though one fetus is severely compromised, and HPL will be increased because of increased placental mass.

INTRAPARTUM MANAGEMENT

A. *Maternal complications*
   1. The incidence of preeclampsia and eclampsia is increased.
   2. Cesarean section is more frequent.
   3. Forceps delivery or version-extraction procedures may lead to extensive lacerations or uterine rupture.
B. *Perinatal complications*
   1. Prematurity
   2. Hypoxia caused by prolapsed cord or premature separation of the placenta after delivery of the first infant
   3. Neurologic injury secondary to version-extraction procedures
C. *Essentials of management*
   1. *Type and crossmatch* two or more units of whole blood, depending on the patient's hemoglobin and hematocrit at the time of admission.
   2. Obtain an abdominal radiograph to determine the position of the fetuses and to assess the presence of interlocking fetal parts or fetal anomalies. If possible an ultrasound determination for biparietal diameter should be performed.
   3. *Each fetus* should be *electronically monitored* using exter-

nal Doppler units connected to separate printout monitors. If membranes have ruptured, the presenting fetus should be monitored internally.
4. Monitor vital signs frequently for the development of preeclampsia.
5. *Induction of labor* using oxytocin is controversial; however, some authorities suggest that the cautious use of oxytocin, assuming continuous electronic monitoring of heart rate and uterine activity, may be employed. Hypertonic and tetanic uterine contractions *must* be avoided.
6. *Dysfunctional labor* should be evaluated using the same criteria used with singleton pregnancy. Oxytocin may be used cautiously if hypotonic dysfunction is diagnosed, again requiring continuous electronic monitoring.

DELIVERY

A. The delivery of twins should take place in a delivery room that can be set up immediately for cesarean section.
B. *Birth-room team*
   1. Obstetrician
   2. Pediatrician
   3. Anesthesiologist
   4. Two nursing teams
C. The route of delivery is determined by the lie, gestational age, and weight of the fetuses. Absolute indications for cesarean section are interlocking or conjoined twins.
D. The route of delivery of the *first* or *leading fetus* should be determined using those principles established for a singleton fetus of a similar lie, gestational age, and weight.
E. Immediately after delivery of the first infant, the presentation of the second infant should be determined by inserting an entire hand into the uterine cavity.
F. The route of delivery of the *second fetus* is controversial. If a cephalic presentation is found, vaginal delivery may be performed. If the second fetus is in a transverse or breech

presentation, total breech extraction or version-extraction may be performed. Because of the significant perinatal morbidity associated with these procedures, cesarean section is advocated in many centers.

G. The interval between delivery of the first and second infant should generally not exceed 30 minutes. After delivery of the first infant, the second infant should be continuously monitored using the external Doppler. If labor appears to be protracted for the second infant, or if irregularity of the fetal heart rate is noted, internal monitoring should be initiated.

H. Cord blood should not be obtained until all infants are delivered, since there is the possibility of common placental circulation.

I. After delivery of the placenta, the patient should be monitored carefully for the development of excessive vaginal bleeding from a hypotonic uterus. Intravenous oxytocin should be administered after delivery of the placenta and for at least two to four hours theralter. If a version-extraction was performed, the uterus should be explored manually for evidence of rupture.

J. If a *cesarean section* is performed, a lower segment vertical uterine incision should be considered, since if there is difficulty in delivery of the second infant, the uterine incision can be extended upward.

K. *Anesthesia for delivery.* If vaginal delivery is performed, the first infant can usually be delivered under a pudendal block and nitrous oxide inhalation. Breech extraction or version-extraction may require uterine relaxation best obtained with general anesthesia.

THREE OR MORE FETUSES

The presence of three or more fetuses significantly increases the incidence of maternal and fetal complications. Premature delivery nearly always occurs. Perinatal mortality and morbidity are increased as a result of prematurity, complicated delivery maneuvers, and fetal hypoxia secondary to either cord prolapse or placental separation. Most authorities believe that pregnancies involving three or more fetuses are best delivered by cesarean section.

BIBLIOGRAPHY

Cetrulo C, Freeman R, Knuppel R: Minimizing the risks of twin delivery. Contemp Obstet Gynecol 9:47, 1977

Crane JP, et al.: Ultrasound growth patterns in normal and discordant twins. Obstet Gynecol 55:678, 1980

Divers W, Hemsell D: The use of ultrasound in multiple gestations. Obstet Gynecol 53:500, 1979

Duncan S, Ginz B, Wahab H: Use of ultrasound and hormone assays in the diagnosis, management and outcome of twin pregnancies. Obstet Gynecol 53:367, 1979

Ferguson WF: Perinatal mortality in multiple gestation: A review of perinatal deaths from 1609 multiple gestations. Obstet Gynecol 23:861, 1964

Jewelewicz R, Vande Wiele R: Management of multifetal gestation. Contemp Obstet Gynecol 6:59, 1975

Misenhimer H, Kaltreider D: Effects of decreased prenatal activity in patients with twin pregnancies. Obstet Gynecol 51:692, 1978

Powers W: Twin pregnancy: Complications and treatment. Obstet Gynecol 42:795, 1973

Ron-El R, et al.: Triplet and quadruplet pregnancies and management. Obstet Gynecol 57:458, 1981

24

Antepartum Bleeding

Jeffrey C. King, M.D.

PRACTICE PRINCIPLES

Approximately 3 percent of all pregnancies are complicated by significant bleeding from the birth canal. The term "significant" is used to differentiate it from "show," which occurs near the onset of most labors. The main causes of antepartum hemorrhage are placenta previa and abruptio placenta. Bleeding may occur from many other causes, but these are relatively unimportant obstetrically. All patients with significant bleeding require hospital admission to rule out placenta previa or placental abruption, since both cause increased morbidity and mortality for mother and fetus.

GENERAL APPROACH TO EVALUATION

A. The *general approach* to patients with late-pregnancy bleeding is to obtain historical information, evaluate overall patient condition, initiate laboratory studies, and begin therapy.

  1. Questions concerning the amount of bleeding, presence and quality of pain, history of previous bleeding, and history of trauma are important.

2. Vital signs should be recorded frequently from both the mother and the fetus (i.e., continuous fetal heart rate monitoring in a viable fetus).
3. Careful physical examination must be performed. *Digital pelvic exam is excluded;* although a carefully inserted speculum may be extremely helpful in evaluating the cause of bleeding.

B. *Standard laboratory tests*
   1. *Maternal.* Hemoglobin and hematocrit, and coagulation studies — prothrombin time, partial thromboplastin time, platelet count, and fibrinogen level. Determination of fibrin split products has been suggested, but one must remember that they are present in about 15 percent of normal pregnancies.
   2. *Fetal.* An APT test may be helpful in determining if the blood loss is fetal or maternal in origin. (Mix vaginal blood with an equal quantity of 0.25 percent NaOH. Fetal blood will not change color, whereas maternal blood will turn light brown.)

C. A continuous urinary drainage catheter is inserted for hourly output determinations and for microscopic urinalysis. A large-bore (16-gauge) intravenous line should be started and an approximate amount of blood should be typed and crossmatched.

PLACENTA PREVIA

A. *Definitions and demographics*
   1. The placenta is implanted, either wholly or partially, in the lower uterine segment.
   2. Generally occurs in *0.5 to 1.0 percent of all pregnancies,* accounting for *30 to 40 percent of cases of antepartum bleeding.*
   3. It appears to be twice as common in the multigravida as in

the primigravida. Other than multiparity and increased maternal age, no additional etiologic factors have been identified.

B. *Classification*

1. *Three degrees of placenta previa* have been recognized depending on the relationship of the placental margin to the internal cervical os.

   a) *Marginal.* The edge of the placenta is at the margin of the internal os.

   b) *Partial.* The internal os is partially covered by placenta.

   c) *Total.* The internal os is completely covered by placenta.

2. *The degree of placenta previa depends on the extent of cervical dilatation at the time of examination.* What appears to be marginal at 2 cm will probably be partial at 6 cm. The fact that the placenta may be implanted in the lower segment makes membrane stripping to stimulate labor a potentially dangerous practice.

C. *Signs and symptoms*

1. The most characteristic sign of placenta previa is *painless, causeless, and recurrent bright red bleeding.*

   a) Although usually slight, the first episode of bleeding may be profuse. It usually will stop spontaneously but can recur when least expected.

   b) The first episode of bleeding occurs at less than 32 weeks in 10 percent, between 32 and 36 weeks in 30 percent, and beyond 36 weeks in 60 percent of patients.

2. *If labor accompanies the painless bleeding,* it is important to note that the uterus relaxes completely between contractions. The fetal presenting part is often high above the pelvic brim. However, *malpresentations are no more frequent when gestational age is adjusted.*

D. *Diagnosis*

1. Placenta previa is suspected on historical data and the

physical examination. It is confirmed by placental localization.

2. *The simplest, most precise, and safest method for placental
localization is ultrasonography.* If the equipment is available, this is the method of choice for investigating a
patient suspected of having a placenta previa. Recent
studies have shown ultrasonography to be 93 to 98
percent *accurate* in placental localization. At genetic
amniocentesis (16 to 18 weeks), almost 10 percent of
patients were diagnosed as having a placenta previa, but
the overwhelming majority converted to a "normal"
placental implantation site by the time of delivery. This
concept of "placental migration" explains the relative
unimportance of the placenta previa diagnosis until 28 to
30 weeks.

3. Other methods for diagnosis, soft-tissue amniography,
placenta isotope scans, and arteriography are of historical
interest only.

E. *Either active or expectant management*

1. *Both gestational age and the amount of bleeding determine
management.* While most cases can be reported into
either active or expected management, some will require
considerable clinical acumen.

2. *Active management*

a) If fetal maturity is documented, the patient should be
delivered by cesarean section.

b) Should the diagnosis be in question, *a "double setup"*
examination is indicated. This is performed in an
operating room with all preparations for cesarean
section having been accomplished. If significant
bleeding jeopardizes the mother or fetus, emergency
delivery by cesarean section is necessary no matter
what the diagnosis. In cases of anterior partial
placenta previa, the uterine incision of choice is a low
vertical.

3. *Expectant management*

a) This course of action may be taken only *when the*

bleeding has been minimal and when the risks of fetal prematurity are high.

    (1) The patient should be hospitalized, confined to bed and intercourse prohibited.

    (2) Blood may be transfused if necessary to maintain the hematocrit at 30 percent or higher.

  b) Significant controversy surrounds the use of *tocolytic agents* in patients with a premature fetus and slight bleeding. Careful use of these agents may settle an irritable uterus and allow continuation of the pregnancy. Obviously, active bleeding contraindicates tocolysis.

  c) These patients are often good candidates for *steroid induction of fetal lung maturation.* Howie and Higgins have shown that the human fetus will respond to maternally administered steroids between 28 and 32 weeks. Prior to 28 weeks there is not enough lung to stimulate and after 34 weeks there is no benefit. The duration of steroid effect is one week, so if delivery is delayed, the dose must be repeated weekly until 32 weeks. When the fetus reaches maturity, a double setup examination should be performed in the operating room. Delivery should then be accomplished by the appropriate means. The work of Brenner is helpful in predicting the delivery interval for patients with symptomatic placenta previa.

4. *Complications. Hemorrhage* can be severe and lead to intrauterine death from anoxia. Following delivery, the eroding trophoblasts may prevent adequate contraction in the lower uterine segment and postpartum hemorrhage may occur. *Rarely, placenta previa is associated with placenta accreta, increta, or percreta.* These conditions, wherein the trophoblasts invade the myometrium to varying degrees, have occasionally resulted in the need for hysterectomy.

F. *Maternal and fetal mortality*

  1. Maternal mortality should approach zero.

2. Fetal mortality is between 8 and 10 percent, principally caused by hypoxia from placental separation and prematurity.

ABRUPTIO PLACENTA

A. *Definitions and demographics*
   1. *Premature separation of a normally implanted placenta from the decidua basalis prior to the third stage of labor* is the most accurate definition of abruptio placenta.
   2. It occurs in *1 to 2 percent* of *all pregnancies* and accounts for *40 to 50 percent* of cases of antepartum bleeding
   3. The primary *etiology* of abruptio placenta is unknown. However, a variety of conditions are associated with it: high multiparity, pregnancy-induced hypertension, short umbilical cord, sudden decompression of the uterus, or trauma. A previous history of abruption is elicited in approximately 10 percent of cases.
B. *Classification* (Fig. 24–1)
   1. The older classification—in which hemorrhage was divided into revealed, concealed, or mixed—has been replaced by a *clinical classification* that depends on the degree of separation and various signs and symptoms. Cases are divided into mild, moderate, and severe placental separation; and generally the amount of hemorrhage parallels the degree of separation. *About 65 percent of cases will be classified as mild,* 23 percent as moderate, and 12 percent as severe abruptio placenta.
   2. *Mild abruption*
      a) Vaginal bleeding is minimal (less than 100 ml).
      b) The uterus may be slightly irritable but remains soft and nontender.
      c) No fetal heart rate abnormalities are presented.
      d) There is no evidence of shock or coagulopathy.
   3. *Moderate abruption*
      a) Bleeding may be moderate (100 to 500 ml).

Class of Abruptio Criteria	Mild (Approx. 65%)	Moderate (Approx. 23%)	Severe (Approx. 12%)
Amount of vaginal bleeding	Less than 100 cc	100-500 cc	Greater than 500 cc
Uterine tone	Slightly irritable Soft, nontender	Increased activity and some tenderness	Tense, tetanic, Tender uterus
FHR pattern	Normal	May be evidence of fetal distress or IUFD	Usually evidence of fetal distress or IUFD
Maternal status	Normal	Mild shock Infrequent coagulopathy	Moderate to severe shock Frequent coagulopathy

Figure 24–1. A clinical classification of Abruptio placentae.

b) Uterine activity and tone are increased; and tenderness is frequently noted.

c) Maternal pulse is elevated, blood pressure lowered, and mild shock may be present.

d) Fetal heart sounds may be present or absent. If the fetal heart sounds are present, monitoring may reveal evidence of fetal distress due to uteroplacental insufficiency.

4. *Severe abruption*

a) External bleeding may be copious (greater than 500 ml) but can be entirely concealed.

b) Moderate to profound shock may be present; evidence of coagulopathy is frequent.

c) The uterus is tense and quite tender to palpation.

d) Fetal demise is frequent.

5. *In cases in which classification is difficult treatment should be as in the severe form.*

C. *Diagnosis*

1. Unfortunately, the diagnosis must be based *solely* on clinical grounds until delivery and inspection of the placental attachment surface is possible.

2. *Ultrasonography* has been advocated, but at least 100 ml of blood would have to be trapped beneath the placenta to be seen ultrasonographically. Bleeding that escapes through the cervix cannot usually be seen as an ultrasonographic abnormality. Recently, some have advocated ultrasonography to examine the entire placental margins in the belief that slight elevation of the margin may be diagnostic.

D. *Signs and symptoms*

1. *Vaginal bleeding* is present in 80 percent of cases, but bleeding may be completely concealed in 20 percent.

2. Sudden onset of constant *pain* that is localized to the lower back and uterus is common with moderate to severe forms. Either generalized or localized *abdominal tenderness* is noted in the more severe cases.

3. *Uterine activity and reactivity* are increased.

4. When bleeding is concealed, an increase in *uterine size* is frequently noted.

5. When fetal membranes rupture, the amniotic fluid is often noted to be bloody, classically called "port wine" stained.

6. *Maternal shock and evidence of fetal compromise parallel the degree of separation.*

7. *Consumptive coagulopathy* is often seen, since placental abruption is its most common cause during pregnancy. Placental separation usually precedes the onset of coagulopathy, but as long as the uterus is unevacuated, the coagulopathy is progressive. While coagulation occurs retroplacentally, the intravascular component is much more significant in terms of altered coagulation factors.

    a) Overt hypofibrinogenemia (less than 150 mg/dl), along with decreased levels of factors V and VIII, prothrombin, and platelets, confirms the diagnosis of coagulopathy.

    b) The presence of increased fibrin split products suggests activation of the thrombolytic pathway to maintain patency of the microcirculation.

E. *Management*

  1. *Mild placental abruption*

    a) *Expectant management* is the treatment of choice when fetal immaturity is present.

    b) However, *it is quite difficult to differentiate mild abruption from placenta previa.* Therefore, the patient should be hospitalized and standard antepartum monitoring techniques such as nonstress tests, estriol determinations, and serial sonography should be instituted. Frequent determinations of hematocrit are necessary to assess the extent of maternal blood loss.

    c) If bleeding increases or fetal maturity is attained, delivery should be accomplished.

  2. *Moderate placental abruption*

    a) The aim of treatment is to *restore blood loss and effect delivery*

       (1) Central venous or Swan-Ganz monitoring can be extremely helpful during replacement therapy.

       (2) Fresh whole blood or packed cells plus fresh frozen plasma or cryoprecipitate is used for replacement. One unit of fresh frozen plasma will increase serum fibrinogen levels by 25 mg percent, while cryoprecipitate contains 0 to 25 gm per unit.

  b) Once the diagnosis is made, *amniotomy* should be performed. Labor usually starts soon after amniotomy, but if there is any delay, an oxytocin infusion should be administered.

  c) The goal is vaginal delivery, but cesarean section is indicated if fetal distress develops and vaginal delivery is not imminent or if progressive hemorrhage jeopardizes either the mother or fetus. Previously, an arbitrary time limit of six hours for delivery was used; however, it has been found that prompt and adequate blood replacement is more important.

  d) Following delivery, coagulation defects return to normal within 24 to 48 hours. However, the platelet count may take up to 10 days to reach its previous level.

3. *Severe placental abruption*

  a) The treatment of this category is essentially the same as for moderate hemorrhage. The extent of bleeding and the effects on both the mother and fetus are, however, greater. A urinary catheter is necessary to assess hourly urinary output. Oliguria is frequently seen, which underscores the necessity of central pressure monitoring.

  b) Fetal demise is common; when it has occurred, cesarean section is rarely necessary except when bleeding cannot be controlled or labor is excessively protracted.

  c) *The importance of aggressive replacement of blood and coagulation factors cannot be overstressed.*

4. *Complications*
   a) *The major complications are those related to hemor-rhagic shock and both intravascular and retroplacental coagulopathy.*
   b) When hemorrhage is severe, some blood may be forced from the placental bed into the muscle fibers toward the uterine serosa. The uterus takes on the appearance of a bruised and edematous organ. This has been described as a *couvelaire uterus;* and because of its extremely poor contractile force, hysterectomy has occasionally been necessary.
   c) Shock may result in *ischemic necrosis to either the kidneys or anterior pituitary.* If the ischemia is of short duration, no changes occur; but when the duration increases, irreversible damage is likely. Cortical necrosis is the most common sequelae of prolonged hypotension. Sheehan's syndrome or panhypopituitarism is rare but may result from prolonged and severe shock due to abruptio placenta.

F. *Maternal and fetal mortality*
   1. Maternal mortality will depend on the time of diagnosis, and the rapidity and skill with which the condition is treated. Generally, the risk appears to be 5 to 10 percent for the most severe cases.
   2. Fetal mortality depends on the extent of placental separation and ranges between 30 and 60 percent.

OTHER CAUSES OF ANTEPARTUM BLEEDING

A. *"Show."* Usually a diagnosis of exclusion, but commonly the blood is dark and mixed with copious mucus. This is the most common cause of a history of "bleeding" in advanced pregnancy.
B. *Cervical*
   1. *Neoplastic* lesions of the cervix are rare, but cytologic sampling is mandatory to rule out carcinoma.

   2. *Severe trichomonas* vaginitis/cervicitis may result in bleeding, but it usually is only a slight pink staining associated with severe vulvar pruritis.

C. *Vasa previa.* The presence of fetal vessels passing over the internal cervical os is defined as vasa previa. Unfortunately, leakage from these vessels cannot be seen with ultrasound and therefore an APT test may be lifesaving for the fetus. The greater risk is during rupture of the membranes. Continuous electronic fetal monitoring may be beneficial for detecting acute fetal distress due to fetal hemorrhage and hypovolemia.

D. *Varicose veins of the vulva.* Though rare, the increased venous presure below the level of the uterus may cause dilation of vulvar vessels. This can result in a feeling of perineal heaviness and occasional spontaneous rupture. Inspection will reveal the source, and pressure will usually stem the flow.

E. *Endocervical polyps.* These may occasionally cause antepartum bleeding, but it is usually limited. Intervention is indicated if bleeding persists or neoplasia is suspected.

F. *Trauma.* Antepartum trauma to the birth canal structures may cause bleeding. Overly vigorous coitus has classically been implicated, although the risks of coitus are questionable.

BIBLIOGRAPHY

Booher D, Little B: Vaginal hemorrhage in pregnancy. N Engl J Med 290:611, 1974

Brenner W, Edelman D, Hendricks C: Characteristics of patients with placenta previa and results of "expectant management." Am J Obstet Gynecol 132:180, 1978

Carp H, Mashiach S, Serr D: Vasa praevia: a major complication and its management. Obstet Gynecol 53:273, 1979

Cotton D, Read J, Paul R, Quilligan E: The conservative aggressive management of placenta previa. Am J Obstet Gynecol 137:687, 1980

Llewellyn-Jones D: Antepartum haemorrhage. In Fundamentals of Obstetrics and Gynaecology. London, Faber, 1979

Naeye R: Placenta previa. Obstet Gynecol 52:521, 1978

Pritchard JA, MacDonald PC: Obstetric hemorrhage. In Williams Obstetrics (16 ed). New York, Appleton-Century-Crofts, 1980, pp 487–526.

Sher G: A rational basis for the management of abruptio placentae. J Repod Med 21:123, 1978

25

Abortion

Section 1
Spontaneous and Induced Abortion in the First and Second Trimester*

Charles R.B. Beckmann, M.D.
Jessica L. Thomason, M.D.

PRACTICE PRINCIPLES

The threat of loss or loss of intrauterine pregnancy is one of the most personally traumatic events that may face a couple and one of the most common clinical situations encountered by the gynecologist. The sensitive and careful management of the various presentations of abortion, salvaging the pregnancy where possible and reducing psychologic and medical morbidity in all cases, then becomes a major goal of good gynecologic care.

INTRODUCTION

Elective second-trimester abortion is a difficult topic, with great controversy in both its medical and legal aspects. Because of this, together with the fact that it is not performed as an

---

*This section appears in both *A Clinical Manual of Obstetrics* and *A Clinical Manual of Gynecology.*

emergency procedure and should be done in a facility where such procedures are performed regularly, limited attention will be devoted to this topic. The reader is referred to several excellent references for detailed discussion and procedural guides.[15,29,71,76] Techniques for dealing with spontaneous abortion in the second trimester, especially dilatation and evacuation and hysterotomy, are given more attention.

A. *Abortion* is the loss or termination of pregnancy prior to *viability*.
   1. If one uses the concept of viability to imply a reasonable potential for extrauterine life, present developments in neonatology cause difficulties in definition and application, especially in the second trimester.[76]
   2. An *abortus* is generally defined as:[29,76]
     a) Less than 500 gm in weight
     b) Less than 20 weeks in gestational age, measured from the first day of the last normal menstrual period (LMP).
     c) From these data The Committee on Terminology of the American College of Obstetrics and Gynecology has proposed defining abortion as "expulsion or extraction of all or part of the placenta or membranes, without an identifiable fetus, or with a liveborn infant or a stillborn infant weighing less than 500 gm. In the absence of known weight, an estimated length of gestation of less than 20 completed weeks (139 days) calculated from the first day of the last normal menstrual period may be used."[29]

B. *Classification of abortion*[72, 73, 76]
   1. *Indication or cause*
     a) *Spontaneous*. Abortion that begins without human intervention. A "miscarriage" in lay terms.[76]
     b) *Elective (induced)*. Abortion initiated by human intervention at maternal request.
     c) *Therapeutic (induced)*.[76] The guidelines of the American College of Obstetrics and Gynecology for

therapeutic abortion define the conditions where abortion may be so classified.

(1) When continuation of the pregnancy may threaten the life of the woman or seriously impair her health. In determining whether or not there is such risk to health, account may be taken of the woman's total environment, actual or reasonably foreseeable.

(2) When pregnancy has resulted from rape or incest. In this case the same medical criteria should be employed in the evaluation of the patient.

(3) When continuation of the pregnancy is likely to result in the birth of a child with grave physical deformities or mental retardation.

d) *Criminal.* Termination initiated by human intervention outside an approved medical facility.

2. *Clinical presentation* (Table 25-1)

   a) *Threatened abortion.* Vaginal bleeding, with or without pain, in a pregnancy before the 20th completed week where clinical judgement suggests that the pregnancy may continue.

   b) *Inevitable abortion.* A clinical diagnosis in cases of vaginal bleeding and crampy lower abdominal pain, in a pregnancy before the 20th completed week, so severe that no hope for salvaging the pregnancy exists.

   c) *Incomplete abortion.* Expulsion of some of the products of conception before the 20th completed week of gestation.[29]

   d) *Missed abortion.* The fetus dies in utero before the 20th completed week of gestation but is retained in utero for eight weeks or more.[29]

   e) *Septic Abortion.* Any infected abortion.[29]

3. *Gestational age.* Usually from the first day of the last normal menstrual period.

   a) *First trimester.* Conception to 12 completed weeks. Often subdivided into early (conception to 6 weeks) and late (7 to 12 weeks).

TABLE 25–1. DIAGNOSIS AND TREATMENT OF THE ABORTIONS

Diagnosis	Threatened Abortion	Inevitable Abortion	Incomplete Abortion	Missed Abortion
SYMPTOMS Crampy, bilateral LQ pain	+/−	++	+++	+/−
Symptoms of pregnancy	+	+	+/−	Usually
Preceding amenorrhea	+	+	+	+
Vaginal bleeding	Spotting	Heavy	Heavy with clots and/or tissue	+/−
PHYSICAL EXAM Cervix open	Usually not	Usually	Yes	+/−
Blood from cervix	Yes (min.)	Yes	Yes	+/−
Tissue/fluid from os	No	No	Yes	+/−
Uterus soft	Yes	Yes	+/−	+/−

Uterus tender	Often	Yes	Yes	Usually not
Abdomen tender	+/−	Usually	Usually	Usually not
LABORATORY TESTS Urinary test—pregnancy	+/−	+/−	+/−	Usually neg., often positive previously
β-hCG by RIA	+	+	+	+/−
Ultrasound exam	Gestational sac if 6 weeks or more with fetal movement	Gestational sac if 6 weeks or more; +/− fetal movement; halo sign +/−	Unnecessary unless ectopic gestation or uterine anomaly suspected	Disorganized cystic or collapsed intrauterine sac; +/− fetus or placenta
TREATMENT	Observation of patient, bed rest, treatment of infection, counseling and support	Evacuation of uterine contents, counseling and support	Evacuation of uterine contents, counseling and support	Evacuation of uterine contents, counseling and support

b) *Second trimester.* Thirteen to 20 completed weeks of gestation.

FIRST-TRIMESTER ABORTION

A. *Prevalence*
   1. At least 10 to 15 percent of pregnancies undergo spontaneous abortion. It is difficult to assess this accurately because of variation in definitions of abortion and their application as well as incomplete and inaccurate record keeping. Finally, with the advent of more sensitive pregnancy testing (radioimmunoassay and radioreceptor assay for human chorionic gonadotropin), it is clear that pregnancy and spontaneous loss (often subclinical) occur far more frequently than previously believed. Thus, the true spontaneous abortion rate may be two or three times that previously suggested.[11,29,75,76,78,79]
   2. It is also difficult to estimate the number of elective first-trimester terminations done in the United States each year. Estimates vary, but perhaps as many as one-quarter to one-third of all pregnancies are terminated electively.[76] The repeat abortion rate may be as high as 20 percent.
B. *Etiology*
   1. In early gestation, in utero demise usually precedes abortions, whereas in late pregnancy this may not be the case. *A specific etiology is often never ascertained.*[76]
   2. *Associated phenomena*
      a) Pathologic ("blighted") ovum[75,76]
      b) Visible embryomal anomalies[76]
      c) Placental anomalies, either intrinsic, metabolic, or implantational[76]
      d) Chromosomal anomalies, present in one-third to one-half of spontaneous abortions[18,75,76,85,90,96]
      e) Increased maternal age[76,85]
      f) Incompatible intrauterine environment, including

uterine anomalies and myomas, although the latter more often causes infertility rather than abortion[76]
  g) Teratogens and mutagens (chemical and microbiological)[76]
  h) Maternal disease (acute or chronic)[76]
  i) Laparotomy[76] (especially if performed before 16 to 20 weeks of gestational age)
  j) Trauma. Often implicated, but unless very extensive, probably plays a small part in the etiology of abortion[76]
  k) Intrauterine devices[1,30,52,76,84,95]
  l) Maternal request (elective abortion)
  m) Radiation exposure[85]
  n) Maternal alcohol use[41,51]
  o) Maternal smoking[41]
  p) Luteal dysfunction[64]
C. Threatened abortion
  1. Very *common*. Estimated to occur in one of three pregnancies[76]
  2. *Symptoms*[29,76]
    a) *Vaginal bleeding (usually minimal spotting)*
      (1) A "physiologic" bleeding, analogous to the placental sign described by Hartman in monkeys, may occur in humans 2½ or 4½ weeks after conception.[43]
      (2) Evaluation for other causes of bleeding must be made, such as cervical polyps, severe vaginal infection (especially *Trichomonas*), cancer, trauma, foreign body, etc.
    b) *Crampy lower quadrant pain may or may not be present.*
      (1) Multiparas may identify this as like "labor" pains.
      (2) Prognosis is worse when pain accompanies the bleeding.
  3. *Physical examination*[29,76]
    a) *Abdomen*. Usually not tender
    b) *Cervix*. Usually closed, although blood will be iden-

tified coming from the os. No signs of labor (effacement or dilatation, nor loss of tissue or fluid).
  c) *Cervical tenderness,* if present, is usually minimal.
  d) Examine for evidence of *vaginal infection* (G.C.
     culture, saline and KOH preparations and PAP
     smear).
4. *Laboratory evaluation*[76]
   a) *Pregnancy test*
      (1) Urinary test. Positive or negative, depending on
          gestational age
      (2) β-hCG by radioimmunoassay. Positive
   b) *Ultrasonography*[17,23,80]
      (1) Gestational sac with smooth contours; absence of
          halo sign; fluid collections unassociated with preg-
          nancy may occasionally be misleading.[51A]
      (2) If greater than six weeks' gestational age with
          fetal heart action or fetal motion on real-time
          scan.
      (3) Be alert for evidence of trophoblastic disease,
          which may present in this manner.
   c) Clean void urine for urinalysis and culture and sen-
      sitivity.
   d) A continued research goal is to establish accurate
      predictions for the outcome of threatened abortion.
      The combined measurement of serum estradiol and
      use of ultrasound shows promise as such an index,[44] as
      do various ultrasound measures used alone. As yet,
      no method is uniformly accepted.[32]
5. *Treatment*[29,76]
   a) *Bed rest* or significant restriction in activity
      (1) Generally accepted as the most common and
          useful therapy.
      (2) Hospitalization is rarely indicated, but may be if
          rest cannot be assured in the home.
   b) *Treat any infection vigorously.*
   c) Progesterone[35,65,76,87]
      (1) Demonstrated as ineffective
      (2) May be teratogenic

   d) Sedation
     (1) Not demonstrated as effective
     (2) May *occasionally* be appropriate if there are other indications concomitant to the threatened abortion that are exacerbated.
   e) *Counseling and assurance*[75]
     (1) An *extremely important* part of the therapy. *Take the time to talk with the patient and her partner, fully explain the situation, and answer all their questions.*
     (2) *Be sure they have means of obtaining care and or counsel during this time* (e.g., answering service).
   f) There is debate about the effectiveness of any measures, the argument being that any patient having real threatened abortion will eventually abort.[76] Nevertheless, therapy as indicated is appropriate.

D. *Inevitable abortion*
  1. *Symptoms*[29,76]
   a) *Excessive vaginal bleeding.* Diagnosis calls for *clinical judgement* based on the amount of bleeding in the context of the balance of the clinical situation.
   b) *Moderate to severe crampy bilateral lower-quadrant pain,* which a multipara may describe as "labor." Often associated with a sensation of pressure or fullness.
  2. *Physical examination*[29,76]
   a) *Abdomen.* Often tender
   b) *Cervix.* Shows signs of labor (effacement and dilatation) with excessive bleeding from the os
     (1) No tissue loss
     (2) Membranes intact. (There is controversy on this point, with some authorities including ruptured membranes in this diagnosis.)
     (3) Cervical tenderness to motion
   c) Uterus remains soft, feeling "pregnant" on examination, but is usually tender to movement.
  3. *Laboratory evaluation*
   a) *Pregnancy tests.* As in threatened abortion

b) *Ultrasound examination*[17,23,80]
  (1) Fetal heart activity and/or fetal motion may or
      may not be present.
  (2) Gestational sac contour may be irregular and its
      diameter smaller than expected for the gestational
      age based on dates.
c) Maternal blood type and Rh

4. *Treatment*
  a) Once the *clinical judgement* that the pregnancy is
     beyond salvage has been made, evacuation of the
     uterine contents by an appropriate method is indi-
     cated.
  b) If the patient is Rh-negative, anti-Rho immunoglobu-
     lin should be given.[3,37,39,59,76,77]

E. *Incomplete abortion*
  1. Loss of the gestation is begun and must be completed
     with medical assistance as described below. (The concept
     of the "complete abortion," where all the products of
     conception are spontaneously expelled, should be dis-
     carded. All patients with incomplete abortion need
     surgical evacuation of the uterus to assure that there are
     no retained tissues.[28])

  2. *Symptoms*
    a) Severe *vaginal bleeding,* with the *passage of blood and
       tissue and/or amniotic fluid*
      (1) If tissue is brought with the patient, it should be
          sent for pathologic evaluation.
    b) *Severe bilateral lower-quadrant pain*
      (1) Often described by a multipara as labor.
      (2) There is often a sensation of fullness or pressure,
          with a desire to "bear down" as the process
          progresses.
      (3) Unilateral pain should alert the physician to the
          possibility of ectopic gestation.

  3. *Physical examination*
    a) *Cervix.* Open and effaced, showing active signs of
       "labor"[29,76]
      (1) Usually tender on palpation

    (2) Blood coming from the os, often with clots

    (3) Evidence of ruptured membranes is common

    (4) Products of conception, either in the vaginal canal or protruding from the os (Fig. 25–1)

    (5) Conceptus and placenta are often expelled simul-

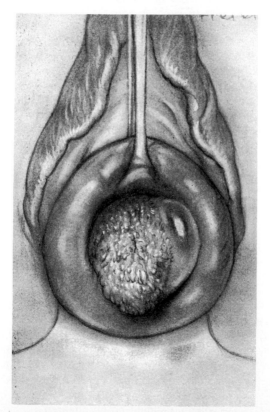

Figure 25–1. Incomplete abortion showing placental fragments extruding from the cervical os. (From Quilligan EJ, Zuspan F: Douglas-Stromme Operative Obstetrics, 4th ed. New York, Appleton, 1982, p 211.)

taneously before the 10th week, separately thereafter

    (6) Retained tissues, especially placental tissue, may
impede myometrial contraction, which constricts
the placental vascular bed and causes hemostasis.
The resulting hemorrhage may be profound, and
appropriate precautions for evaluation and treatment of such an eventuality are indicated. Immediate removal of large pieces of protruding
tissue at initial examination (by traction with a
ring forceps) may reduce the bleeding significantly.

  b) *Uterus.* May be somewhat firmer and smaller than
expected for the gestational age. This is because of
loss of part of the products of conception.

  c) *Abdomen.* Usually tender

4. *Laboratory evaluation*

  a) *Pregnancy test.* As in threatened abortion

  b) *Ultrasonography.* Unnecessary unless ectopic gestation or uterine anomaly is suspected[63]

  c) *Blood type and Rh of mother*

  d) *Complete blood count*

  e) Other laboratory tests as clinically indicated, including:

    (1) Sickle cell status of black patients

    (2) Any clinical suspicion of coagulopathy warrants
appropriate evaluation, including, minimally,
platelet count, PT/PTT.

5. *Treatment*[29,76]

  a) *Evacuation of uterine contents*[76]

    (1) This may be done on an inpatient or outpatient
basis, depending on facilities. More advanced
pregnancies, and those in which there is excessive
hemorrhage (especially with anemia or hypovolemia) should be hospitalized.

    (2) If the patient is febrile, broad-spectrum antibiosis
should be begun, before the procedure if possible,

but after appropriate cultures (aerobic and anaerobic) are taken.

   (3) All tissues should be sent for pathologic examination, to identify the gestation and to screen for trophoblastic changes.[24]

b) It should be emphasized to the patient and her husband that most spontaneous first-trimester abortions are nonrecurring. *Counseling and appropriate reassurance at the time of pregnancy loss are key aspects of complete therapy.*[71,76]

c) *Dilatation, suction, and curettage*[29,75,76,93]

   (1) Gross fetal or placental identification is often difficult due to maceration of the tissues by evacuation procedures or delay from the time of in utero demise.

   (2) Both dilatation and curettage and suction and curettage are used in the first trimester, both in induced and spontaneous abortions. In either case, morbidity caused by uterine perforation, cervical laceration, hemorrhage, and incomplete abortion increases after the 12th week of completed gestation.

   (3) Suction instead of sharp curettage has been shown to reduce the complication rate, lower operative blood loss, and shorten operative time.[7,71] The need for extensive sharp curettage (with the possibility of denuding the decidua basalis and causing hemorrhage or Ashermans syndrome) is lessened. There is little advantage, however, to a blunt rather than sharp curette, since it is the surgical technique rather than the instrument that causes most problems.

   (4) Details of dilatation and suction or curettage may be found in several excellent texts, to which the reader is referred.[29] A brief outline is offered as a general guide.

   (5) *Dilatation and suction or curettage.* Following

appropriate preoperative evaluation and preparation, the anesthesia of choice is administered. The bladder should be empty, with catheterization if necessary to ensure that the bladder is empty.[66] Perineal shaving is unnecessary, as no decrease in infectious or surgical morbidity in shaved patients has been demonstrated.[29] A careful bimanual examination under anesthesia is performed. A weighted vaginal speculum or a Graves bivalve speculum is placed, the cervix identified, and the vagina and cervix cleaned with an antiseptic solution such as povidone-iodine (Betadine). If the patient is awake, the Graves speculum may be more comfortable and hence preferable.[93] The anterior lip of the cervix is then grasped with a tenaculum, ring forceps, or Allis clamp and pulled outward gently to lengthen and straighten the endocervical canal and, to some extent, the uterine cavity. Care must be taken not to place the tenaculum too high so as to impinge on the bladder or to pull too hard so as to pull the tenaculum through the cervical tissue, lacerating it. A second tenaculum may be used if significant traction is anticipated. The uterus is then carefully measured with a uterine sound, first within the endocervical canal, and then part way into the uterine cavity (Fig. 25–2). This helps determine the need for dilatation, as well as further estimating the size and direction of the uterine cavity, which will aid in the subsequent instrumentation.[7,53] Pratt or Hegar dilators are then *slowly* used as needed to dilate the cervix sufficiently to allow instrumentation and removal of the products of conception (Fig. 25–3). Laceration of the cervix may be avoided by the slow and gentle use of these instruments. *There is no rush* to complete dilatation.

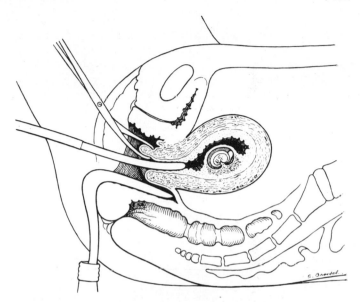

Figure 25–2. Sounding of the uterus with weighted vaginal speculum in place and anterior lip of the cervix grasped with a tenaculum. (From Quilligan EJ, Zuspan F: Douglas-Stromme Operative Obstetrics, 4th ed. New York, Appleton, 1982, p 184.)

If a vacuum suction is to be used, it is inserted, without the suction being engaged. The suction machine has previously been set up and tested to show that it maintains an appropriate amount of suction (usually 50 to 60 mm Hg). An intravenous infusion of oxytocin is begun "piggyback" into the main intravenous line as the suction procedure is begun (20 to 40 units of oxytocin in one liter of solution is usually sufficient). This oxytocin infusion is maintained during the procedure and for a few hours afterward. Blood loss is significantly reduced and uterine tone increased,

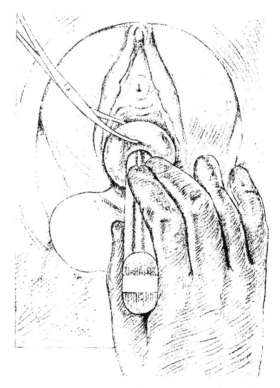

Figure 25–3. Dilatation of the cervix. (From Quilligan EJ, Zuspan F: Douglas-Stromme Operative Obstetrics, 4th ed. New York, Appleton, 1982, p 185.)

the latter decreasing the chances of uterine perforation of the pregnancy-softened uterine wall.[29,56] Suction is then applied, and the suction tip is gently revolved about the inside of the uterine cavity to remove the products of conception (Fig. 25–4). This may need to be done several times to remove all of the tissue. Sufficient repetition is usually indicated by the absence of retrieval of

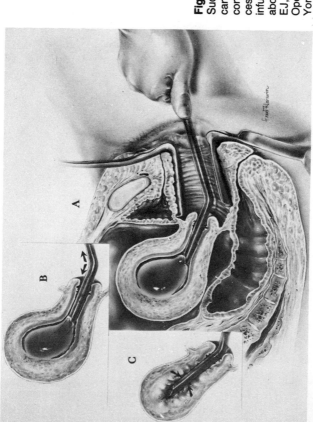

Figure 25–4. Suction curettage. A. Suction tip inserted through cervical canal. B. Suction applied, with uterine contraction due to the suction process as well as intravenous oxytocin infusion. C. Empty uterus contracted about the suction tip. (From Quilligan EJ, Zuspan F: Douglas-Stromme Operative Obstetrics, 4th ed. New York, Appleton, 1982, p 186.)

tissue, a frothy bloody return, and a "rough scratchy" ("gritty") feeling on the tip of the suction catheter against the uterine wall.[93] Sometimes, tissue pieces too large to pass the cannula are encountered (Fig. 25–5). These are easily removed with an ovum or other forceps, whereupon the suction procedure may be completed. Such pieces should be checked for routinely at the end of these procedures. The size of the suction tip chosen will vary with the gestational age, the estimated size of the uterus, and the amount of dilatation accomplished. Tips vary from 7 to 12 mm in diameter.[93]

Sharp curettage may be used to check for

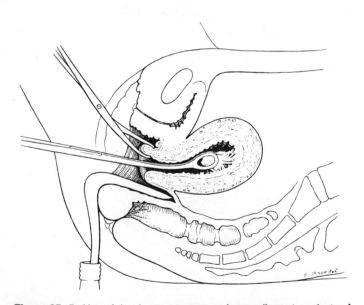

Figure 25–5. Use of ring forceps to remove large adherent products of conception. (From Quilligan EJ, Zuspan F: Douglas-Stromme Operative Obstetrics, 4th ed. New York, Appleton, 1982, p 199.)

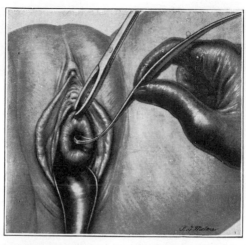

Figure 25–6. Introduction of the curette. Note that in order to avoid excessive pressure application by the curette, the instrument is held between the thumb and forefinger. (From Pritchard J, MacDonald P: Williams Obstetrics, 16th ed. New York, Appleton, 1980, p 606.)

retained products, or as a primary method of removal. In the latter case, blood loss is increased somewhat. In either case, the sharp curette is gently introduced into the uterine cavity and pulled out under mild pressure in smooth, even strokes (Fig. 25–6). Excessive pressure may lead to perforation or denuding of the basalis. To help avoid this, the curette should be held in thumb and forefinger only, so that excessive pressure cannot be exerted. After the products of conception are removed, all implementation is removed, and the sites of the traction or tenaculum insertion on the cervix are checked to ensure that there are no lacerations and that any bleeding is ceasing. *A second careful bimanual examination at the end of the procedure is essential,* to help check for completeness of procedure, trauma (as a developing hematoma), and for adnexal abnormality (as in a combined gestation).

(6) *Dilatation may be difficult,* especially in nulliparous or older patients. This is also more common in elective and some missed abortions compared with the treatment of the inevitable or incomplete abortion. *The use of laminaria tents* may help with this procedure, as well as reducing the incidence of cervical trauma or laceration.[68] Made from the stems of a seaweed (*Laminaria japonica*), laminaria are small sterile "sticks" of material that are carefully placed into the endocervical canal and then beyond so that their tips just pass the internal os but without rupturing the membranes (Fig. 25–7). They come in three sizes, small (3 to 5 mm in diameter) medium (6 to 8 mm), and large (8 to 10 mm). The size that may be tightly fit, but not forced, through the os is chosen. Over the next 8 to 12 hours the hygroscopic ("water-seeking") seaweed slowly expands (often three to five times its original diameter),[93] facilitating a slow and minimally traumatic dilatation. Often sufficient dilatation is accomplished by this method alone. If not, there is often little mechanical dilatation left to be done.[29] Concerns about an increased incidence of infection with the use of laminaria have proven unjustified.[93]

d) *Hysterotomy* may very rarely be indicated in failed dilatation or suction and curettage,[76] but not as a routine method for abortion.[69]

e) *Hysterectomy* may be indicated if there is concomitant uterine or other disease that, *of itself,* would warrant hysterectomy.[5,54,94] It is not a usual primary method of abortion.[83]

f) There are *no* routinely effective medical methods of first-trimester abortion.

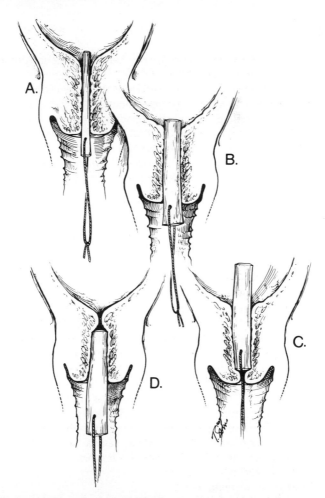

Figure 25–7. Insertion of laminaria. A. Laminaria immediately after being gently, but tightly, placed so that the inner end is just past the internal os. B. The water-swollen laminaria and cervix that has been dilated as a result. C. Laminaria placed too far into the uterine cavity. Dangers here include inadvertent premature rupture of the membranes as well as difficulty in retrieval of the laminaria. D. Laminaria not inserted far enough to dilate the internal os. (From Pritchard J, MacDonald P: Williams Obstetrics, 16th ed. New York, Appleton, 1980 p 604.)

g) If the patient is Rh-negative, anti-Rho immunoglobu-lins should be given.[3,37,39,59,76,77]

h) Patients experiencing *recurrent spontaneous abortion* should undergo vigorous evaluation, including couple karyotyping, since the incidence of chromosomal anomalies and other medical problems in this group is higher than that of the general population.[18,34,75,90,96]

i) In many centers, *prophylactic antibiotics* (commonly oral tetracycline) are given at the time of elective first-trimester termination. The goal is to reduce the incidence of postabortal endometritis and pelvic in-flammatory disease and their possible effects on fertility.[46,88]

j) *Elective first-trimester abortion* follows the same pre-cepts as above. *Simultaneous sterilization* by tubal ligation may be performed without increased risk beyond that associated with the sterilization proce-dure itself.[22,83]

F. *Missed abortion*[29,76]

1. Defined as retention of a dead fetus for more than eight weeks, during the first half of pregnancy.[76]

2. *Symptoms*

a) Initially the patient may "feel pregnant," often fol-lowed by an episode diagnosed as threatened abor-tion. Thereafter, amenorrhea may persist, but the subjective signs of pregnancy may wane.[76]

b) Some patients have minimal vaginal spotting.

c) Other patients may have no symptoms and/or persist in "feeling" pregnant.

3. *Physical examination*

a) Failure of fetus to grow in accordance with length of amenorrhea, and often regression in uterine size as the process progresses (absorption of amniotic fluid plus fetal maceration).[76]

b) Rarely, minimal vaginal bleeding.

c) Cervix will not show signs of labor (effacement and/or dilatation).

4. *Laboratory evaluation*
    a) *Pregnancy tests*
        (1) Urinary. May be negative initially or may progress from positive to negative
        (2) Radioimmunoassay for β-hCG. Falling titer, but usually positive
    b) *Ultrasonography*[17,23,80]
        (1) Disorganized cystic intrauterine sac with or without fetal pole or placental tissue identification. No fetal motion will be present.
        (2) To identify hydatidiform changes that mandate further measures.[29]
5. *Treatment*
    a) *Missed abortion will often terminate in a spontaneous incomplete abortion.*
    b) *If it does not, uterine evacuation is indicated.*
    c) Expectant management, because of the possible medical complications, as well as the emotional trauma to the patient, is no longer acceptable.
    d) Because there is often confusion about the diagnosis of pregnancy and then of in utero demise, patients are placed under great emotional strain. Emotional support and, often, expectant counseling are essential to complete therapy.[29]

G. *Criminal abortion*[29]
1. *The diagnosis is entertained based on an index of suspicion raised by:*
    a) *Coherence and believability of the patient's history*
    b) Patient's emotional status
    c) Time and circumstances of presentation
    d) Appearance of patient and those who accompany her
2. *Physical and laboratory examination*
    a) *Same as for incomplete abortion with the following additions:*
        (1) *Careful examination for trauma* of any kind, but especially as follows:
            (a) External genitalia

      (b) General body. Especially of abdomen and back/buttocks; watch for signs of acute abdomen associated with perforation of the uterus or viscera or of blunt trauma.

      (c) Vagina/perineum. Look especially for signs of perforation, laceration, and abrasion.

      (d) Cervix. Look especially for signs of trauma such as tenaculum puncture sites or other signs of instrumentation.

  (2) Gonorrhea, aerobic, and anaerobic *cultures* and *a Gram stain* should be taken from the endocervix.

  (3) *Supine anterior-posterior and lateral and standing* anterior-posterior *radiographs* of the abdomen and pelvis should be made to search for foreign objects or bowel perforation with a gas bubble under the diaphragm.

3. *Treatment*

  a) *Uterine evacuation* and treatment as in incomplete abortion

  b) *Broad-spectrum antibiosis*

  c) Additional radiologic, and if necessary surgical, evaluation of any suspected trauma

  d) Whether to *report* a suspected criminal abortion depends on the philosophy of the individual physician, the rules of the health care facility, and the legal statutes governing criminal abortion.

H. *Septic abortion*[29,76]

  1. *Definition. Any infected abortion*

    a) Anaerobic and aerobic organisms are usually both involved, including streptococcus, staphylococcus, *Escherichia coli., Bacteriodies* species, *Proteus vulgaris, Neisseria gonorrhea,* and, rarely, *Clostridia* species.[13]

  2. May occur with any abortion, but more frequently seen in neglected incomplete abortion and criminal abortion.[13,76]

  3. Septic bacterial shock is a feared complication, that, if not treated vigorously, may prove fatal.

4. *Treatment.* Completion of the abortion as with incomplete abortion by appropriate means of evacuation, medical support as clinically indicated in cases of shock, culturing, and vigorous antibiosis.[13,76] Antibiosis should, if possible, be begun before evacuation. Many antibiotic regimens have proven effective, e.g., clindamycin and gentamicin. In any event, coverage for aerobic and anaerobic organisms is essential.

5. *The possibility of* Clostridia *species infection* must be especially kept in mind because of its rapid onset with septicemia, intravascular hemolysis, shock, and renal failure.[29]

6. Hysterectomy is seldom necessary unless indicated by extensive uterine damage,[76] absolute refractoriness to therapy, or worsening shock or septicemia.[29]

I. *Diagnosis and treatment of complications*[29,76,93,100]

  1. *Incomplete abortion*

    a) Surgical completion of evacuation of uterine contents

    b) Appropriate culturing and antibiosis

  2. *Uterine perforation*[67,97]

    a) Incidence. Estimated at 0.8 to 1.5/1000 abortions, as many perforations are either unrecognized or unreported.[7,49,66,76]

    b) Physician inexperience and severe anteflexion or retroflexion of the uterus are cited as the most common causes of uterine perforation.[76] Careful preprocedure bimanual examination, appropriate use of the uterine sound to ascertain the exact direction of the endocervical canal, and careful, gentle dilatation and instrumentation will reduce these causes of error.[7,53]

    c) When perforation is suspected, prompt cessation of the procedure (if in progress) and evaluation of the possible perforation (site, maternal status) and gestation (abortion not begun, complete, incomplete) is made. *Table 25–2 suggests a clinical classification of*

TABLE 25–2. CLINICAL CLASSIFICATION AND TREATMENT OF UTERINE PERFORATION DURING ABORTION

Clinical Classification	Treatment
A. *Immediate recognition with cessation of the procedure* (suspected or actual perforation by any instrument including suction cannula with no suction applied)	
1. *Completed abortion.* Perforation after contents of uterus completely evacuated	Inhospital observation of clinical status, serial CBCs, for at least 48 hr.
2. *Intact sac.* Gestation undisturbed	As above, then readmit in about 2 weeks for repeat surgical evacuation.
3. *Incomplete abortion.* Perforation occurs during evacuation; uterus partially emptied.	Immediate diagnostic laparoscopy. Laparotomy and repair if needed. Completion of abortion, either transcervically under laparoscopic observation or, if laparotomy, via uterine rent if transcervical approach inappropriate.

B. *Delayed recognition after operative manipulation* (suction or curettage). No abdominal contents identified. Uterine evacuation may have been attempted before possible perforation was recognized.
   1. *Complete abortion*
   2. *Intact sac*
   3. *Incomplete abortion*

All require immediate diagnostic laparoscopy with laparotomy if indicated (bowel trauma, uncontrolled bleeding, etc.) B.2, B.3: Abortion may be completed as in case A.3.

C. *Perforation with identification of abdominal contents* (bowel, omentum, fat, etc.)
   1. *Completed abortion*
   2. *Intact sac*
   3. *Incomplete abortion*

All require immediate laparotomy and surgical repair as needed. C.2, C.3: Abortion may be completed as in case A.3.

(Adapted from Walden W, Birnbaum S: Contemp Obstet Gynecol 15:47, 1980. By permission.)

such perforations and their therapy. The use of diagnostic laparoscopy has reduced the need for laparotomy by more than one-half.[7,8,49,53,66,76,93,97]

3. *Infection*[29]
   a) *Endometritis/PID*[71]
      (1) Culture and appropriate antibiosis
      (2) Examine the patient for retained products of conception; when in doubt, repeat dilatation or suction and curettage is indicated after antibiosis is begun.
    b) *Chronic cervicitis.* Sometimes associated with cervical laceration
    c) *Sepsis.* An infrequent but serious complication, with a death-to-case rate for septic abortion estimated at about 0.5 deaths/100,000 legal and spontaneous abortions.[36A]
4. *Failure to recognize simultaneous ectopic pregnancy*
5. *Anesthetic reaction*
6. *Uterine synechiae* (Asherman's syndrome)
7. *Cervical incompetence*
8. *Cervical scarring and stenosis*
9. *Cervical laceration*[93]
   a) *External laceration.* Most commonly caused by a tearing action by a tenaculum. One or two hemostatic sutures usually suffice to repair this type of laceration.
   b) *Laceration of the internal os.* Felt to be associated with too vigorous or rapid dilatation, or dilatation at increased gestational age. The latter suggests that elective transcervical abortion should be performed at as early a gestational age as possible.[42,86]
10. *Postabortal syndrome*[29,67,93]
    a) Variously called postabortal syndrome, postabortal hematometra, postabortal uterine atony, and "re-do syndrome."
    b. Although the cervix has remained open, blood clots collect within the uterine cavity (sometimes quickly, sometimes after several days), causing a swollen, tender uterus associated with fever and crampy pain.

Oxytocics may help,[81] but re-evacuation is the treatment of choice. Antibiosis is indicated. Hospitalization may be indicated.

11. *Failed abortion with continuation of pregnancy.*[93] A rare outcome. One series estimated an incidence of 0.071/100 cases (46 cases in a series of 65,045 elective first-trimester terminations).[33]
12. *Hemorrhage*[29]
13. *Uterine rupture*[74]
14. *Ureteral injury*[6]
15. *Amniotic fluid embolism and disseminated intravascular coagulation*[92]
16. *Failed abortion because of uterine anomalies*[63]

SECOND-TRIMESTER ABORTION

A. *Elective and therapeutic*
   1. Because of the many problems associated with second-trimester termination of pregnancy, including medicolegal and psychosocial as well as purely medical, *such procedures are best done in facilities where they are performed routinely.* In such a setting an experienced staff will avoid many of the errors experienced by a staff exposed to these procedures on an intermittent basis.[42,71,75]
   2. If second-trimester termination is considered, documentation of gestational age by ultrasound is a wise precaution.[70,93]
B. *Technique*[29,76,93]
   1. *Dilatation and evacuation*[20]
      a) In the United States one opinion has been that transcervical uterine evacuation should not be performed beyond 12 completed weeks of gestation.[19,29]
      b) Many operators, however, disagree, suggesting that morbidity and mortality are much decreased with dilatation and evacuation as compared to other sec-

ond-trimester techniques until 16 weeks of completed gestational age.[16,21A,38,40,45,93] The use of the technique is increasing steadily.[21A]

c) The technique is similar to that in first-trimester dilatation and suction or curettage except that surgical forceps are usually needed to remove fetal parts, especially the calvarium.[93] Laminaria are used extensively, since greater cervical dilatation is usually required.

2. *Oxytocin infusion*

a) Of little value until cervical dilatation has begun.[76]

b) Potential problems[76] include failure of intended effect, water intoxication,[60,61] and rarely uterine rupture[74] (most often in grandmultiparas).

c) Often used in conjunction with other methods to good effect.[9,14,82]

3. *Intraamniotic hyperosmotic solutions* (hypertonic saline, hyperosmolar urea)[14,29,48,71,76]

a) In many centers, hypertonic saline has been shown to be especially effective[9,41] and is still popular, although the use of prostaglandins is supplanting its use.

b) The procedures carry significant risks, however:[42,71,76,82]

   (1) Sepsis

   (2) Hyperosmolar crisis

   (3) Disseminated intravascular coagulation[12,58,81,89]

   (4) Water intoxication[55]

   (5) Fever

   (6) Myometrial necrosis (especially associated with inadvertant intramyometrial injection)[36,98]

   (7) Uterine rupture

   (8) Cervical and vaginal fistulae[36,62]

   (9) Retained placenta

4. *Prostaglandins*[29,76,93]

a) *Intraamniotic prostaglandin $F_{2\alpha}$ $(PGF_{2\alpha})$*[2,31,62]

   (1) A method often used for advanced second-trimester termination,[71] this route of administration for $PGF_{2\alpha}$ is successful in most cases within 48

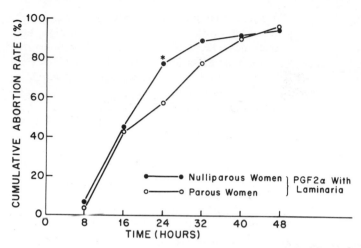

Figure 25–8. Cumulative abortion rate (percent) after the use of intraamnionic prostaglandin $F_{2\alpha}$ plus laminaria. (From Pritchard J, MacDonald P: Williams Obstetrics, 16th ed. New York, Appleton, 1980, p 610.)

hours, with a mean time to abortion of 20 to 31 hours. One estimate suggests 86 percent will abort completely, 12.2 percent incompletely, and 1.8 percent will fail to abort[57,71] (Fig. 25-8). In the event of failure, uterine malformation may be the cause, and evaluation for it should be made so that appropriate therapy may be begun if indicated. Ultrasonography plays a key role in this evaluation.[57]

(2) Without augmentation (usually with oxytocin), about 15 to 20 percent of patients require a second injection.[93]

(3) Oxytocin administration, especially after membranes are ruptured, reduces evacuation time significantly. Great care must be taken, however, in the administration of this combination.[2,71]

(4) Use of laminaria also reduces evacuation time.

Whether they are inserted before or after injection varies with the operator and institution, but placement 12 to 24 hours before injections appears most efficacious.[31,62,71,93]

(5) Has been used in various multiple combinations, including intraamniotic urea,[50] oxytocin,[76] and laminaria.[76,91]

(6) To avoid transient fetal survival, combinations of $PGF_{2\alpha}$ and saline have been used to good effect. However, they do have the disadvantage of exposing the patient to some degree of the risks of hypertonic saline that are not inherent in the use of prostaglandins alone.[10,93]

(7) 15(S)-15-Methyl-prostaglandin F_2 (an artificial methylated analog of $PGF_{2\alpha}$) has been found useful, both as an intravaginal preparation and intramuscularly, in second-trimester termination and in the failed transvaginal second-trimester termination by other methods (intraamniotic prostaglandin, saline, etc.).[53A,56B]

b) *Prostaglandin E_2 (PGE$_2$) vaginal suppositories*

(1) Especially useful in missed abortions of advanced gestational age and in intrauterine fetal demise in advanced pregnancy.[2,4,25]

(2) Available in 10-mg suppositories, placed every two to four hours.

(3) Augmentation with oxytocin, especially after membrane rupture, is helpful in many cases. If used, careful monitoring of the severity of contractile activity is important.

(4) 15(S)-15-Methyl-prostaglandin E_2 (an artificial methylated analog of PGE_2) has been found useful, intravaginally and intramuscularly, in second-trimester termination.[56A]

c) *Adverse reactions common to prostaglandins*[42,71,76,93]

(1) Cervical or vaginal laceration and fistulae formation[62]

(2) Infection

(3) Delayed or incomplete abortion (especially retained placenta)

(4) Uterine rupture[81A]

(5) Nausea, emesis, and diarrhea (prophylactic medication is indicated — prochlorperazine, diphenoxylate)

(6) Hypotension

(7) Tachycardia

(8) Disseminated intravascular coagulation

(9) Hemorrhage

(10) Hyperthermia

d) Asthma is a contraindication to the use of prostaglandins for abortion.[93]

e) Since retention of fetal, or more commonly placental, tissue occurs, *a routine exploration of the vagina, cervix, and uterine cavity after completion of the procedure is indicated.* This allows identification and correction of complications in many of these areas.[36,49,62,71,93]

5. *Laminaria*[29,42,76]

a) Technique previously discussed

b) Often used in conjunction with other methods, both dilatation and evacuation and prostaglandin administration

6. *Hysterotomy*[29,69,76]

a) Occasionally indicated when maternal status prohibits the use of other methods of abortion, but *outdated* as a primary method of abortion[69]

b) Used in the event of failed transcervical abortion

c) Because of the vertical uterine scar, *further pregnancies must be delivered by cesarean section*[76]

d) A desire for permanent sterilization is not an indication to use hysterotomy as a primary method of abortion

e) *Basic technique*

(1) Following an appropriate preoperative evaluation and preparation, including determination of maternal blood type and Rh and the type and

crossmatching of blood, the patient is brought to the operating room and the anesthesia of choice is administered. The abdomen is then opened in the usual manner, exposing the uterus, ovaries, and fallopian tubes, which should be carefully inspected.

(2) Prior to uterine incision, a dilute oxytocin solution infusion is begun "piggyback" into the main IV line.

(3) A small vertical incision is made in the uterus. If there is a question of involving the bladder, a "bladder flap" may be created, although this is usually unnecessary. To avoid unnecessary additional blood loss, a small amount of oxytocin in sterile saline solution may be injected directly along the proposed incision line.

As small an incision as possible is made, and it is carried down slowly until the placenta and membranes are encountered. These should not be opened, if possible, so that the contents may be removed intact. The incision is then expanded as needed with scalpel or bandage scissors. The index finger is then carefully introduced between the products of conception and uterine wall, which are separated by blunt dissection until they are expelled through the uterine opening. The cavity should then be explored to ascertain that there is no remaining tissue. A sharp curette or ring or ovum forceps may be used if needed (Figs. 25–9, 25–10).

The uterine incision is then closed in layers. Whether two or three layers are used depends on the depth of the incision wall, but the first layer should be of interrupted suture introduced about half-way between the endometrial and serosal surfaces and exiting just above the endometrial surface, being placed at about 0.5-cm intervals. The outer layer(s) may be closed at the operator's discretion (Fig. 25–11).

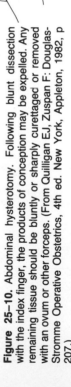

Figure 25–9. Abdominal hysterotomy. After careful vertical incision of the uterus such that the bag of waters has not been breeched, the index finger is used to perform a gentle blunt dissection of the products of conception from the uterine cavity. (From Quilligan EJ, Zuspan F: Douglas-Stromme Operative Obstetrics, 4th ed. New York, Appleton, 1982, p 207.)

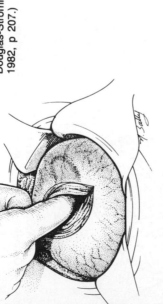

Figure 25–10. Abdominal hysterotomy. Following blunt dissection with the index finger, the products of conception may be expelled. Any remaining tissue should be bluntly or sharply curettaged or removed with an ovum or other forceps. (From Quilligan EJ, Zuspan F: Douglas-Stromme Operative Obstetrics, 4th ed. New York, Appleton, 1982, p 207.)

624

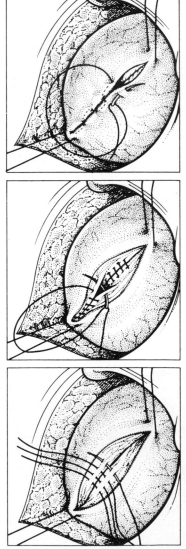

Figure 25–11. Abdominal hysterotomy. Repair of uterine incision in layers. (From Quilligan EJ, Zuspan F: Douglas-Stromme Operative Obstetrics, 4th ed. New York, Appleton, 1982, p 207.)

f) The *most common complications* are hemorrhage, infection, peritonitis, thrombophlebitis, and embolism.

g) This procedure has the highest morbidity and mortality rate of all abortion procedures, and should be used only when all other methods have been exhausted.[69]

7. *Hysterectomy*[5,29,54,76,83,94]

a) *Indications*

(1) Uterine or other gynecologic pathology that *by itself,* would have warranted the procedure

(2) Serious irreparable damage to the uterus

(3) Hemorrhage control following abortion by another method

b) *The technique* is that of cesarean hysterectomy. In the event that the operation is done for uterine trauma, careful attention to anatomy is imperative, especially the bladder and ureters.

c) The complications are those of hysterectomy, with increased risk of involvement of bladder and ureter.

8. Maternal blood type and Rh should be determined and Rh immunoglobulin administered if indicated.[3,37,39,59,76,77]

9. All tissues retrieved should be sent to the pathology lab for dating and for screening of trophoblastic changes.[24]

C. *Optimal setting*

1. Second-trimester termination is technically difficult and fraught with risk.

2. It should be performed only in medical facilities where the following are available:[93]

a) Staff experienced in the procedures and identification of the complications

b) Facilities to deal adequately and immediately with all possible complications

c) A well-organized pre- and postabortion counseling system[15]

d) A well-organized medical follow-up system

3. *Patients undergoing second-trimester termination procedures should never be left unattended, both for medical and psychosocial reasons.*

MORBIDITY AND MORTALITY

A. *Morbidity*
   1. The *risk of morbidity* in all abortions is decreased by medical attention at an early gestational age by competent experienced staff in an approved facility.[15,42,76,93]
   2. Present data suggest an *incidence of abdominal surgical procedures* coincident to abortion of about 3.9/1000 cases, including all causes, both related and unrelated to the abortion itself.[49]
   3. *Suggested adverse effects on future pregnancies* after abortion (especially elective) include midtrimester spontaneous abortion, preterm delivery, infertility, and low-birth-weight infants. Controversy exists over these associations and their interpretation.[6,21,26,27,47,86,99]

B. *Mortality*
   1. The *risk of mortality* from elective abortion is about *0.6 to 1.0/100,000* up to 8 weeks of gestation, doubling for each additional 2 weeks of gestation thereafter,[29,42,49,71,76] as compared to a present maternal mortality rate of 8 to 10/100,000 live births.[93] Thus, abortion and maternal mortality rates are probably equal at about 14 to 16 weeks of completed gestational age, with the value for abortion exceeding that for continued pregnancy thereafter.[49]
   2. Dilatation or suction and curettage carries the lowest risk, followed by intraamniotic injection of $PGF_{2\alpha}$ or intravaginal PGE_2, and then hysterotomy/hysterectomy. Both the procedures and the gestational age determine the individual risk.[93]

MEDICOLEGAL AND SOCIAL ISSUES

Before the Supreme Court decision of *Roe* v. *Wade* in 1973, most abortions were "therapeutic," or presented as some type of incomplete abortion. Since then, elective abortion has become a major part of the reproductive control pattern in the United States. Great controversy presently exists about the many issues relating to abortion. The ultimate outcome of the deliberations over these is uncertain, but whatever decisions emerge will have a tremendous impact on women's health care in years to come.[76,93]

Generally, state laws leave abortion decisions in the first trimester to the patient and her physician, whereas regulations of abortion in later pregnancy vary widely and are constantly changing.[76] Physicians who consider performing any elective abortions should fully review the regulations in their practice locality.[15]

When considering elective abortion, questions about gestational age should be answered by ultrasound examination if possible.[70,71,93] Further, pathologic examination of the retrieved products of conception to document the pregnancy and to rule out trophoblastic disease is indicated.[71]

REFERENCES

1. Alvior GT: Pregnancy outcome with removal of intrauterine devices. Obstet Gynecol 41:894, 1973
2. Anderson GG, Steege JF: Clinical experience using intraamniotic prostaglandin $F_{2\alpha}$ for trimester abortion in 600 patients. Obstet Gynecol 46:591, 1975
3. Ascari WQ: Abortion and maternal Rh immunization. Clin Obstet Gynecol 14:625, 1971
4. Bailey CD, Newman C, Ellinas SP, Anderson GC: Use of prostaglandin E_2 vaginal suppositories in intrauterine fetal death and missed abortion. Obstet Gynecol 45:110, 1975
5. Ballard C: Therapeutic abortion and sterilization by vaginal hysterectomy. Am J Obstet Gynecol 118:891, 1974
6. Barton J, Grier E, Mutchnik D: Uretero uterine fistulae as a complication of elective abortion. Obstet Gynecol (Suppl 1) 52:815, 1976
7. Ben-Baruch G, Menezek J, Shalev J, et al.: Uterine perforation during curettage. Perforation rates and postperforation management. Isr J Med Sci 16:821, 1980
8. Berek J, Stabblefield P: Anatomic and clinical correlates of uterine perforation. Am J Obstet Gynecol 135:181, 1979

9. Berger G, Edelman D, Kerenyi T: Oxytocin administration, instillation-to abortion time, and morbidity associated with saline instillation. Am J Obstet Gynecol 121:941, 1975

10. Bortman M: Use of combination prostaglandin $F_{2\alpha}$ and hypertonic saline for midtrimester abortion. Prostaglandins 12:625, 1976

11. Braunstein G, Karow W, Gentry W, Wade M: Subclinical spontaneous abortion. Obstet Gynecol (Suppl 1) 50:41S, 1977

12. Brown FD, Davidson E, Phillips LL: Coagulation changes after hypertonic saline infusions for late abortions. Obstet Gynecol 39:358, 1972

13. Burkman R, Atienza M, King T: Culture and treatment results in endometritis following elective abortion. Am J Obstet Gynecol 128:556, 1977

14. Burnette L, King T, Atienza M, Bell W: Intra-amniotic urea as a midtrimester abortifacient: Clinical results and serum and urinary changes. Am J Obstet Gynecol 121:7, 1975

15. Burr W, Schultz K: Delayed abortion in an area of easy accessibility. JAMA 244:44, 1980

16. Cadesky K, Ravinsky E, Lyons E: Dilation and evacuation: A preferred method of midtrimester abortion. Am J Obstet Gynecol 139:329, 1981

17. Cadkin A, Sabbagha R: Ultrasonic diagnosis of abnormal pregnancy. Clin Obstet Gynecol 20:265, 1977

18. Carr DH: Cytogenetic aspects of induced and spontaneous abortions. Clin Obstet Gynecol 15:203, 1972

19. Conger S, Tyler C, Pakter J: A cluster of uterine perforations related to suction curettage. Obstet Gynecol 40:551, 1972

20. Cates W: D & E after 12 weeks: safe or hazardous? Contemp Obstet Gynecol 13:23, 1979

21. Cates W: Late effects of induced abortion. Hypothesis of knowledge? J Reprod Med 22:207, 1979

21A. Cates W, Grimes D: Deaths from second trimester abortion by dilatation and evacuation: Causes, prevention, facilities. Obstet Gynecol 58:401, 1981

22. Cheng M, Rochat R: The safety of combined abortion-sterilization procedures. Am J Obstet Gynecol 129:548, 1977

23. Chilcote W, Asokan S: Evaluation of first trimester pregnancy by ultrasound. Clin Obstet Gynecol 20:253, 1977

24. Cohen B, Burkman R, Rosenshein N, et al.: Gestational trophoblastic disease within an elective abortion population. Am J Obstet Gynecol 135:452, 1979

25. Corson S, Bolognese R: Vaginally administered prostaglandin E_2 as a first and second trimester abortifacient. J Reprod Med 14:43, 1975

26. Daling JR, Emanuel I: Induced abortion and subsequent outcome of pregnancy in a series of American women. N Engl J Med 297:1241, 1977

27. Daling J, Spadoni L, Emanuel I: Role of induced abortion in secondary infertility. Obstet Gynecol 57:59, 1981

28. Danforth D: Obstetrics and Gynecology, 3rd ed. Hagerstown, Md., Harper & Row, 1977, p 331

29. Douglas RG, Stromme WB: Operative Obstetrics, 3rd ed. New York, Appleton-Century-Crofts, 1976, Chap 6

30. Dreishpoon IH: Complications of pregnancy with an intra-uterine contraceptive device in situ. Am J Obstet Gynecol 121:412, 1975

31. Duenhoelter J, Grant N, Jimenez J: Concurrent use of prostaglandin $F_{2\alpha}$ and laminaria tents for induction of midtrimester abortion. Obstet Gynecol 47:469, 1976

32. Eriksen P, Philipsen T: Prognosis in threatened abortion evaluated by hormone assays and ultrasound scanning. Obstet Gynecol 55:435, 1980

33. Fielding W, Lee S, Friedman EA: Continued pregnancy after failed first trimester abortion. Obstet Gynecol 52:56, 1978

34. Genest P: Chromosome variants and abnormalities detected in 51 married couples with repeated spontaneous abortions. Obstet Gynecol Surv 35:368, 1980

35. Goldzieher JW: Double-blind trial of a progestin in habitual abortion. JAMA 188:651, 1964

36. Goodlin R, Newell J, O'Hare J, et al.: Cervical fistula, a complication of midtrimester abortion. Obstet Gynecol 40:82, 1972

36A. Grimes D, Cates W, Selik R: Fatal septic abortion in the United States, 1975–1977. Obstet Gynecol 57:739, 1981

37. Grimes D, Geary F, Hatcher R: Rh immunoglobulin after ectopic pregnancy. Am J Obstet Gynecol 140:246, 1981

38. Grimes D, Hulka J, McCutchen M: Midtrimester abortion by dilatation and evacuation versus intra-amniotic instillation of prostaglandin $F_{2\alpha}$: A randomized clinical trial. Am J Obstet Gynecol 137:785, 1980

39. Grimes D, Ross WC, Hatcher RA: Rh immunoglobulin utilization after spontaneous and induced abortion. Obstet Gynecol 50:261, 1977

40. Grimes D, Schultz K, Cates C, et al.: Midtrimester abortion by dilatation and evacuation: a safe and practical alternative. N Engl J Med 296:1141, 1977

41. Harlap S, Shiono P: Alcohol, smoking and incidence of spontaneous abortions in the first and second trimester. Obstet Gynecol 36:209, 1981

42. Harman C, Fish D, Tyson J: Factors influencing morbidity in termination of pregnancy. Am J Obstet Gynecol 139:333, 1981

43. Hartman CG: Uterine bleeding as an early sign of pregnancy in the monkey (*Macaca rhesus*) together with observation on fertile period of menstrual cycle. Bull Hopkins Hosp 44:155, 1929

44. Hertz J, Mantoni M, Svenstrup B: Threatened abortion studied by estradiol-17β in serum and ultrasound. Obstet Gynecol 55:324, 1980

45. Hodari A, Peralta J, Quiroga P, Gerbi E: Dilatation and curettage for second trimester abortions. Am J Obstet Gynecol 127:850, 1977

46. Hodgson J, Major B, Portmann K, et al.: Prophylactic use of tetracycline for first trimester abortions. Obstet Gynecol 45:574, 1975

47. Hogue CJR: Review of postulated fertility complications subsequent to pregnancy termination. In Sciarra JJ, Zatuchni GI, Speidel JJ (eds): Risks, Benefits, and Controversies in Fertility Control. Hagerstown, Md., Harper & Row, 1978, p 356

48. Herenyi T, Mandelman N, Sherman D: Five thousand consecutive saline inductions. Am J Obstet Gynecol 116:593, 1973

49. King T, Atienza M, Burkman R: The incidence of abdominal surgical procedure in a population undergoing abortion. Am J Obstet Gynecol 137:530, 1980

50. King TM, et al.: The synergistic activity and intra-amniotic prostaglandin $F_{2\alpha}$ and urea in the midtrimester election abortion. Am J Obstet Gynecol 120:704, 1974

51. Kline J, Stein Z, Shrout P, et al.: Drinking during pregnancy and spontaneous abortion. Obstet Gynecol Surv 36:209, 1981

51A. Laing F, Filly R, Marks W, Brown T: Ultrasonic demonstration of endometrial fluid collection unassociated with pregnancy. Ultrasound 137:471, 1980

52. Last PA: Pregnancy and the intrauterine contraceptive device. Contraception 9:439, 1974

53. Laufe L, Kreutner A: Vaginal hysterectomy: A modality for

therapeutic abortion and sterilization. Am J Obstet Gynecol 110:1096, 1971

53A. Lauersen N: A new abortion technique: intravaginal and intramuscular prostaglandin. Obstet Gynecol 58:96, 1981

54. Lauersen N, Birnbaum S: Laparoscopy as a diagnostic and therapeutic technique in uterine perforation during 1st trimester abortions. Am J Obstet Gynecol 117:522, 1973

55. Lauersen N, Birnbaum S: Water intoxication associated with oxytocin administration during saline-induced abortion. Am J Obstet Gynecol 121:2, 1975

56. Lauersen N, Conrad P: The effect of oxytocic agents on blood loss during first trimester suction curettage. Obstet Gynecol 44:428, 1974

56A. Lauersen N, Secher N, Wilson K: Midtrimester abortion induced by serial intramuscular injections of 15(S)-15-methyl prostaglandin E2 methyl ester. Am J Obstet Gynecol 123:665, 1975

56B. Lauersen N, Wilson K: The effects of intramuscular injections of 15(S)-15-methyl-prostaglandin $F_{2\alpha}$ in failed abortions. Fertil Steril 28:1044, 1977

57. Lauersen N, Wilson K, Zervoudakis K, et al.: Management of failed prostaglandin abortion. Obstet Gynecol 47:473, 1976

58. Lemkin S, Kattlove H: Maternal death due to DIC after saline abortion. Obstet Gynecol 42:233, 1973

59. Leong M, Duby S, Kinch R: Fetal-maternal transfusion following early abortion. Obstet Gynecol 54:424, 1979

60. Leventhal JM, Reid D: Oxytocin-induced water intoxication with grand mal convulsions. Am J Obstet Gynecol 102:310, 1968

61. Lilien AA: Oxytocin-induced water intoxication. A report of maternal death. Obstet Gynecol 32:171, 1968

62. Lowensohn R, Ballard C: Cervicovaginal fistula: An apparent increased incidence with prostaglandin $F_{2\alpha}$. Am J Obstet Gynecol 119:1057, 1974

63. McArdle C: Failed abortion in a septate uterus. Am J Obstet Gynecol 131:910, 1978

64. McDonough P, et al.: Overall evaluation of recurrent abortion. In Givens JR (ed): The Infertile Female. Chicago, Yearbook Medical, 1979, p 385

65. Matsunaga E, Shiota K: Threatened abortion, hormone therapy, and malformed embryos. Obstet Gynecol Surv 35:521, 1980

66. Nathanson BN: Management of uterine perforation suffered at elective abortion. Am J Obstet Gynecol 114:1054, 1972

67. Nathanson BN: The postabortal pain syndrome: a new entity. Obstet Gynecol 41:739, 1972

68. Newton BW: Laminaria tent: relic of the past or modern medical device? Am J Obstet Gynecol 113:442, 1972

69. Nottage B, Liston W: A review of 70 hysterotomies. Br J Obstet Gynecol 82:310, 1975

70. O'Brien G, Queenan J, Campbell S: Assessment of gestational age in the second trimester by real time ultrasound measurement of the femur length. Am J Obstet Gynecol 139:540, 1981

71. Palomaki J: Abortion techniques: What are their risks and complications. Contemp Obstet Gynecol 9:73, 1977

72. Parsons L, Sommers S: Gynecology, 2nd ed. Philadelphia, Saunders, 1978, Chap 27

73. Parsons L, Sommers S: Gynecology, 2nd ed. Philadelphia, Saunders, 1978, Chap 26

74. Peyser M, Toaff R: Rupture of uterus in the first trimester caused by high-concentration oxytocin drip. Obstet Gynecol 40:371, 1972

75. Poland B, Miller J, Jones D, Trimble B: Reproductive counseling in patients who have had a spontaneous abortion. Am J Obstet Gynecol 127:685, 1977

76. Pritchard J, MacDonald P: Williams Obstetrics, 16th ed. New York, Appleton-Century-Crofts, 1980, Chap 24

77. Queenan JT: Modern Management of the Rh Problem, 2nd ed. Hagerstown, Md., Harper & Row, 1977, p 256

78. Rasor J, Braunstein G: A rapid modification of the Beta-hCG radioimmunoassay. Obstet Gynecol 50:553, 1977

79. Rosal T, Saxena B, Landesman R: Application of a radioreceptorassay of human chorionic gonadotropin in the diagnosis of early abortion. Fertil Steril 26:1105, 1975

80. Sanders RJ, James AM: Ultrasound in Obstetrics and Gynecology. New York, Appleton-Century-Crofts, 1977

81. Sands R, Burnhill M, Hakim-Elahi E: Postabortal uterine atony. Obstet Gynecol 14:595, 1974

81A. Sawyer M, Lipshitz J, Anderson G, Dilts P: Third-trimester uterine rupture associated with vaginal prostaglandin E_2. Am J Obstet Gynecol 140:710, 1981

82. Schiffer M, Parter J, Clahr J: Mortality associated with hypertonic saline abortion. Obstet Gynecol 42:759, 1973

83. Schulman H: Major surgery for abortion and sterilization. Obstet Gynecol 40:738, 1972

84. Shine RM, Thompson JF: The in situ IUD and pregnancy outcome. Am J Obstet Gynecol 119:124, 1974

85. Simpson JL: What causes chromosomal abnormalities and gene mutations? Contemp Obstet Gynecol 17:99, 1981

86. Slater P, Davies A, Harlap S: The effect of abortion method of the outcome of subsequent pregnancy. J Reprod Med 26:123, 1981

87. Smith C, Gregori C, Breen J: Ultrasonography in treated abortion. Obstet Gynecol 51:173, 1978

88. Sonne Holm S, Heisterberg L, Hebjorn S: Prophylactic antibiotics in first trimester abortions: a clinical controlled trial. Am J Obstet Gynecol 139:693, 1981

89. Stander RW, et al.: Changes in maternal coagulation factors after intra-amniotic injection of hypertonic saline. Obstet Gynecol 37:660, 1971

90. Stenchever MA, Jarvis JA: Cytogenetic studies in reproductive failure. Obstet Gynecol 37:83, 1971

91. Strauss JH, Wilson M, Caldwell D, et al.: Laminaria use in midtrimester abortion induced by intra-amniotic prostaglandin $F_{2\alpha}$ with urea and intravenous oxytocin. Am J Obstet Gynecol 134:260, 1979

92. Stromme W, Fromke V: Amniotic fluid embolism and disseminated intravascular coagulation after evacuation of missed abortion. Obstet Gynecol (Suppl 1) 52:76S, 1978

93. Stubblefield P: Current technology for abortion. Curr Probl Obstet Gynecol 2(4), 1978

94. Stumpf P, Ballard C, Lowensohn R: Abdominal hysterectomy for abortion sterilization. Am J Obstet Gynecol 136:714, 1980

95. Tatum H, Schmidt F, Jain A: Management and outcome of pregnancies associated with copper T intrauterine contraceptive device. Am J Obstet Gynecol 126:809, 1976

96. Tsenghi C, Metaxoutou-Stavridaki C, Strataki-Benetou M, et al.: Chromosome studies in couples with repeated spontaneous abortions. Obstet Gynecol 47:463, 1978

97. Walden W, Birnbaum S: Classifying perforations that occur during abortion. Contemp Obstet Gynecol 15:47, 1980

98. Wentz AC, King T: Myometrial necrosis after therapeutic abortion. Obstet Gynecol 40:315, 1972

99. World Health Organization Task Force on Sequelae to Abortion: Gestation, birth-weight, and spontaneous abortion in pregnancy after induced abortion. Lancet 1:142, 1979

100. Wulff G, Friedman M: Primary diagnosis of complications by gestational age from LMP. Obstet Gynecol 49:351, 1977

Section 2
The Incompetent Cervical Os

Jessica L. Thomason, M.D.
Charles R.B. Beckmann, M.D.

DEMOGRAPHICS

- *Definition:* Cervix unable to retain intrauterine pregnancy until term
- *Incidence:* 1/125[1] to 1/2000 pregnancies[2], multiparous and primiparous

ETIOLOGY

A. *History of cervical trauma*
   1. *Major cause,* occurring in 30 to 50 percent of patients
   2. *Spontaneous.* Laceration during delivery; subsequent fistula formation
   3. *Surgical history.* Dilatation and curettage or evacuation, conization, amputation, tracheloplasty, etc.
   4. *Obstetrical operative delivery.* Midforceps, breech, Dührssen's incisions
   5. *Abortions.* Repeaters of first-trimester abortions have *no* increased incidence.[3]

B. *Congenital anomalies*
   1. *Spontaneous* (congenital). Increased with uterine, cervical, or vaginal abnormalities

    2. *Idiopathic.* Increased incidence with diethylstilbestrol exposure in utero[4]
C. *Other* (doubtful importance)[2]
    1. Abnormal circulation in isthmical region of cervix
    2. Bacterial flora, different from "normal patients"

DIAGNOSIS OF INCOMPETENT CERVICAL OS

A. Rule out other reasons for midtrimester loss, i.e., syphilis, amnionitis, abnormal placentation, submucus fibroids
B. *Diagnosis* is suggested by:
    1. Previous midtrimester loss
    2. Classic history of "painless labor" in the midtrimester
    3. "Heavy feeling" in pelvis
    4. "Bearing down" or "pressure" in upper vagina
    5. Blood-stained, mucoid discharge
    6. Profuse watery discharge
C. *Nonpregnant state*
    1. Physical exam to rule out abnormalities of cervix and vagina
    2. Passage of #8 Hegar (#15 to 17 Pratt) dilator easily through cervical os
    3. Hysterosalpingogram
        a) Rules out uterine cavity abnormalities
        b) Measures isthmus. If $\geq$ 6 to 7 mm, diagnosis is made
D. *Pregnant state*
    1. Symptoms, as discussed above
    2. Physical exam
        a) Absence of labor
        b) Evidence of cervical effacement and/or dilatation
        c) Intact membranes bulging through cervix

TREATMENT METHODS

A. *Nonpregnant state*
    1. Lash procedure (Fig. 25–12)[5,18]
        a) Surgical excision of cervical abnormality
        b) Vaginal delivery possible after procedure

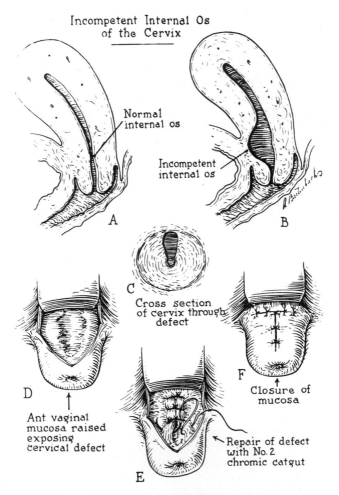

Incompetent Internal Os
of the Cervix

Normal internal os

Incompetent internal os

A

B

C
Cross section
of cervix through
defect

D
Ant. vaginal
mucosa raised
exposing
cervical defect

E
Repair of defect
with No. 2
chromic catgut

F
Closure of
mucosa

Figure 25–12. The Lash procedure (From Lash AF, Lash SR: Am J Obstet Gynecol 59:68, 1950. By permission.)

B. *Pregnant state*
1. Nonsurgical approach
   a) *Bed rest,* with hydration, in deep Trandelenburg position
   b) *Pessary.*[6] Placement needed in first trimester; often multiple size changes needed
   c) *Baylor balloon.* Need minimal effacement for placement
2. Surgical (cerclage) approach
   a) Vaginal approach
      (1) *McDonald.*[8,11] Purse-string suture at internal os (Fig. 25–13).
      (2) *Shirodkar.*[9] Dissection of bladder and vaginal mucosa to internal os and suture placement (Fig. 25–14)
      (3) *Wurm.* Two mattress sutures placed at right angles through internal os (Fig. 25–15)
      (4) *Modifications.* All basically tighten internal cervical os
   b) Abdominal approach
      (1) *Benson and Durfee.*[13] Exploratory laparotomy needed to place suture, subsequent cesarean section needed for delivery
      (2) *Modifications.*[14] All require cesarean section for delivery
3. Hormonal therapy. Worthless, may have teratogenic effect[15,16,17]

RESULTS OF THERAPY

A. *Nonpregnant state*—Lash procedure
1. Vaginal delivery possible after procedure[10]
2. Future fertility not decreased[16]
B. *Pregnant state*
1. Nonsurgical
   a) Lower fetal survival rates

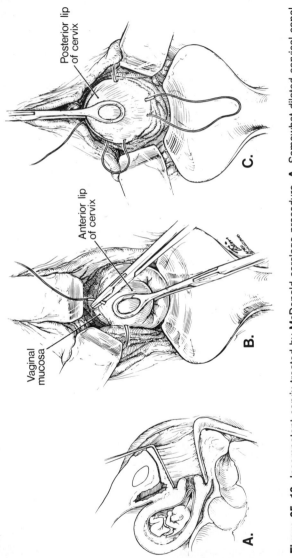

Figure 25–13. Incompetent cervix treated by McDonald cerclage procedure. **A.** Somewhat dilated cervical canal and beginning prolapse of membranes (arrow). **B.** Start of the cerclage procedure with a suture of number 2 proline being placed superiorly in the body of the cervix very near the level of the internal os. **C.** Continuation of the placement of the suture in the body of the cervix so as to encircle the os (*Continued*).

Posterior lip of cervix

Anterior lip of cervix

Vaginal mucosa

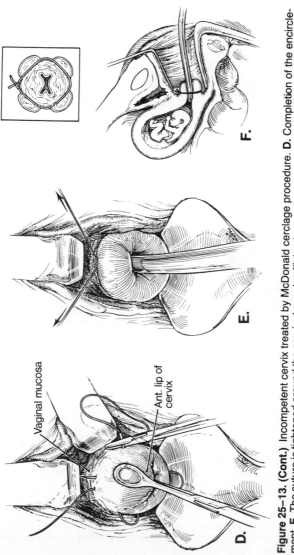

Figure 25–13. (Cont.) Incompetent cervix treated by McDonald cerclage procedure. **D.** Completion of the encirclement. **E.** The suture is tightened around the cervical canal sufficiently to reduce the diameter of the canal to a few mm and is then securely tied. In the illustration a *small* dilator has been placed just through the level of ligation to maintain patency of the canal when the suture is tied. **F.** The effect of the suture placement on the cervical canal is apparent. (From Pritchard J, MacDonald P: Williams Obstetrics, 16th ed. New York, Appleton, 1980, pp 599–600.)

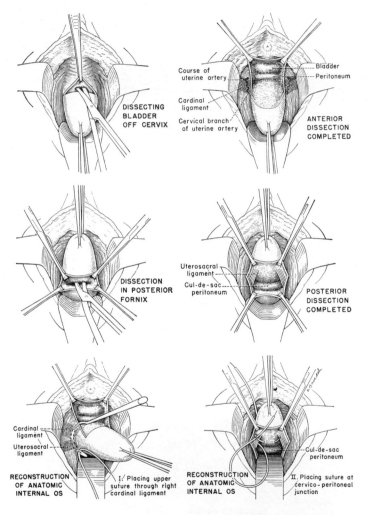

Figure 25–14. Preconceptional Shirodkar procedure. (From Quilligan EJ, Zuspan F: Douglas-Stromme Operative Obstetrics, 4th ed. New York, Appleton, 1982, pp 155–57.)

641

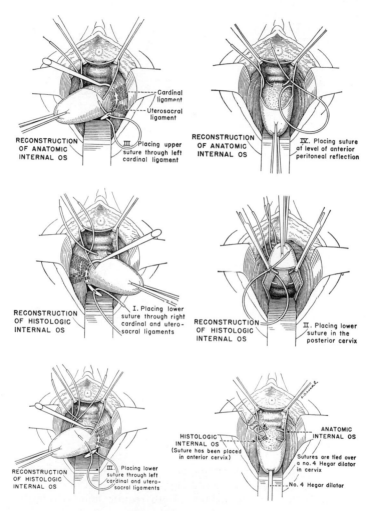

Figure 25–14. (Cont.)

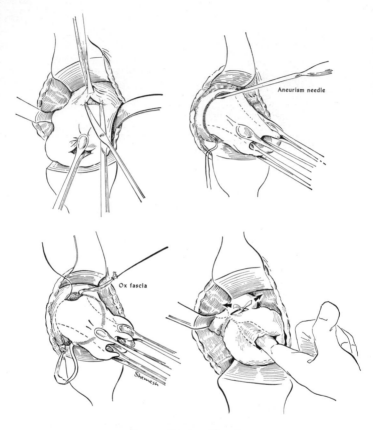

Figure 25–14. (Cont.)

b) No study comparing bed rest, hydration alone versus
   cerclage has been done
c) Pessary and balloon. Both require minimal effacement and dilatation and therefore patient selection is
   more difficult
2. Surgical (cerclage)
   a) Fetal survival rates
      (1) Prior to procedure 20 to 50 percent[19–27]

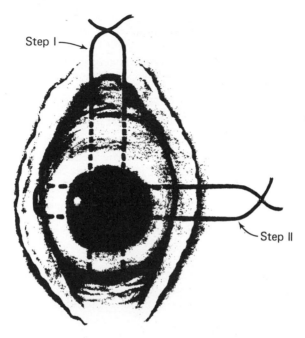

Figure 25–15. The Wurm procedure. (From Hefner J, et al.: Obstet Gynecol 18:16, 1961.)

　　(2) Post procedure 70 to 90 percent
　b) Timing of operation
　　(1) Suture placement early in gestation has led to better survival rates[19,27–29]
　　(2) Less dilatation and less effacement at cerclage placement correlates with a higher success rate
　c) Type of suture
　　(1) No differences in survival between McDonald and Shirodkar procedures are noted[19]
　　(2) Greater blood loss and a higher cesarean section rate are seen with Shirodkar procedures[12,19,26]
　d) Type of anesthesia. No difference in fetal survival with general versus local anesthesia[28]

    e) Antibiotics. No difference in amnionitis whether or
        not these drugs are used[27]
    f) Cesarean section
        (1) Necessary if abdominal cerclage placed
        (2) Rate is increased in all types of cerclage

COMPLICATION OF CERCLAGE

A. *Premature labor, premature delivery.* Bed rest for 24 hours
    after procedure is indicated; tocolytic agents may be useful.
B. *Suture displacement.* Some patients require multiple suture
    placements; this is not contraindicated.
C. *Infection — major problem*
    1. Immediate removal of suture is indicated.
    2. Types of infection include chorioamnionitis, suture line
       infection, and sepsis.
D. *Rupture of membranes*
    1. During suture placement. Terminate procedure im-
       mediately
    2. Spontaneous in later gestation. Immediate removal of
       suture is indicated.
E. *Bleeding*
F. *Leukorrhea.* Must rule out ruptured membranes; sometimes
    helped by vaginal creams after pathogens causing vaginitis
    ruled out
G. *Vesicovaginal fistula.* Rare complication
H. *Cervical laceration from the suture during labor.* Documenta-
    tion of exact EDC indicated to allow elective cutting of
    suture prior to date of anticipated delivery
 I. *Uterine rupture during labor.* Avoided if patient not allowed
    to labor with suture in place

CONTRAINDICATIONS TO CERCLAGE

• Labor: Rule out by electronic fetal monitoring and
minimal physical examinations
• Uterine bleeding

- Ruptured membranes: Infection too hazardous
- Almost fully dilated cervix: Technically difficult
- Hydramnios: Rule out by sonography
- Fetal anomalies: Rule out by sonography

REFERENCES

1. Jennings CL: Temporary submucosal cerclage for cervical incompetence: Report of forty-eight cases. Am J Obstet Gynecol 113:1097,1972
2. Little B, Tenny B: Incompetent cervical os. Clin Obstet Gynecol 6:403, 1963
3. Daling JR, Emanuel I: Induced abortion and subsequent outcome of pregnancy in a series of American women. N Engl J Med 297:1241, 1977
4. Nunley WC, Kitchin JD: Successful management of incompetent cervix in a primigravida exposed to diethylstilbestrol in utero. Fertil Steril 31:217, 1979
5. Lash AF, Lash SR: Habitual abortion: The incompetent internal os of the cervix. Am J Obstet Gynecol 59:68, 1950
6. Vitsky M: Simple treatment of the incompetent cervical os. Am J Obstet Gynecol 81:1194, 1961
7. Yosowitz EE, Haufrect F, Kaufman RH, Goyette RE: Silicone-plastic cuff for the treatment of the incompetent cervix in pregnancy. Am J Obstet Gynecol 113:233, 1972
8. McDonald IA: Suture of the cervix for inevitable miscarriage. J Obstet Gynecol Br Emp 64:346, 1957
9. Shirodkar VN: A new method of operative treatment for habitual abortions in the second trimester of pregnancy. Antiseptic 52:299, 1955
10. Hefner JD, Patow WE, Ludwig JM: A new surgical procedure for the correction of the incompetent cervix during pregnancy: The Wurm procedure. Obstet Gynecol 18:616, 1961
11. Shaalan, MK: A simple midcervical cerclage operation for cervical incompetence during pregnancy. Am J Obstet Gynecol 107:969, 1970
12. Curet, LB, Killer W, Olsen RW: Temporary submucosal cervical cerclage. Obstet Gynecol 55:392, 1980
13. Benson RC, Durfee RB: Transabdominal cervicouterine cerclage during pregnancy for the treatment of cervical incompetency. Obstet Gynecol 25:145, 1965

14. Watkins RA: Transabdominal cervico-uterine suture. Aust NZ J Obstet Gynecol 12:62, 1972

15. Heinonen OP, Slone D, Monson RR, Hook BB, Shapiro S: Cardiovascular birth defects and antenatal exposure to female sex hormones. N Engl J Med 296:67, 1977

16. Nora JJ, Nora AH, Blu J, et al: Exogenous progestogen and estrogen implicated in birth defects. JAMA 240:837, 1978

17. Block MF, Rahhal DK: Cervical incompetence. A diagnostic and prognostic scoring system. Obstet Gynecol 47:279, 1976

18. Lash AF: Fertility and reproduction following repair of the incompetent internal os of the cervix. Fertil Steril 11:531, 1960

19. Harger JH: Comparison of success and morbidity in cervical cerclage procedures. Obstet Gynecol 56:543, 1980

20. Cushner IM: The management of cervical incompetence by purse-string suture. Am J Obstet Gynecol 87:882, 1963

21. Hofmeister FJ, Schwarts WR, Vondrak BF, Martens W: Suture reinforcement of the incompetent cervix. Am J Obstet Gynecol 101:58, 1968

22. Nishijima S: Antepartum cervical cerclage operations. Am J Obstet Gynecol 104:272, 1969

23. Bacchus MY, Hay DM: Shirodkar suture: A review of 10 years experience. Am J Obstet Gynecol 108:250, 1970

24. Robboy MS: The management of cervical incompetence: UCLA experience with cerclage procedures. Obstet Gynecol 41:108, 1973

25. Lipshitz J: Cerclage in the treatment of incompetent cervix. S Afr Med J 49:2013, 1975

26. Ritter HA: Surgical closure of the incompetent cervix: 15 years experience. Int J Obstet Gynecol 16:194, 1978

27. Kuhn RJP, Pepperell RJ: Cervical ligation: A review of 242 pregnancies. Aust NZ J Obstet Gynecol 17:79, 1979

28. Peters WA, Thiagarajah S, Harbert GM: Cervical cerclage: Twenty years experience. South Med J 72:933, 1979

29. McDonald IA: Incompetence of the cervix. Aust NZ J Obstet Gynecol 17:34, 1977

26

Disorders of the Placenta, Umbilical Cord, and Amniotic Fluid

Jeffrey W. Ellis, M.D.

PRACTICE PRINCIPLES

Many anomalies of the placenta, umbilical cord, and membranes, as well as of the amniotic fluid, are trivial. Some, however, are pathologic and lead to a wide variety of disorders whose evaluation and treatment are as varied as the conditions themselves.

PLACENTA

A. *Size*
   1. *Normal.* At term, the placenta is 15 to 20 cm in diameter, 1.5 to 3.0 cm in thickness, and weighs 450 to 550 gm (one-sixth the weight of the fetus).
   2. *Variations*
      a) *Decreased size* is usually associated with maternal vascular compromise caused by hypertensive disease

or longstanding severe diabetes. The fetus is often either small for gestational age or growth-retarded, maintaining a placental:fetal ratio of 1:5 to 1:7.

b) *Increased size* is associated with erythroblastosis fetalis, syphilis, and class A–C diabetes. The placental:fetal ratio is often 1:2 to 1:3.

B. *Shape and configuration*

1. *Normal.* A single, round to oval disk

2. *Variations*

a) *Placenta bipartita or tripartita.* The placenta is incompletely divided into two or three lobes. Vessels cross between the lobes before uniting in the umbilical cord.

b) *Placenta duplex or triplex.* The lobes of the placenta are completely separated. Vessels do not cross between the lobes and unite only immediately before entering the umbilical cord.

c) *Placenta succenturiata.* Small accessory lobes are found in the membranes at a distance from the periphery of the main placenta. Blood vessels course through the membranes to connect the accessory lobe to the main placenta.

3. *Clinical management.* In the course of delivery of a placenta with variations in configuration, vessels may be torn and one or more lobes may be retained in the uterus. After delivery of the placenta, the placental edges, membranes, and umbilical cord should be thoroughly examined for the presence of open, lacerated vessels. Manual exploration of the endometrial cavity should be performed to remove retained lobes.

C. *Structural variations and disorders*

1. *Placenta circumvallata.* A white fibrous ring is present on the fetal surface at varying distances from the placental margin. The ring is composed of a double fold of amnion and chorion. Vessels on the fetal surface terminate at the ring.

a) *Etiology.* Thought to occur when the decidua basalis is insufficient to meet the increasing nutritional requirements of the fetus. Villi at the periphery then grow out laterally.

  b) *Clinical significance.* Most often an incidental finding with no effect on the course of pregnancy. May be associated with irregular antepartum bleeding, premature labor, and a chronic, watery vaginal discharge (hydrorrhea).

2. *Placenta membranacea.* The placenta is thin and membranous, occupying the entire surface of the chorion. The entire uterine cavity may be covered by placenta.

  a) *Etiology.* The chorion laeve fails to undergo atrophy, presumably due to a persistent rich blood supply in the decidua capsularis.

  b) *Clinical significance*
    (1) The internal os may be completely or partially covered by placenta. Antepartum bleeding similar to that encountered with placenta previa can occur. Management is similar to that of placenta previa.
    (2) The third stage of labor may be prolonged, requiring manual removal.
    (3) Placental separation is often incomplete, resulting in immediate or delayed postpartum bleeding. Manual removal or curettage will be required.

3. *Placental infarcts.* Irregular white to yellow areas of varying size and consistency may be found in most term placentas.

  a) *Etiology*
    (1) Vascular thrombosis
    (2) Fibrin deposition

  b) *Clinical significance.* In most cases, the functional capacity of the placenta is unaltered. Maternal hypertensive disease and diabetes may be associated with large areas of infarction that significantly reduce placental functional capacity.

4. *Placental calcification.* Areas of calcification may be spread throughout the placenta, appearing as fine white granules or plaques.

    a) *Etiology*. A late phase of degeneration of villi commonly found in the term placenta

    b) *Clinical significance*. None

5. *Placental cysts*. Thin-walled cysts varying in size up to 5 to 6 cm may be found on the fetal surface. They contain yellow or blood-tinged fluid.

    a) *Etiology*. Formed as a result of obliteration of trophoblastic elements by fibrinoid degeneration

    b) *Clinical significance*. None

6. *Amnion nodosum*. Yellow or gray-white nodules up to 2 to 5 mm in size are found on the fetal surface, usually near the insertion of the umbilical cord. They contain varying amounts of fibrin and desquamated fetal cells.

    a) *Etiology*. Unknown

    b) *Clinical significance*. Often associated with oligohydramnios and multiple congenital anomalies: renal agenesis, polycystic kidneys, urethral obstruction, pulmonary hypoplasia. The pediatric service should be notified if amnion nodosum is suspected.

D. *Placental tumors*

  1. *Chorioangioma*. Vascular proliferations varying in size up to 7 to 8 cm are found throughout the placenta.

    a) *Etiology*. Blood vessels and stroma originating in the chorionic mesenchyme proliferate in a benign pattern without relation to the developing villi.

    b) *Clinical significance*. Normally an incidental finding. Large tumors have been associated with hydramnios and antepartum bleeding.

  2. *Metastatic tumors*. Tumor metastases in the placenta are rare, though they may occur in the presence of any malignancy that has hematogenous spread.

  3. *Trophoblastic proliferations*

E. *Placenta accreta, increta, or percreta*

F. *Placental infection*

  1. *Chorioamnionitis*

  2. *Syphilis*. The placenta is large, pale, and greasy in appearance. Microscopically, there is a reduction in the number of blood vessels as a result of endarteritis and

stromal proliferation. Spirochetes may be demonstrated by dark-field examination.

3. *Tuberculosis.* Characteristic tuberculous lesions of the placenta are uncommon even in the presence of active maternal disease. Bacilli may be found in the absence of tubercles.

UMBILICAL CORD

A. *Length*
   1. *Normal.* The average cord is 55 cm at term
   2. *Variations.* From 2 cm to 200 cm
      a) *Short cord*
         (1) *To allow normal delivery,* the cord must be of sufficient length to extend from the placental site to the vulva: at least 32 to 35 cm if the placenta is at the fundus, at least 20 cm if the placenta is low-lying. The cord may become relatively short if extensive coiling around the fetus has occurred.
         (2) *Complications.* Delayed descent of the fetus, detachment of the placenta, rupture of the cord, umbilical hernia, uterine inversion
      b) *Long cord.* Complications include cord prolapse and fetal entanglement
B. *Physical variations*
   1. *Knots*
      a) *True knots* occur as a result of fetal motion, with the fetus passing through a loop of cord. Vessel pulsation normally prevents tightening. During descent of the fetus, the knot may tighten, however, leading to vascular obstruction.
      b) *False knots* represent kinking of vessels and areas of thickened Warton's jelly. They have no clinical significance.
   2. *Coiling (entanglement).* The cord is often coiled around portions of the fetus, usually the neck (nuchal cord) or an extremity. This affects the fetus only if the cord becomes

relatively short or if the cord tightens, compromising circulation. A pattern of variable deceleration of the fetal heart rate may be noted during labor. Fetal death rarely occurs. At delivery, it may be necessary to unwrap or transect a nuchal cord to prevent excessive traction. Intertwining of the cords of monoamniotic twins with resulting circulatory compromise may cause the death of one or both fetuses.

3. *Torsion.* Varying degrees of twisting of the cord are common and are due to fetal movement. Rarely, extensive twisting will cause vascular compromise and fetal death.

4. *Cysts of the cord.* Cysts of varying size may be found along the length of the cord. True cysts are remnants of the umbilical vesicle or allantois. False cysts may attain large size and result from liquefaction of Wharton's jelly.

C. *Cord insertion*

1. *Normal.* The cord is inserted at or near the center of the placenta. The umbilical vessels are completely contained within the substance of the cord.

2. *Variations*

a) *Battledore placenta.* The cord inserts at the margin of the placenta. This has no clinical significance.

b) *Velamentous insertion*

(1) The vessels of the cord separate from the cord at varying distances from the placenta. The vessels course unprotected through the membranes before entering the margin of the placenta. This insertion is found in 1 percent of singleton pregnancies, 9 percent of twin pregnancies, and in nearly 100 percent of triplet pregnancies.

(2) *Clinical significance*

(a) Unprotected vessels may tear or rupture during labor, leading to extensive fetal blood loss.

(b) *Vasa previa* is a condition where the umbilical vessels of a velamentous insertion cross over the internal os and lie below the presenting part of the fetus. Compression by the presenting part during labor may lead to vascular compromise, evidenced by fetal heart rate irregularity. Spontaneous or artificial membrane rupture may tear the vessels, leading to extensive fetal blood loss.

D. *Vascular anomalies*

1. *Normal.* The umbilical cord contains two arteries and one vein.

2. *Variations*

a) *Single umbilical artery*

(1) *Incidence.* One percent of singleton pregnancies and 5 percent of multiple gestations are associated with a single umbilical artery.

(2) *Clinical significance.* Twenty to 30 percent of cases are associated with multiple, severe congenital anomalies of the genitourinary, cardiovascular, and musculoskeletal systems. The pediatric service should be notified if a single umbilical artery is discovered.

b) *Varices.* Varices of the umbilical cord are common and usually have no clinical significance. Large varices may rupture if the cord undergoes excessive traction.

c) *Common placental circulation.* Vascular communications (artery to artery, artery to vein, vein to vein) occur commonly in monochorionic placentas of monozygotic twins.

(1) *Artery-to-artery anastomosis* may lead to:

(a) Acute blood volume shifts between fetuses during delivery.

(b) Loss of blood from the second fetus if the cord of the first fetus is allowed to bleed after delivery.

(2) *Arteriovenous anastomoses* may lead to significant complications due to unequal perfusion of the fetuses.

(3) *Hypoperfused fetus.* Anemia, hypotension, microcardia, retarded growth, oligohydramnios.
(4) *Hyperperfused fetus.* Polycythemia, hypertension, cardiac hypertrophy, hydramnios.

AMNIOTIC FLUID

A. The normal production and exchange of amniotic fluid is a complex mechanism that involves a critical balance between mother and fetus. Amniotic fluid volume normally increases progressively during pregnancy until approximately 34 weeks' gestation, when volume slowly begins to decline.
B. *Hydramnios (polyhydramnios)*
1. A condition characterized by the accumulation of excessive quantities of amniotic fluid, usually greater than 2000 ml. The fluid may accumulate either acutely or chronically. Hydramnios occurs in 0.2 to 0.7 percent of pregnancies.
2. *Associated maternal and fetal conditions.* Hydramnios occurs as a result of disturbances in amniotic fluid circulation. Fetal swallowing of amniotic fluid and fetal urination are critical in maintaining normal circulation and thus normal volume.

	Presumed Etiology
1. *Idiopathic* (30 to 40 percent)	
2. *Diabetes mellitus*	Unknown
3. *Fetal Anomaly* Anencephaly, spina bifida	Increased transudation of fluid across exposed meninges; impaired fetal swallowing and absence of antidiuretic hormone

	Presumed Etiology
Esophageal atresia, duodenal atresia, tracheo-esophageal fistula	Impaired fetal swallowing, bowel obstruction
4. *Erythroblastosis fetalis*	Increased placental mass; impaired fetal swallowing due to edema
5. *Multiple gestation* (usually monoamniotic)	Unequal fetal perfusion (one fetus will have oligohydramnios)

3. *Symptoms.* Symptoms normally do not become significant until the amniotic fluid volume exceeds 3000 ml. Symptoms result from the pressure exerted on adjacent organs by the enlarging uterus.
   a) *Abdominal pain* is due to overstretching of the uterus and abdominal wall.
   b) *Dyspnea, acute respiratory distress, and cyanosis* are due to excessive elevation of the diaphragm, leading to decreased ventilation.
   c) *Leg edema and vulvar edema* are due to compression of venous return.
4. *Clinical presentations*

	Acute Hydramnios	**Chronic Hydramnios**
Incidence	2 percent of cases; usually occurs at 20 to 24 weeks gestation	98 percent of cases; usually occurs at 28 to 32 weeks gestation
Symptoms	Severe	Mild to severe
Weight gain	Often 10 to 12 pounds in 4 weeks	Often 2 to 8 pounds in 4 weeks

5. *Diagnosis*
   a) *Suspect hydramnios* when:
      (1) There is sudden increase in size of the uterus.
      (2) Uterus is significantly larger than would be predicted for the gestational age.
      (3) Uterus is tensely distended and fetal parts are difficult to palpate.
      (4) Auscultation of the fetal heart rate is difficult.
   b) *Diagnostic studies*
      (1) *Ultrasonography.* In hydramnios, total intrauterine volume will be significantly increased. Multiple gestations, fetal hydrops, and congenital anomalies may also be detected.
      (2) *Amniography.*
         (a) The injection of a radiopaque substance into the amniotic cavity will allow radiographic demonstration of neural tube defects and gastrointestinal obstruction.
         (b) *Technique*

            1. Determine placental location by ultrasound.

            2. Using the standard techniques of amniocentesis, withdraw amniotic fluid to ensure an intraamniotic position of the needle.

            3. The amniotic fluid removed may be evaluated for lecithin/sphingomyelin ratio, creatinine, bilirubin, and α-fetoprotein levels.

            4. Inject 15 to 20 ml of Hypaque-75 into the amniotic cavity.

            5. Thirty to 60 minutes after injection, obtain supine and lateral radiographs of the abdomen.

            6. The external surfaces of the fetus will be outlined, aiding the diagnosis of gross neural tube defects.

7. Gastrointestinal obstructions and swallowing defects will be noted by the failure of normal passage of the radiopaque dye into the fetal intestines.

6. *Management*
   a) *General principles*
      (1) Evaluate and treat possible underlying causes: diabetes, erythroblastosis fetalis.
      (2) Determine the presence of congenital anomaly by ultrasonography or amniography. Inform the pediatric service if an anomaly is detected.
      (3) Assess the patient's symptoms. Severe respiratory compromise and abdominal pain will require hospitalization. Mild to moderate symptoms can often be managed on an outpatient basis.
   b) *Acute hydramnios*
      (1) Hospitalization is usually required due to the severity of symptoms.
      (2) If evaluation of the fetus reveals an anomaly incompatible with life, delivery should be accomplished by induction with oxytocics.
      (3) In the presence of a normal fetus or a fetus with a surgically correctable anomaly, maternal symptoms should be relieved and the pregnancy allowed to continue.
      (4) *Technique of therapeutic amniocentesis*
         (a) Determine placental location by ultrasonography.
         (b) Using the standard techniques of amniocentesis, an inside-the-needle catheter is inserted into the amniotic cavity. A 14-or 16-gauge inside-the-needle catheter or a suprapubic cystostomy needle-catheter unit may be used. The catheter is threaded into the amniotic cavity and the needle is withdrawn.
         (c) Fluid should be withdrawn slowly at a rate not exceeding 500 ml/hour.

    (d) Generally, no more than 1500 ml should be withdrawn in a 24-hour period. A sudden decrease in intraamniotic volume has been associated with placental abruption.

    (e) This procedure may be repeated every two to three days as necessary to relieve symptoms.

    (f) Complications of therapeutic amniocentesis are intrauterine infection, placental abruption, and premature labor. Some centers will administer standard doses of labor-inhibiting agents after therapeutic amniocentesis.

    (g) Since large amounts of protein are removed by amniocentesis, the patient should receive a high-protein diet.

  (5) Severe symptoms refractory to these treatment measures require termination of the pregnancy.

c) *Chronic hydramnios*

  (1) *Mild to moderate symptoms* can be treated on an outpatient basis, with the patient maintaining bed rest with elevation of the head of the bed. Decreased fluid intake, salt restriction, and diuretics have proven ineffective.

  (2) *Severe symptoms* will require hospitalization. If the fetus is mature or if a severe fetal anomaly is detected, the fetus should be delivered. If the fetus is normal and immature, bed rest and therapeutic amniocentesis are indicated until fetal maturity.

d) *Complications of labor and delivery*

  (1) Several serious complications of labor and delivery are associated with hydramnios. Operating room facilities and at least two units of whole blood should be immediately available when a patient with hydramnios is in labor. Perinatal mortality approaches 50 percent due to prematurity, severe congenital anomalies, intrauterine asphyxia due to prolapsed cord or placental

abruption, and complications of erythroblastosis fetalis and diabetes. A pediatrician should be present for all deliveries and equipment for recuscitation immediately available.

(2) *Premature labor* is commonly associated with hydramnios (usually the acute form). Standard protocols for management of premature labor should be followed. Labor should not be inhibited in the presence of placental abruption or severe fetal anomaly.

(2) *Dysfunctional labor* is due to overdistention of the myometrium. The slow removal of 1000 to 1500 ml of fluid by amniocentesis may be followed by normal labor.

(4) *Abnormal presentation* is common as a result of increased fetal mobility within the overdistended uterus. The route of delivery is determined by obstetric factors.

(5) *Umbilical cord prolapse* may occur due to poor adaption of the presenting part to the pelvic inlet. An immediate vaginal examination should be performed after spontaneous rupture of the membranes. Amniotomy should be avoided in the presence of an unengaged presenting part.

(6) *Placental abruption* may occur when the intrauterine surface suddenly diminishes in size after membrane rupture. Continuous electronic monitoring of the fetus and frequent assessment of maternal vital signs are mandatory.

(7) *Postpartum hemorrhage* may occur as a result of uterine atony secondary to overdistention. Oxytocics should be administered intravenously after delivery of the placenta, and the patient should be carefully monitored for the development of uterine atony.

C. *Oligohydramnios.* A condition characterized by a decreased volume of amniotic fluid

1. *Associated maternal and fetal conditions*

	Presumed Etiology
1. Fetal renal agenesis, polycystic kidneys, ureteral or urethral stricture	Decreased or absent fetal urination
2. Postmaturity	Unknown
3. Rupture of membranes	Fluid loss exceeds production
4. Amnion nodosum	Unknown
5. Multiple gestation	Common placental circulation; underperfused twin has decreased urinary output

2. *Complications.* If oligohydramnios occurs early in pregnancy, amniotic adhesions and pressure from the surrounding uterus may cause serious deformity or amputation of extremities.
3. *Diagnosis*
   a) *Suspect* oligohydramnios when:
      (1) The uterus is smaller than would be predicted for the gestational age.
      (2) The uterus is firm and the fetus is easily palpated.
   b) *Diagnostic studies.* Ultrasonography will reveal a significant reduction in amniotic fluid volume.
4. *Management.* Postmaturity and ruptured membranes should be appropriately evaluated and treated. For all other cases, no specific treatment is required. *The*

pediatric service should be notified of any patient with oligohydramnios so that appropriate studies may be performed after birth to detect congenital anomalies.

BIBLIOGRAPHY

Benirschke K: The Pathology of the Human Placenta. New York, Springer-Verlag, 1967

Browne EJ: On the abnormalities of the umbilical cord which may cause antenatal death. J Obstet Gynecol Br Emp 32:17, 1925

Ellis J: Disorders of the umbilical cord, placenta, membranes, and amniotic fluid. Curr Probl Obstet Gynecol 4(7):1–41, 1981

Fox H: Pathology of the Placenta. Philadelphia, Saunders, 1978

Jacoby H, Charles D: Clinical conditions associated with hydramnios. Am J Obstet Gynecol 94:910, 1966

Queenan J, Gadow E: Polyhydramnios: chronic versus acute. Am J Obstet Gynecol 106:625, 1970

Spellacy W, Gravem H, Fisch R: The umbilical cord complications of true knots, nuchal coils, and cords around the body. Am J Obstet Gynecol 94:1136, 1966

Torpin R: The Human Placenta. Springfield, Ill., Charles C. Thomas, 1969

27

Postpartum Hemorrhage

Charles R.B. Beckmann, M.D.

PRACTICE PRINCIPLES

Despite the decreases in morbidity and mortality resulting from modern intensive care management techniques, excessive postpartum bleeding remains one of the most feared and serious complications of pregnancy. Because it often presents suddenly, without warning, optimal management depends on appropriate preparation (especially in the face of known risk factors) and a thorough knowledge of the various causes of postpartum hemorrhage and of their pathophysiology and treatment.

POSTPARTUM HEMORRHAGE

Demographics

A. *Definitions*
    1. Classical definition by [39,41]
        a) *Time interval* between delivery of the baby (stage II) and onset of excessive bleeding
            (1) *Immediate.* During stage III or in the first 24 hours of the puerperium

      (2) *Delayed.* From the second postpartum day to six weeks thereafter,[47] the time when normal involution is completed[16]

   b) *Amount of blood loss,* defined as greater than 500 ml blood loss

      (1) Careful measurement of blood loss at normal delivery shows the average loss to be 550 to 700 ml (1000 to 1500 ml at cesarean section)[34,38]

      (2) The *estimated blood loss* (EBL) at delivery is usually *underestimated,* often by significant amounts, especially if there is simultaneous blood loss from an episiotomy or laceration[38,41]

  2. The "legal definition" of 500 ml blood loss remains the standard,[41] but in physiologic terms, a woman probably should not be considered to have a true postpartum hemorrhage until she loses more blood than that normally lost at delivery. Such designation also depends on the antepartum hematocrit of the patient, as well as on her general state of health. A normal patient may lose a volume of blood equivalent to the increase normal to pregnancy without ill effects, whereas an anemic patient may show such effects sooner.[38,39]

  3. Postpartum hemorrhage is most easily (and correctly) diagnosed in the third stage of labor or in the immediate puerperium. Slow, steady puerperal vaginal bleeding over several days is easily mistermed a "heavy lochia rubra," until the total blood loss is large enough to cause recognizable effects. Attention to the blood loss throughout the puerperium will avoid this error.[41]

B. *Incidence*

  1. The overall incidence is *estimated at 1 to 5 percent of deliveries.*[14,41,42] Estimates comparing immediate and delayed postpartum hemorrhage indicate the former is more common.[13]

  2. Postpartum hemorrhage is a recurrent phenomena in 10 to 25 percent of cases with one previous postpartum hemorrhage and in a far greater percentage if there has been more than one previous episode.[8,12,47]

C. *Morbidity and mortality*
   1. The "total" *morbidity* of postpartum hemorrhage in-cludes that of its associated causes and the effect of the hemorrhage (if any) on them, as well as the "actual" morbidity of the hemorrhage and its therapy.[34,39]
      a) Severe shock associated with postpartum hemorrhage may result in some degree of pituitary ischemia resulting in its dysfunction and to partial panhy-popituitarism. This is called Sheehan's syn-drome.[10,17,18,44]
      b) It is difficult to give a value for morbidity, because of definitional problems for both hemorrhage and mor-bidity. Certainly, it must be significant, even in the 1980s.
   2. *Mortality* is relatively rare in modern times, but is still a leading cause of maternal mortality when it does occur. This is an especially important datum when it is recog-nized that postpartum hemorrhage should be preventable in many cases, or anticipated so that catastrophic out-come may be avoided.

Pathophysiology

A. Postpartum hemorrhage results from uterine atony, ob-stetric lacerations, and retained products of conception. The *differential diagnosis* of postpartum hemorrhage involves the entities that comprise each category.[12,30,41]
   1. *Uterine atony* (approximately 7/10 cases) [16,41]
      a) Labor
         (1) Prolonged labor[9]
         (2) Stimulated labor (induced or augmented)
         (3) Rapid labor[9,47]
      b) Uterus
         (1) Overdistention (multiple gestation, polyhy-draminos, fetal macrosomia, etc.)[47]
         (2) Anomalies
         (3) Myomas (especially submucous)[47]
         (4) Primary atony (no demonstrable cause)
         (5) Subinvolution[13,16]

    c) Anesthesia
      (1) General (especially halogenated agents, most especially halothane)[9,31]
      (2) Regional anesthesia, especially if associated with hypotension.
    d) Iatrogenic
      (1) Operative delivery
      (2) Status after uterine surgery (myomectomy, anomaly repair, cesarean section)
    e) Uterine inversion
    f) Amniotic fluid embolism
2. *Obstetric lacerations.* Approximately 2 in 10 cases[41]
    a) Bleeding from lacerations of the vulva, vagina, cervix, and uterus or from an episiotomy or extension thereof, should be identified and surgically repaired.
    b) Hematomas, when near or on the visible surfaces, are easily identified, while deeper ones may be occult, accounting for a dangerous amount of blood loss before recognition.
    c) Uterine rupture is a rare cause.
3. *Retained tissue* (fetal, placental, etc.). Approximately 1 in 10 cases,[41] although it becomes more common in delayed postpartum hemorrhage.[13]
    a) Placenta previa
    b) Placental abruption
    c) Abnormally adherent placenta (placenta accreta)
    d) Trapped placenta
    e) Retained placental tissue (retained secundies), often a recurrent phenomena[8]
    f) Retained succenturiate lobe[47]
    g) Infection[13]
      (1) Endometritis (primary or secondary to retained products of conception)
      (2) Chorioamnionitis
    h) Angular pregnancy[27]
    i) Large placenta (e.g., diabetes)
4. Additional rare causes of postpartum hemorrhage include coagulation defects such as von Willebrand's

disease, [35,39] anticoagulation therapy, thrombocytopenic purpura, and leukemia.[41]

B. *Normal placental separation*[3,39]

1. *Placental separation* is primarily a mechanical shearing of the placenta from the uterus along the soft, fragile, spongy decidual plane.[3,9] Its main cause is the rapid change in size between the placenta and the placental bed of the uterus, the placenta being relatively fixed in size compared to the uterus, which is rapidly shrinking in size as it contracts. As this occurs, two basic processes are allowed:

   a) The placenta is freed to pass out of the uterus. (Classically described as by "Duncan's mechanism," where blood escapes past the uterus as it is expelled, or by "Schultz's mechanism," when blood collects behind the placenta and is lost at once as the placenta is expelled.)[9]

   b) The myometrium is no longer constrained in an expanded state by an attached placenta and is free to contract down on the spiral arteries, the primary mechanism by which postpartum hemostasis is affected.[16]

   c) With these events the normal involutionary process commences.[16]

2. Normal placental separation is thus dependent on normal:

   a) Placental implantation

   b) Placental development and maturation

   c) Uterine structure and contractility (including response to natural oxytocics)

   d) Spontaneous uterine evacuation of the placenta by uterine contraction and decrease in size, and thereby mechanical arterial constriction.[16]

3. *Third-stage timing — retained placenta*[9,14]

   a) Seventy-five percent of placentas will separate and be expelled within 3 minutes, and 95 percent within 10 minutes.

   b) A placenta may be considered retained after 15 to 20

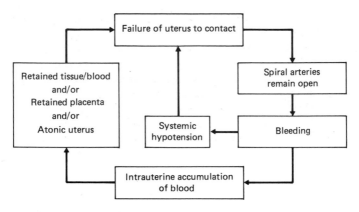

Figure 27–1. Pathophysiologic cycle of postpartum hemorrhage.

minutes (sooner if hemorrhage ensues and therapy is begun).

C. The *cycle of pathophysiologic events in postpartum hemorrhage* is essentially the same whether it starts with uterine atony or retained tissue.[41]

D. *The three key interventions in the treatment of postpartum hemorrhage* thus include:
   1. Uterine evacuation
   2. Enhancement of uterine contractility
   3. Maintenance of systemic blood pressure

Management

A. *Prevention*
   1. By *recognition of the risk factors* for postpartum hemorrhage (i.e., the elements of its differential diagnosis) and appropriate preparation when recognized, many postpartum hemorrhages may be avoided, at best, or at least minimized in extent and effect. Indeed, strict adherence to this basic precept is the most important step that may be taken to reduce the morbidity and mortality of

postpartum hemorrhage.[8,14,41] Because of the postpartum patient's youth and hence resilient cardiovascular system, which can compensate for significant blood loss, and because she has an additional "reserve" composed of the additional blood volume of pregnancy, a "normal" pulse and blood pressure may be misinterpreted in the face of significant blood loss until the critical point at which these mechanisms are no longer capable of "shielding" the patient from profound shock—which then may rapidly ensue.[39]

2. *Minimal preparation* includes knowledge of a recent hematocrit, placement or immediate availability of a large-bore intravenous line, immediately available anesthesia and operating room capability, and immediately available blood in sufficient quantity.

3. *Use of oxytocics*
   a) *Oxytocin* has been administered by many routes and in many doses during the last moments of stage II and in stage III to facilitate placental separation and expulsion or expulsion of placental fragments, as well as for uterine contraction and thereby spiral artery constriction. Many different regimens are used, all of which are acceptable as long as they do not begin prior to the delivery of the head nor involve intravenous bolus administration. (The former may adversely affect the baby by causing a tetanic uterine contraction, causing uteroplacental dysfunction or dystocia; the latter, the mother by causing cardiac effects.)[14] Typical regimens include:
      (1) 10 units IM at delivery of the fetal shoulder.
      (2) 20 units in 1 liter of fluid begun by IV drip on delivery of the fetal shoulder or baby.
   b) *When oxytocin is combined with gentle uterine massage, normal completion of the third stage of labor is usually accomplished.*[14,39,41]
   c) *Ergonovine (Ergotrate)* and *methylergonovine (Methergine)* have been used in many routes and

dosages, causing powerful uterine spasm. While highly effective, continued bleeding and uterine atony "requiring" the use of this agent usually means that further evaluation is actually needed. Because of its hypertensive effects, it is contraindicated in hypertensive patients.

4. *Manual exploration of the uterus* after placental expulsion has been condemned by some [9,11,47] as an unnecessary invasion of the uterus[46] predisposing to infection and praised by others as a useful means to avoid retained placental fragments and to identify unsuspected uterine pathology without an increased infection rate.[6,13,21,41,46] *Manual exploration of the uterus probably carries no increased risks if done with aseptic technique and is useful where there is clinical suspicion of retained placenta.* Its routine use is problematic and is best left to the clinical discretion of the physician.[41]

5. *Routine manual removal of the placenta* has been advocated,[9,25] but considering its risks[11,19,40] and the rates of spontaneous expulsion of the placenta, *its use on a routine basis is unjustified.*[11,19,41] Delay in delivery of the placenta after spontaneous separation, however, is an open invitation to hemorrhage (the maneuver of Brandt is most useful to assist in placental expulsion after spontaneous separation).[3,41]

6. The criteria for use of *ultrasound examination* to detect retained placental tissue and hence help select those patients who need dilatation and curettage from those who would benefit from direct therapy for uterine atony are under development.[28,30,42,43]

B. *Initial management*

1. Upon recognition of postpartum hemorrhage, the following sequence of events should be initiated:[39,41]

   a) Frequent vital signs

   b) Rapid administration of IV fluids—preferably normal saline or lactated Ringer's with dextrose—via at least one large-bore catheter (16 gauge or larger).

c) If shock seems imminent, or is present, a second large-bore IV line should be begun and a rapid infusion of colloid or albumin initiated.

d) A central venous pressure line is indicated if shock is present, placed either via the subclavian or antecubital routes.

e) Crossmatching of at least four units of whole blood — more if indicated — and initiation of transfusion as soon as the blood is available.[41] If blood loss is massive, the use of uncrossmatched O-negative blood may be lifesaving and should not be avoided if the clinical situation warrants its use.[39]

f) Immediate consultation with the anesthesia staff and the collection of staff sufficient to avoid delays in care are essential[39]

g) Continuous administration of IV oxytocin[39]

2. Careful *reinspection* by speculum and bimanual examination should be done. Any lacerations previously unidentified should be treated. Any retained tissue and blood clots easily accessible with finger or ring or ovum forceps should be removed, as that immediate decrease in intrauterine volume may significantly decrease blood loss. *The key to the successful completion of these steps is attaining proper exposure at examination,* i.e., use of sufficient anesthesia to allow full exposure of all structures.

3. Thereafter, *bimanual compression and massage* of the uterus should be carried out (Fig. 27–2). This, in combination with intravenous administration of oxytocin, is usually sufficient to cause contraction of the enlarged boggy uterus.

4. *If there is suspicion of retained tissue,* a complete dilatation and curettage should be performed as soon as feasible.[13,42] Care must be taken, however, not to perform an overly aggressive curettage, causing Asherman's syndrome.[1,41] The endometrium appears to be especially vulnerable to such damage between the 14th and 24th

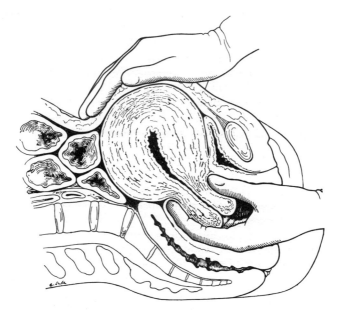

Figure 27–2. Manual compression and massage of the uterus. (From Quilligan EJ, Zuspan F: Douglas-Stromme Operative Obstetrics, 4th ed. New York, Appleton, 1982, p 758.)

days puerperal and the 8th to 14th days postabortal,[16,41] although this is the time period when "delayed" postpartum hemorrhage is most likely to occur.[47]

5. Other regimens, including uterine packing[24,29,39,41] and hot intrauterine lavage[15] have been advocated. While they are probably effective in some cases, their proper use is reserved to situations when a physician very experienced in their use is available, and hence is probably limited.[29,39]

6. Recent experience with the use of prostaglandins in the treatment of postpartum hemorrhage caused by uterine atony has been encouraging. The IM injection of PG $F_{2\alpha}$

or its 15-methyl analogue or the placement of a vaginal suppository containing PG ϵ_2 or its 15-methyl analogue in the posterior fornix may be very effective.[7,22,33,39,45,48]

C. In some cases, such initial conservative management is unsuccessful, and hemorrhage continues. If this occurs, *operative intervention* is indicated.

1. The wishes of the patient concerning her reproductive capabilities (i.e., uterus) should be ascertained beforehand. If the patient wishes to maintain her reproductive capability, every reasonable effort should be made to preserve her uterus so long as such effort does not place the patient in undue jeopardy.

2. Following stabilization of the patient, insofar as possible,[39] general anesthesia should be administered and a last careful speculum and bimanual examination be performed, with repair of any injury noted. A final dilatation (if needed) and curettage should then be done, followed again by compression and massage of the uterus combined with simultaneous oxytocic therapy. These maneuvers will occasionally suffice.

3. If bleeding continues, laparotomy is indicated.

D. *Management at laparotomy*

1. While vigorous treatment of systemic hypotension should continue, *a decrease in arterial pulse pressure to the uterus will often result in diminution or cessation of hemorrhage.* Several techniques, some "temporary" and some more "prolonged" are available, all of which decrease the pulse pressure without stopping uterine blood flow entirely and thus arrest the hemorrhage yet preserve the uterus.[4,5,38,41] Even if no attempt is to be made to preserve the uterus, the "temporary" techniques should be used to reduce the blood loss while hysterectomy is being performed.

2. *"Temporary" methods*

a) All these techniques involve *vascular compression to cause a reduction in pulse pressure.*

b) *Manual compression of the aorta* against the spine has been successfully employed and has the advantage of being easy and quick once the abdomen is open. A variation is the use of a Harris aortic compressor designed to facilitate aortic compression.[20]

c) Use of a *tourniquet,* either about the uterus and adnexae or about the uterus by passing the tourniquet through a hole created adjacent to the uterus in the avascular part of the broad ligament. Various items have been used as the tourniquet, the most popular being a Foley catheter.[2,41]

3. *"Prolonged" methods*

a) *Ligation of major trunks of the vascular supply of the uterus* has proven a very effective therapy. While the abundant collateral blood supply quickly (within one hour) reestablishes nearly normal blood flow to the uterus, the period of decreased arterial pulse pressure is effective in many cases.[4,5,32,41]

b) *Techniques*

(1) *Uterine artery ligation* is done by passage of a heavy suture from front to back under the pulsatile uterine artery, exiting in the posterior inferior avascular part of the broad ligament. The immediate response will be a blanching of the uterus and, if successful, a cessation of bleeding. *It is important to note that the uterus may remain boggy or contract only slightly, a situation not to be misinterpreted as failure. Cessation of hemorrhage is the criteria of success or failure.*[36,41,49]

(2) *Ligation of the hypogastric arteries* has been a traditional method and is also very successful. Its main disadvantage is that it requires relatively more surgical skill and time to perform for most operators.[4,5,38,39,41]

4. *Hysterectomy* is the final method, stopping the hemorrhage by removing its source. Occasionally the patient may be so unstable that operative time should be minimized, one of the few indications for supracervical hysterectomy.

PLACENTA ACCRETA

Definitions

A. Under certain circumstances abnormal placentation occurs such that the decidual layer either fails to form or forms incompletely and trophoblastic tissue gains direct access to the myometrium. *Abnormal adherence or invasion of the placenta to the myometrium* results.[3,5,7] Difficulty in retrieval of such placental tissue in the third stage of labor often leads to postpartum hemorrhage secondary to retained tissue and uterine atony.

B. *Classification* of abnormally adherent placenta[3,5,6,9,14,26]
   1. *By degree of adherence or invasion* of placenta to the myometrium
      a) *Placenta accreta:* to but not into the myometrium
      b) *Placenta increta:* into but not through the myometrial thickness
      c) *Placenta percreta:* through the myometrial thickness
   2. *By the fraction of placenta involved. Incomplete* (partial, focal) or *complete* (total)
   3. Unless trophoblastic tissue invades extrauterine structures, classification beyond abnormally adherent placenta is probably more useful for pathologic description than in clinical use. *Placenta accreta is a term well established in the literature and often used for all the variants of abnormally adherent placenta.*[5,8]

Demographics

A. *Incidence*
   1. Estimates range from 1/500 to 1/100,000 births.[3,5,6,9,14] Based on these data, a reasonable estimate for recognized and reported cases is *1/5,000 to 1/10,000 births.* The incidence does increase with advanced maternal age and multiparity.[3,5,9]
   2. The actual incidence is probably higher, and unknow-

able, as many instances of incomplete abortion, "temporarily" retained placenta, and difficult manual removal of retained placenta actually represent an abnormally adherent placenta.[3,8] This problem is often augmented by the requirement of microscopic demonstration of placental tissue adherent to or infiltration of the myometrium by placental villi.[5,14]

B. *Morbidity and mortality*

1. *Morbidity is increased,* the degree inestimable as discussed.

2. *Mortality*
   a) Maternal: 9 to 12 percent[5,6,10]
   b) Fetal: 10 percent[5]

Pathophysiology

A. Various explanations of abnormal placentation have been offered. All involve two basic elements: (1) deficient or absent decidua, and (2) abnormal invasive activity of trophoblastic tissue.[3,5]

1. *Trophoblast.* In normal placentation the trophoblast implants and invades the decidua in the first trimester, then stops. Various mechanisms for this "selective invasion and cessation of invasion" have been postulated, including responses to the changing neurohumoral milieu of pregnancy, a dysfunctional self–non-self recognition system for the uteroplacental unit, etc. Aberrations of these mechanisms are proposed as etiologies.[5,8,12,13] Placenta membranacea is also a rare associated cause.[14]

2. *Decidua.* Various defects of the decidua, either intrinsic or caused by underlying uterine pathology, have been suggested.
   a) Abnormal decidual tissue
   b) Previous placenta accreta (history of indicated manual placental removal, postpartum hemorrhage with dilatation and curettage for retained tissue)[2,3,5,8,14]
   c) Uterine fibroids (especially submucous)[3,5,8]
   d) Placenta previa[1,5,8,11,12]

    e) Previous cesarean section (or hysterotomy)[3,5,8,9]

    f) Uterine anomalies[5,8]

    g) Previous uterine surgery (myomectomy, repair of anomaly, cornual resection, tubal implantation)[3,5,8,9]

    h) Trophoblastic disease, especially if treated with cytotoxic drugs[13]

    i) Endo(myo)metritis[3,5,8,14]

    j) Overly vigorous uterine curettage[3,5,8–10,14]

    k) Cornual placental implantation[5]

    l) Anomalous placenta[5]

B. Considering the low reported (and thus presumed "serious") incidence of placenta accreta compared to the combined frequencies of the various suggested etiologic associations, most such associations probably have little validity. Those which evidently do include:

    1. *Overly vigorous curettage* with extensive damage to the endometrium and inner myometrium,[3–5] whether for gynecologic indication or postabortally or postpartum. *Asherman's syndrome* has an especially prominent association.[4]

    2. *Placenta previa.* Placenta previa occurs in about 1 percent of pregnancies but has an associated accreta of some degree between 15 and 25 percent of the time.[1,3–5,8,9,11,12] Placenta previa accreta is usually not recognized until the third-stage problems characteristic of accreta develop. Antepartum bleeding is common but is associated with the previa rather than the accreta.[1,9]

    3. *Uterine scars* resulting from cesarean section or reconstructive uterine surgery, causing defects in the myometrium/endometrium[3,5,14]

C. If the entire placenta is adherent to the uterus, hemorrhage may be minimal as long as the pathologic uteroplacental unit is intact, the main problem being the inability to remove the placenta.[9,10] Postpartum (and postabortal) hemorrhage ensues when:

    1. In a complete placenta accreta when vain attempts to find a nonexistent decidual cleavage plane results in bleeding from torn vessels.[5,6]

2. In an incomplete or partial placenta accreta for the same reasons as in the complete placenta accreta, plus the inability of the uterine part where the placenta was implanted normally and separated to contract and affect hemostasis. This situation usually leads to the most severe hemorrhage.[5],[9]

3. Uterine inversion is an associated complication.[5],[9]

D. In most cases placenta accreta seems to have no untoward effect on the antepartum course, labor, or the newborn prior to delivery.[5],[9],[12] An exception may be an increased likelihood of uterine rupture.[5],[9]

Diagnosis

A. Usually discovered clinically when spontaneous placental separation does not occur, when it is manually impossible to find the cleavage plane and affect placental separation, or with the onset of postpartum hemorrhage.[5],[8],[10],[14]

B. The diagnosis may be suggested on ultrasound examination.

C. Antepartum bleeding and hemorrhage are common with placenta accreta previa, but not with placenta accreta alone.[5],[9] Uterine rupture is more likely if the trophoblastic invasion of the myometrium is extensive.[9]

Management

A. *Hysterectomy* is indicated in most circumstances:[3],[8-10],[12]

1. Total abdominal hysterectomy is the treatment of choice in most cases.

2. If extrauterine structures have been invaded, surgical therapy appropriate to the situation is indicated.

3. Supracervical hysterectomy is sometimes indicated when the patient's clinical status is so unstable as to preclude the longer definitive procedure.

B. *Conservative therapy* has been successfully employed in situations where the patient is stable and has expressed the desire to avoid sterilization via hysterectomy, understanding the considerable risks of hemorrhage and infection.[3],[6],[10]

1. A wide range of therapies have been tried, most involving removal of as much placental tissue as possible followed by uterine packing and oxytocic therapy.[5] The new prostaglandin therapies may have a place in such a regimen.
2. Successful outcomes have been reported, with subsequent pregnancies in some cases.[3,14]
3. Because of the paucity of experience with conservative management and the considerable risks involved, such management should be reserved for exceptional cases and attempted only by physicians experienced in the techniques involved.[10,11]

AMNIOTIC FLUID EMBOLISM

A. *Demographics*
   1. *Incidence*. Difficult to estimate because of the difficulty in establishing confirmed diagnosis except at autopsy; probably *between 1/10,000 and 1/30,000 live births*.[3,5]
   2. *Morbidity and mortality*. Amniotic fluid embolism is a very morbid process, until recently thought to be fatal in most cases. Although vigorous management may salvage some patients, it nevertheless presently accounts for *10 to 15 percent of maternal deaths*.[3,5,10,11,13]
   3. Patients are at *higher risk for amniotic fluid embolism* when they:[14]
      a) Are older (greater than 30)[1,3–5,11]
      b) Are multiparous[1,3–5,11]
      c) Have large infants[1,5]
      d) Demonstrate postdatism[3]
      e) Have extended, hypertonic and/or stimulated labor[1,3–5,11]
      f) Have intrauterine fetal demise[3,5,11]
      g) Experience premature placental separation [may be a key association, since it may explain how amniotic fluid (and debris) gains entry to the circulation][3,11]

B. *Pathophysiology*

  1. The route of entry of the particulate laden amniotic fluid into the circulation remains obscure. Premature placental separation is probably involved in most cases, with a transient tear in the chorioamniotic membrane.[3,9]

  2. The particulate matter contained in the amniotic fluid initiates the *physiologic sequences of amniotic fluid embolism* by causing mechanical obstruction in the distal pulmonary arterial tree. The acute pulmonary hypertension that ensues induces reflex vasoconstriction of the pulmonary and coronary arteries via the vagus nerve, as well as causing acute cor pulmonale and right heart failure. Decreasing blood flow to the left heart leads to decreased cardiac output and progressive systemic hypotension. The ventilation-perfusion ratio is deranged, resulting in hypoxia: this in turn stimulates tachypnea. Bronchospasm and increased mucous formation worsens the situation.[3,7]

  3. *Vaginal hemorrhage* occurs in about *40 to 50 percent* of patients, usually with a coagulopathy characterized primarily by *hypofibrinogenemia.*[1,3]

  4. *Pathology*

    a) Special stains for *mucin, fat,* and *fetal squames* (especially mucicarmine and Alcian green) will demonstrate their presence in lung specimens *at postmortem examination.*[1,3]

    b) *Diagnosis with patient survival* is more difficult. An early suggestion was right cardiocentesis and blood smear for fetal squames, etc., a procedure whose risks forestalled wide acceptance.[1,3,5,6] With the advent of modern managements including central venous pressure (or Swan-Ganz) line placement, access to the necessary blood samples may become acceptable, allowing diagnosis more readily. Nile blue stains of sputum may demonstrate fetal squames.[4]

C. *Diagnosis*

  1. *Amniotic fluid embolism may present*[3]

    a) Abruptly as sudden cardiopulmonary arrest, preceded

in some cases by a short interval of respiratory distress and/or acute apprehension. Even with vigorous modern resuscitation techniques, these patients have a poor prognosis.

b) Gradually, with the pathophysiologic sequences proressing steadily in severity until the patient is unstable.

2. *Signs and symptoms*[3,11,12]
   a) Dyspnea, cyanosis, tachypnea
   b) Hypotension (shock) systemically, and tachycardia
   c) Apprehension
   d) Excessive vaginal bleeding (40 to 50 percent of cases)
   e) Convulsions (usually grand mal type)

3. *Laboratory findings*
   a) Amniotic fluid particulate matter (fetal squames, lanugo, fat cells, mucin, meconium) in trachael samples or in blood from the right heart.[1,3–5,11]
   b) Arterial blood gases showing hypoxemia and acidosis.[3]
   c) Chest x-ray film shows no characteristic early signs; later, if the patient survives, findings of pulmonary edema and congestion may be seen.[4,5,8,11]
   d) The electrocardiogram (ECG) may show rapidly developing evidence of right heart strain.
   e) Hemogram may show anemia, especially if preexisting or if there is an ongoing massive blood loss.
   f) Coagulation studies
      (1) Hypofibrinogenemia is the only consistent finding, occurring in about 50 percent of cases surviving long enough to develop the process.[1,7,11]
      (2) If hemorrhage ensues, full-blown disseminated intravascular coagulation with its characteristic laboratory findings may be manifest.
   g) Lung scanning may be useful in diagnosis.[2,5]

D. *Treatment*
   1. *Survival is possible in some cases, the likelihood increasing with the speed with which vigorous management is begun. Delay is fatal.*
   2. Upon reasonable suspicion of amniotic fluid embolism:[3]
      a) *100 percent oxygen under positive pressure,* first by

mask, then via endotracheal intubation as soon as possible.[1,11] Serial evaluations of the patient are simultaneously begun, including blood pressure, pulse, ECG monitoring, ABGs, etc.

b) Placement of a *central venous line* (or even better, Swan-Ganz catheter), allowing access to cardiac function data. The *postplacement chest x-ray* may also serve as the baseline study.

c) Administration of the following is suggested:
   (1) *Atropine* to block vagal effects and reduce pulmonary secretions (0.4 mg IV)[1]
   (2) *Digoxin* to facilitate cardiac function (according to standard rapid digitalization regimens)
   (3) *Papaverine hydrochloride* to reduce arterial vasospasm (50 to 100 mg IV over several minutes, repeat q2h)[1]
   (4) *Isoproterenol* to augment cardiac contractility and cause bronchiolar dilatation (0.2 mg IV, 1-ml ampule of 1:5000 solution, followed by an IV infusion, initially at 0.3 µg/kg/minute)[7]

d) Other potentially useful medications
   (1) *Aminophylline* to facilitate bronchodilation. It must be used very cautiously in the face of hypotension.[3]
   (2) *Vasopressors,* which may increase blood pressure by vasoconstriction and exert a direct inotropic effect. *Mephentermine* by monitered IV infusion (30 mg in 100 ml sterile normal saline) is one such agent, especially useful because of its potent inotropic effect.[3]
   (3) *Steroids*

e) *Amniotomy* should be done if membranes are intact to prevent further amniotic fluid embolism.[1,3]

f) *Rotating limb tournequets* may be used to reduce venous return.[3]

g) If, despite all efforts, the patient's condition continues to deteriorate, with demise a likely outcome, *cardiopulmonary bypass* may be tried.[3,5]

    h) *Vaginal hemorrhage* associated with documented *hypofibrinogenemia* may be treated by
      (1) *Fibrinogen replacement*
      (2) Administration of a *fibrinolysin inhibitor* such as ε-aminocaproic acid (5 gm slow IV followed by 1 gm hourly up to 30 gm per 24 hours).[3,5] *Heparin* is recommended by some authors for syndrome resembling disseminated intravascular coagulation that often ensues.[4,5]
    i) Plasma expanders — albumin, colloid, or blood — should be administered only for specific indications, and not as a "general treatment" for systemic shock.[3]

UTERINE INVERSION

A. *Definition. Situation, puerperal or nonpuerperal, in which the uterus is "turned inside out."*[1,18]
B. *Classification*
  1. Classification is important because the choice of therapy is based on an evaluation of *the duration and degree of inversion.*
  2. *Classification by degree of inversion*[1,12,20]
    a) *Incomplete.* Uterine corpus does not extend beyond the external cervical os.
    b) *Complete.* Uterine corpus has extended beyond the external cervical os.
  3. *Classification by duration of inversion*[1,12,3A,20]
    a) *Acute*
      (1) Puerperal: Immediately after delivery
      (2) In either case, puerperal or nonpuerperal, before formation of a contraction ring
    b) *Subacute*
      (1) Begins with establishment of cervical "contraction ring," where the cervix contracts about the uterine body that has passed through its opening. A "ring" is thereby formed from the body of the cervix.

      (2) Formation usually about *30 minutes* after inversion.

   c) *Chronic*. Inversion of greater than four weeks duration.

C. *Incidence*
1. The incidence of inversion is uncertain, because of:
   a) Variation in reporting. Lack of reporting the situation may be due to the mistaken thought that it is always iatrogenic.[1,16]
   b) Lack of recognition
2. The incidence in the literature varys from 1/4000 to 1/250,000, while a *reasonable estimate is 1/25,000 deliveries*.[3,13,14]

D. *Demographics*[1]
1. Average age 25 years, 60 percent between 21 and 30 years old
2. Fifty to 60 percent are primigravidas

E. *Etiology*
1. A *common misconception* is that uterine inversion is always a preventable iatrogenic problem. This does not seem to be true, although uterine inversion can certainly be caused by too vigorous management of the third stage (i.e., excessive pulling on the umbilical cord to affect placental delivery).[3,13,16,21]
2. *Two conditions are necessary for uterine inversion.*
   a) Cervical dilatation. There must be an opening through which the uterine portion may invert.
   b) A portion of the uterine fundus must "reflex" sufficiently such that it may be deformed from its normal configuration, invert, and pass through the cervical opening. Once begun, the uterine part "leading" the inversion is felt to act as a "foreign body," which the remainder of the uterus "perceives" as such and acts to expel.[3,4,10,11]
   c) In addition, many authors feel that the degree of "suddenness" of uterine emptying is crucial, such that uterine inversion is most likely when uterine emptying is very rapid.[2]

3. *Proposed etiologic or causal relationships*
  a) *Puerperal*[1,13,14,20]
     (1) *Predisposing factors*
        (a) Fundal implantation of the placenta is considered by many to be essential for uterine inversion.[3,16] Certainly, such placental positioning may predispose to uterine inversion, as in a case of inappropriate umbilical cord traction.[3A]
        (b) Abnormal placental implantation, e.g., placenta accreta, such that any movement to placental delivery will "automatically" cause uterine inversion.
        (c) Congenital weakening or anomalies of the uterine wall that cause a given uterine body to be especially susceptible to inversion at the anomalous points.[16] This is the concept of "congenital predisposition," which many hold to be valid, and on this basis argue that many uterine inversions during third stage are unavoidable regardless of the third-stage management.[6]
        (d) Weakening of the uterine wall at the site of normal placental attachment and separation, leading to poor or ineffective contractile activity at that site. The "foreign body" argument is then applied to this area.
        (e) Uterine anomalies[16]
        (f) Protracted labor is suggested by many authors, although others doubt this is a major predisposing factor.[21]
        (g) Previous inversion[21]
        (h) Intrapartum use of $MgSO_4$[16A]
     (2) *Exciting causes (third-stage mismanagement)*[16]
        (a) Too vigorous manual placental removal
        (b) Application of excessive umbilical cord tension in attempting to affect placental separation and removal[3A]

      (c) Application of excessive pressure on the uterus from abdominal massage in attempts to affect placental separation and expulsion or in the treatment of the atonic postpartum uterus.[14A]

      (d) Excessive increase in intraabdominal pressure, as when a patient is asked to bear down to facilitate placental delivery or in vigorous coughing or sneezing.

   b) *Nonpuerperal*[13,17]

      (1) Uterine myomas, especially the pedunculated submucous type,[16] are probably the most common cause of nonpuerperal inversion.[3]

      (2) Uterine carcinoma

      (3) Uterine anomalies

      (4) Idiopathic inversion[3]

F. *Diagnosis*

  1. *Cardinal findings*[13,18,21]

   a) *Pain*

   b) *Shock,* often seemingly disproportionate to the situation[3]

   c) *Hemorrhage,* also seemingly disproportionately severe to the situation,[15] although recent authors have questioned the emphasis on unusual severity[21]

   d) *Vaginal mass*

   e) Where the uterus is palpable abdominally, palpation of a "dimple" (*the inversion cup*)[3] (Fig.27–3).

   f) Sensation of bearing down or of delivery[16]

  2. Because early diagnosis (and rapid treatment) is of great importance, the value of postpartum cervical inspection is emphasized by most authors. Some suggest that cervical inspection and uterine manual exploration should be routine,[13] especially in the face of unexplained shock or hemorrhage.[16]

  3. In the *chronic phase,* pressure sensations plus irregular menses and/or excessive vaginal discharge may be the only symptoms, especially if the inversion is partial and

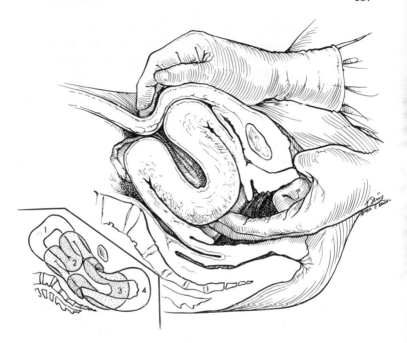

Figure 27–3. Diagnosis of uterine inversion by abdominopelvic examination. (From Pritchard J, MacDonald PC: Williams Obstetrics, 16th ed. New York, Appleton, 1980, p 888.)

the uterus does not extrude past the introitus.[2,16] Urinary symptoms may also be present, especially frequency and urgency.[3]

G. *Treatment*

   1. *Shock*

      a) *Rapid onset of severe shock, seemingly out of proportion to blood loss or the amount of pain that seems to be present, is characteristic.*

      b) *The vigorous, immediate treatment for shock is mandatory*[14]

2. *Hemorrhage*
   a) *Hemorrhage is characteristic, as is its gross underesti-mation. Blood transfusion should be started as soon as possible after diagnosis, with typed blood only if the patient was anemic prior to the event.*
3. *Techniques for uterine replacement*[17]
   a) In the *acute phase,* replacement may often be easily accomplished by *manual reposition of the uterus,* the Johnson technique,[9,13,20] (Fig. 27–4) if performed within a few minutes of inversion; it is facilitated by

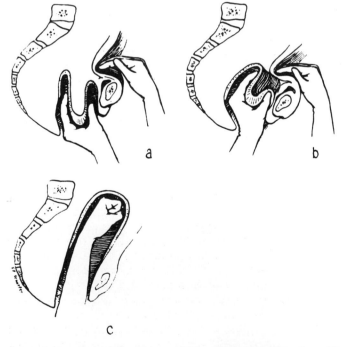

Figure 27–4. Manual uterine reposition. (From Schaefer: Surg Clin North Am 599, 1949.)

early administration of general anesthesia, which provides uterine relaxation as well as anesthesia.[1] The fingers of the vaginal hand are steadily pressed superiorly, progress monitored in part by the abdominal hand. This lifting action also raises the uterus, allowing the broad ligaments to assist passively in reposition. When inversion has been reversed, the vaginal hand, in fist form, is left inside the uterus, which is encouraged to contract by oxytocic administration via intravenous drip and manual massage. After contraction is well established, the hand may be removed. Afterward, careful manual exploration of the uterus and inspection of the cervix and vagina are essential to avoid missing lacerations caused by the inversion or repositioning.[14] *Placental detachment should be affected, if possible, before reposition is attempted.*[3,6,20,21] Great care should be taken if halothane anesthesia is used to help with uterine relaxation, as it may aggravate hemorrhage. Oxytocic agents should be withheld during the acute phase reposition efforts.[13,18]

b) In the *subacute phase,* three techniques should be attempted, in the following order:

(1) *Manual repositioning,* probably best tried at this stage under general anesthesia.[1]

(2) *Huntington procedure.* Under general anesthesia, via an abdominal incision, sequential application of clamps is made on the "inner" margins of the inversion cup, with traction being applied to these in an attempt to "pull" the uterus back through the inversion cup formed by the cervical contraction ring.[1,7,8,13] Countertraction on the cervix per vagina may help in repositioning.[16]

(3) *Haultain procedure* (Fig. 27–6) is attempted upon failure of the Huntington procedure. An incision is made in the posterior aspect of the cervical construction ring, and the uterus is forced back through the newly created space by vaginal

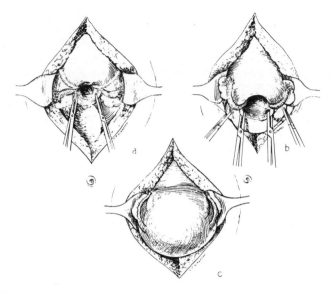

Figure 27–5. Steps in the Huntington procedure. (From Schaefer: Surg Clin North Am 599, 1949.)

pressure applied by an assistant. The incision is then closed in the uterus.[5]

c) In the *chronic phase,* evaluation must first be made of the status of the uterine tissues. If they have been inverted for a long time and are not vital, the patient is best served by hysterectomy. If, however, the tissues are viable, and the patient wishes to preserve her reproductive capability, the Huntington and then the Haultain procedure may be tried in sequence. Manual reposition is usually ineffectual at this stage.[17] There is, in addition, the vaginal approach of Spenilli,[19] which has proven successful in some situations.[1,13]

d) In all cases, failure at all attempts at uterine reposition should be followed by hysterectomy.

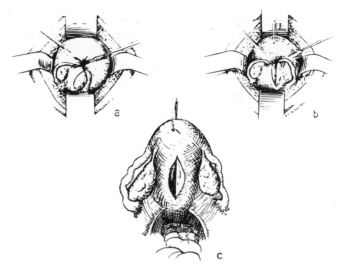

Figure 27–6. Steps in the Haultain procedure. (From Schaefer: Surg Clin North Am 599, 1949.)

    e) Prophylactic antibiotics have been suggested for all cases.[13,21]

H. *Morbidity and mortality*

  1. Morbidity and mortality are directly related to the duration of the inversion-replacement interval; the longer the interval, the greater the risk and vice versa.[14]

  2. *Main causes of morbidity*[13]

    a) Recurrence. The incidence is uncertain, but probably ranges from 5 to 25 percent.[3,20]

    b) Urinary retention. An indwelling Foley catheter should be placed after reposition.

    c) Sepsis. Broad-spectrum antibiotic therapy should be begun after reposition.

    d) Anemia

    e) Pituitary necrosis secondary to shock (Sheehan's syndrome)

    f) Pulmonary embolism[17]

    g) Intestinal damage by strangulation during the inversion. If there is evidence of bowel involvement in the inversion, the bowels should be carefully inspected and their function carefully monitored in the reposition period.

3. *Mortality*. Uterine inversion is a major surgical emergency that used to claim nearly one-quarter of patients suffering this condition. With *early recognition and prompt total therapy,* mortality should now be minimal.[2,21] Thus, rapidity of therapy is crucial within the first 48 hours, after which mortality declines rapidly, even in the unrecognized state.[11]

REFERENCES

Postpartum Hemorrhage

1. Asherman JG: Traumatic intra-uterine adhesions. J Obstet Gynaecol Br Emp 57:892, 1950

2. Bieren R, McKelway W: The use of a tourniquet in uterine surgery. Am J Obstet Gynecol 71:433, 1956

3. Brandt ML: The mechanism and management of the third stage of labour. Am J Obstet Gynecol 25:662, 1933

4. Burchell RC: Physiology of internal iliac artery ligation. J Obstet Gynaecol Br Commonw 75:642, 1968

5. Burchell RC, Mengert WF: Internal iliac artery ligation: a series of 200 patients. Int J Gynaecol Obstet 7:85, 1969

6. Cacciarelik R: The third stage of labor, a plea for manual removal of the placenta. Am J Obstet Gynecol 57:351, 1949

7. Corson SL, Bolognese RJ: Postpartum uterine atony treated with prostaglandins Am J Obstet Gynecol 129:918, 1977

8. Dewhurst CJ, Dutton WAW: Recurrent abnormalities of recurrent hemorrhage the third stage of labour. Lancet 2:764, 1957

9. Dieckmann WJ, O'Dell LD, Williger VM, et al.: The placental stage and postpartum hemorrhage. Am J Obstet Gynecol 54:415, 1947

10. DiZerega G, Kletzky O, Mishell D: Diagnosis of Sheehan's syndrome using a sequential pituitary stimulation test. Am J Obstet Gynecol 132:348, 1978

11. Doolittle H: Routine manual inspection of the postpartum uterus, a study of the late effects. Obstet Gynecol 9:422, 1957

12. Doran JR, O'Brien SA, Randall JH: Repeated postpartum hemorrhage. Obstet Gynecol 5:186, 1955

13. Duckman S, Suarez J, Andia C: Delayed postpartum hemorrhage. Obstet Gynecol 36:568, 1970

14. Fliegner J: Third stage management: how important is it? Obstet Gynecol Surv 582

15. Fribourg S, Rothman L, Rovinsky J: Intrauterine lavage for control of uterine atony. Obstet Gynecol 41:876, 1973

16. Gainey HL, Nicolay KS, Lapi A: Noninvolution of the placental site: clinical and pathological studies. Am J Obstet Gynecol 69:558, 1955

17. Grimes H, Brooks M: Pregnancy in Sheehan's syndrome, report of a case and review. Obstet Gynecol Surv 35:481, 1980

18. Haddock L, Vega L, Aguilo L, Rodriquez O: Adrenocortical, thyroid, and human growth hormone reserve in Sheehan's syndrome. Johns Hopkins Med J 131:80, 1972

19. Halsey H: Manual removal of the placenta. Am J Obstet Gynecol 64:38, 1962

20. Harris LJ: A new instrument for control of hemorrhage by aortic compression; a preliminary report. Can Med Assoc J 91:128, 1964

21. Hawkins R: Exploration of the uterus following delivery. Am J Obstet Gynecol 49:1094, 1955

22. Hayashi R, Castillo M, Noah M: Management of severe postpartum hemorrhage due to uterine atony using an analogue of prostaglandin $F_{2\alpha}$. Obstet Gynecol 58:426, 1981

23. Hertz RH, Sokol R, Dierker L: Treatment of postpartum uterine atony with prostaglandin E_2 vaginal suppositories. Obstet Gynecol 56:129, 1980

24. Hester JD: Postpartum hemorrhage and reevaluation of uterine packing. Obstet Gynecol 45:501, 1975

25. Hoffman R: Routine manual removal of the placenta. Am J Obstet Gynecol 68:645, 1954

26. Irving F, Hertig A: A study of placenta accreta. Surg Gynecol Obstet 64:178, 1937

27. Jansen R, Elliott P: Angular intrauterine pregnancy. Obstet Gynecol 58:167, 1981

28. Lee C, Madrazo B, Crukker B: Ultrasonic evaluation of the postpartum uterus in the management of postpartum bleeding. Obstet Gynecol 58:227, 1981

29. Lester WM, Bartholomew RA, Colvin ED, et al.: Reconsideration of uterine pack in postpartum hemorrhage. Am J Obstet Gynecol 93:321, 1965

30. Malvern J, Campbell S: Ultrasonic scanning of the puerperal uterus following secondary postpartum hemorrhage. J Obstet Gynecol Br Commonw 80:320, 1973

31. Marx G, Kim Y, Lin C, Halevy S, Schulman H: Postpartum uterine pressures under halothane or enflurane anesthesia. Obstet Gynecol 51:695, 1978

32. McDonough PG, Emich JP Jr, Schwartz RH: Interval before appearance of collaterals following hypogastric ligation. Obstet Gynecol 25:213, 1965

33. Nelson G: Prostaglandins and reproduction. Curr Probl Obstet Gynecol 4:10, 1981

34. Newton M: Postpartum hemorrhage. Am J Obstet Gynecol 94:711, 1966

35. Noller KL, Bowie EJW, Kempers RD, et al.: Von Williebrand's disease in pregnancy. Obstet Gynecol 41:865, 1973

36. O'Leary JL, O'Leary JA: Uterine artery ligation in the control of intractable postpartum hemorrhage. Am J Obstet Gynecol 94:920, 1966

37. Oxhorn H: Human Labor and Birth, 4th ed. New York, Appleton, 1980

38. Pritchard J, Baldwin R, Dickey J, Wiggins K: Blood volume changes in pregnancy and the puerperium. Am J Obstet Gynecol 84:1271, 1962

39. Pritchard J, MacDonald P (eds): Williams Obstetrics, 16th ed. New York, Appleton, 1980

40. Queenan JT, Nakanoto M: Postpartum immunization: the hypothetical hazard of manual removal of the placenta. Obstet Gynecol 23:392, 1964

41. Quilligan E, Zuspan F: Operative Obstetrics, 4th ed. New York, Appleton, 1982

42. Rome R: Secondary postpartum hemorrhage. Br J Obstet Gynaecol 82:289, 1975

43. Sanders R, James E: Ultrasonography in Obstetrics and Gynecology. New York, Appleton, 1980, pp 311–320

44. Sheehan H, Murdock R: Postpartum necrosis of the anterior pituitary: Pathological and clinical aspects. Br J Obstet Gynaecol 45:456, 1938

45. Takagi S, Yoshida T, Togo Y, et al.: The effects of intramyometrial

injection of prostaglandin $F_{2\alpha}$ on severe postpartum hemorrhage. Prostaglandins 12:565, 1976

46. Thierstein S, Jahn H, Lange K: Routine third-stage exploration of the uterus. Obstet Gynecol 10:269, 1957

47. Thorsteinsson V, Kempers R: Delayed postpartum bleeding. Am J Obstet Gynecol 107:565, 1970

48. Toppozada M, El-Bossaty M, El-Rahman H, El-Din A: Control of intractable atonic postpartum hemorrhage by 15-methyl prostaglandin $F_{2\alpha}$. Obstet Gynecol 58:327, 1981

49. Waters E: Surgical management of postpartum hemorrhage with particular reference to ligation of uterine arteries. Am J Obstet Gynecol 64:1143, 1952

Placenta Accreta

1. Abitol MD, Daichman I, Mackles A: Placenta accreta associated with placenta previa. Obstet Gynecol 12:209, 1958

2. Begneaud W, Dougherty CM, Mickal A: Placenta accreta in early gestation: Report of two cases. Am J Obstet Gynecol 92:267, 1965

3. Breen J, Neubecker R, Gregori C, Franklin J: Placenta accreta, increta, and percreta, a survey of 40 cases. Obstet Gynecol 49:43, 1977

4. Demowski WP, Greenblatt RB: Asherman's syndrome and risk of placenta accreta. Obstet Gynecol 34:288, 1969

5. Fox H: Placenta accreta, 1945–1969. Obstet Gynecol Surv 27:475, 1972

6. Harer WB: Placenta accreta: Report of eight cases. Am J Obstet Gynecol 72:1309, 1956

7. Irving FC, Hertig AT: A study of placenta accreta. Surg Gynecol Obstet 64:178, 1937

8. Luke RK, Sharpe JW, Greene R: Placenta accreta. The adherent or invasive placenta. Am J Obstet Gynecol 95:660, 1966

9. Pritchard J, MacDonald P: Williams Obstetrics, 16th ed. New York, Appleton, 1980

10. Quilligan EJ, Zuspan F (eds): Douglas-Stromme Operative Obstetrics, 4th ed. New York, Appleton, 1982

11. Rubenstein AI, Lash SR: Placenta previa accreta. Am J Obstet Gynecol 87:198, 1963

12. Tamis AB, Tamis RH: Placenta previa accreta. Obstet Gynecol 25:120, 1965

13. Van Thiel DH: Partial placenta accreta in pregnancies following

chemotherapy for gestational trophoblastic neoplasms. Am J Obstet Gynecol 112:54, 1972

14. Weeks LR, Grieg LB: Placenta accreta: a twenty year review. Am J Obstet Gynecol 113:76, 1972

Amniotic Fluid Embolism

1. Aguillon A, Andjus T, Grayson A, Race G: Amniotic fluid embolism: a review. Obstet Gynecol Surv 17:619, 1962
2. Altchek A, Lituak RS: Amniotic fluid pulmonary embolism. Obstet Gynecol 27:885, 1966
3. Anderson D: Amniotic fluid embolism, a re-evaluation. Am J Obstet Gynecol 98:336, 1967
4. Chung A, Merkatz I: Survival following amniotic fluid embolism with early heparinization. Obstet Gynecol 42:809, 1973
5. Gregory M, Clayton E: Amniotic fluid embolism. Obstet Gynecol 42:236, 1973
6. Gross P, Benz EJ: Pulmonary embolism by amniotic fluid. Surg Gynecol Obstet 85:315, 1947
7. Halmagyi D, Starzecki B, Shearman R: Experimental amniotic fluid embolism: mechanism and treatment. Am J Obstet Gynecol 84:251, 1962
8. Kircher KF, Roberts WD, Tye JG: Nonfatal amniotic fluid embolism. Am J Roentgen 98:434, 1966
9. Learly OC, Hertig AT: The pathogenesis of amniotic fluid embolism. N Engl J Med 243:588, 1950
10. Nichols GP, Raney GH: Postpartum confusion: Heart failure in amniotic fluid embolism. Arch Intern Med 117:807, 1966
11. Peterson E, Taylor H: Amniotic fluid embolism, an analysis of 40 cases. Obstet Gynecol 35:787, 1970
12. Russell WS, Jones WN: Amniotic fluid embolism: a review of the syndrome and report of 4 cases. Obstet Gynecol 26:476, 1965
13. Scott MM: Cardiopulmonary considerations in nonfatal amniotic fluid embolism. JAMA 183:989, 1963
14. Steiner PE, Luschbaugh CC: Maternal pulmonary embolism by amniotic fluid as a cause of obstetric shock and unexpected deaths in obstetrics. JAMA 117:1245, 1941

Uterine Inversion

1. Bell J, Wilson GF, Wilson LA: Puerperal inversion of the uterus. Am J Obstet Gynecol 66:767, 1953

2. Bunke JW, Hofmiester FJ: Uterine inversion—Obstetrical entity or oddity. Am J Obstet Gynecol 91:934, 1965

3. Das P: Inversion of the uterus. J Obstet Gynaecol Br Emp 47:525, 1940

3A. Douglas RG, Stromme WB (eds): Operative Obstetrics. New York, Appleton, 1982, Chap 19

4. Gordon OA: A contribution to the etiology and treatment of puerperal inversion of the uterus. Am J Obstet Gynecol 32:399, 1936

5. Haultain F: The treatment of chronic uterine inversion by abdominal hysterectomy, with a successful case. Br Med J 2:974, 1901

6. Henderson J, Alles RW: Puerperal inversion of the uterus. Am J Obstet Gynecol 56:133, 1948

7. Huntington JL: Acute inversion of the uterus. Boston Med Surg J 184:376, 1921

8. Huntington JL, Frederick FC, Kellog FS: Abdominal reposition in acute inversion of the uterus. Am J Obstet Gynecol 15:34, 1928

9. Johnson AB: A new concept in the replacement of the inverted uterus and a report of nine cases. Am J Obstet Gynecol 57:557, 1949

10. Jones WC: Reports of two cases of postpartum inversion of the uterus with discussion of the pathogenesis of obstetrical inversion. Am J Obstet Gynecol 69:982, 1914

11. Jones WC: Inversion of the uterus. With report of a case occurring during the puerperium and causes by a fibroid. Surg Gynecol Obstet 16:632, 1913

12. Kellog FS: Puerperal inversion of the uterus. Classification for treatment. Am J Obstet Gynecol 18:815, 1929

13. Kitchin JD, Thiagarajah S, May HV, Thornton W: Puerperal inversion of the uterus. Am J Obstet Gynecol 123:51, 1975

14. Lee W, Baggish M, Lashgari M: Acute inversion of the uterus. Obstet Gynecol 51:144, 1978

15. McCullagh W: Inversion of the uterus—A report of three cases and an analysis of 233 recently recorded cases. J Obstet Gynaecol Br Emp 32:280, 1925

16. Moir J, Myerscough P: Accidents and complications of the immediate postpartum period—uterine inversion. In Baeliere, Trindal, and Cassel (eds): Operative Obstetrics. 1971, pp 896–910

16A. Platt L, Druzin M: Acute puerperal inversion of the uterus. Am J Obstet Gynecol 141:187, 1981

17. Pride G, Shaffer R: Nonpuerperal uterine inversion. Obstet Gynecol 49:361, 1977

18. Pritchard J, MacDonald P: Williams Obstetrics, 16th ed. New York, Appleton, 1980

19. Samarra K: Puerperal inversion of the uterus, with reference to pregnancy following Spinelli's operation. J Obstet Gynaecol Br Commonw 72:426, 1965

20. Schaefer G, Veprovsky ED: Inversion of the uterus. Surg Clin North Am, April, 1949, p 599

21. Watson P, Besch N, Bowes W: Management of acute and subacute puerperal inversion of the uterus. Obstet Gynecol 55:12, 1980

28

Operative Obstetrics
Jeffrey W. Ellis, M.D.

PRACTICE PRINCIPLES
Most labors proceed to spontaneous vaginal delivery. Operative intervention, however, may be necessary for fetal and/or maternal indications.

CESAREAN SECTION
Cesarean section is an operative procedure in which the infant, placenta, and membranes are delivered through an incision in the abdominal and uterine walls.

A. *Indications. Cesarean section is indicated when delivery of the fetus is required and vaginal delivery or delay in delivery would injure the fetus or mother.* The following *indications* for cesarean section are discussed in detail in individual chapters (See Index):
   1. *Fetopelvic disproportion* (cephalopelvic disproportion, CPD). May be due to fetal macrosomia, congenital anomaly, pelvic contraction or distortion, pelvic soft-tissue mass, or a combination of these.
   2. *Dysfunctional labor with failure to progress*
   3. *Abnormal presentation.* Transverse lie, locked twins, and some cases of breech, brow, and face presentations.

4. *Potentially weak uterine scars* from a previous cesarean section, myomectomy, unification procedure, perforation, or rupture.
5. *Fetal distress* unresolved by conservative measures when delivery is not imminent.
6. *Umbilical cord prolapse* when delivery is not imminent.
7. *Placenta previa*
8. *Abruptio placentae* complicated by fetal distress or severe hemorrhage
9. *Ruptured uterus*
10. *Previous colporrhaphy or fistula repair*
11. *In cases where immediate delivery is indicated with a cervix unfavorable for rapid delivery.*
12. *Failed induction of labor*
13. *Active genital herpes infections* if membranes have been ruptured less than four hours or if the patient is in active labor with unruptured membranes.
14. *Failed forceps delivery*
15. *Multiple gestations* involving three or more fetuses
16. *All infants less than 1500 gm* (controversial)
17. *All infants greater than 4000 gm* (controversial)
18. An infant with a biparietal diameter greater than 10.0 cm (controversial)

B. *Classification of cesarean sections*
1. Classical (vertical corporeal)
2. Lower-segment transverse
3. Lower-segment vertical
4. Extraperitoneal
5. Cesarean hysterectomy

C. *Classical cesarean section*
1. *Technique.* The uterine incision is made vertically in the midline in the upper, contractile segment. Closure of the incision requires three or more layers of either continuous or interrupted suture. The incision cannot be reperitonealized, since it lies well above the vesicouterine peritoneum.
2. *Indications.* The generally accepted indications for class-

ical cesarean section are:

a) Transverse lie
b) Anterior placenta previa
c) Extensive varicosities of the lower uterine segment
d) Distortion of the lower uterine segment by myomata
e) Inaccessibility of the lower uterine segment because of dense adhesions or an adherent bladder
f) In cases of carcinoma of the cervix, the lower uterine segment and cervix should not be entered if subsequent radical surgery or radiation therapy is planned.

3. *Disadvantages/complications*

a) Increased thickness of the myometrium leads to more intraoperative blood loss and greater difficulty in uterine closure.
b) Reperitonealization is not possible, leading to possible continuous leakage of uterine contents and adhesions of bowel and omentum to the uterine incision.
c) Spontaneous rupture of the incision before and during labor is more frequent than with lower-segment incisions. It is generally agreed that *in the presence of an upper-segment incision, all subsequent pregnancies should be delivered by cesarean section.*

D. *Lower-segment transverse cesarean section (LSTCS)*

1. *Technique.* The vesicouterine peritoneum is incised transversely and the bladder is separated from the lower uterine segment by blunt dissection. A 3- to 4-cm transverse incision is made in the lower segment. The incision is carried laterally, curving slightly upward, using either blunt-nosed scissors or by tearing with the fingers. The incision is closed in two layers using a running stitch of an absorbable suture. The vesicouterine peritoneum is reapproximated using a running stitch of an absorbable suture.

2. *Indications.* In most cases, an LSTCS is the procedure of choice for the following reasons:

a) Because the lower uterine segment is thin, intraoperative bleeding is reduced and closure of the uterine incision is generally uncomplicated.

   b) The uterine incision is covered by vesicouterine peritoneum, decreasing the possibility of leakage of uterine contents into the peritoneal cavity. This is especially important when intrauterine infection is present. Adhesions of bowel and omentum to the uterine incision are decreased.

   c) This incision has the lowest incidence of subsequent rupture.

3. *Disadvantages/complications.* The position and size of the uterine incision may make delivery of the fetus difficult, e.g., transverse lie. The transverse incision may extend laterally, leading to transection of one or both uterine arteries. Uncontrolled bleeding or expanding broad ligament hematoma may require hypogastric artery ligation or hysterectomy.

E. *Lower-segment vertical cesarean section (LSVCS)*

1. *Technique.* The technique is similar to the low-segment transverse incision; however, the uterine incision is made vertically in the lower segment. The vertical incision can be extended easily into the upper segment if necessary to facilitate atraumatic delivery.

2. *Indications*

   a) Premature pregnancies when the lower segment is poorly developed

   b) Cases of abnormal presentation or multiple gestation when a difficult delivery is anticipated (transverse lie, breech, locked twins, congenital anomaly)

3. *Disadvantages/complications*

   a) The upper uterine segment may be entered. This carries the disadvantage of the classical incision.

   b) Downward extension of the incision may cause entry into the vagina, with subsequent bacterial contamination, or entry into the bladder.

F. *Extraperitoneal cesarean section*

1. *Technique.* The primary rationale for this procedure is

that the peritoneal cavity is not entered. Once the abdominal fascia has been divided, the parietal peritoneum is bluntly separated from the overlying fascia. The dissection is carried down to the level of the bladder. The visceral peritoneum is then separated from the bladder by blunt or sharp dissection. The bladder is separated from the lower uterine segment and pushed downward. A low-segment transverse or vertical uterine incision is made.

2. *Indications.* In cases of infected uterine contents, leakage into the peritoneal cavity is prevented, thus decreasing the incidence of peritonitis and abscess formation. *This procedure is rarely performed today because of increasingly effective antibiotics.*

3. *Complications/disadvantages*
   a) The procedure is technically difficult and time-consuming. Inadvertent entry into the peritoneal cavity often occurs.
   b) Bladder and ureteral injury may occur during dissection of the visceral peritoneum.

G. *Cesarean hysterectomy*
   1. *Technique.* An LSVCS is performed in the usual fashion. The uterine incision is closed using one layer of a running, locking stitch. Alternately, the uterine incision is approximated using sponge forceps. A hysterectomy is performed in the usual fashion. Since the vascular structures are considerably dilated, meticulous sharp dissection and individual ligation of vessels is mandatory to prevent hemorrhage. Large pedicles should be avoided.
   2. *Indications*
      a) Uncontrolled uterine hemorrhage
      b) Ruptured uterus that cannot be repaired
      c) Grossly infected uterus
      d) *Carcinoma in situ* of the cervix or severe dysplasia diagnosed before pregnancy in a patient requesting sterilization

e) Symptomatic benign disease of the uterus in a patient requesting sterilization

3. *Complications/disadvantages*
   a) Excessive blood loss
   b) Bladder and ureteral injuries
   c) Operative time increased by 30 minutes or more
   d) Bleeding into the ovarian pedicle may require salpingo-oophorectomy.
   e) Cervical tissue may be retained due to difficulty in determining the cervicovaginal junction.

H. *Management of postcesarean pregnancies*
   1. *Basic principles*
      a) A uterine scar may be weaker than the surrounding myometrium and therefore prone to rupture during subsequent pregnancies.
      b) There is no satisfactory method for determining the integrity and strength of the uterine scar before or during labor.
      c) Rupture of the uterus is an obstetric emergency that may lead to death of both the fetus and mother.
   2. *Vaginal delivery*
      a) *Patient selection.* Criteria used in selecting patients for vaginal delivery after cesarean section differ among medical centers. *The following criteria are commonly used when considering a trial of labor and possible vaginal delivery in a patient with a previous cesarean section.*
         (1) The indication for the original cesarean section is nonrecurring (not performed for disproportion).
         (2) The patient has had only one previous cesarean section, for which the incision was confined to the lower segment.
         (3) The patient has had an uncomplicated vaginal delivery of a term-sized infant preceding the cesarean section (controversial).
         (4) The present fetus is no larger than the largest infant successfully delivered vaginally (controversial).

b) *Contraindications*
   (1) More than one previous cesarean section (some controversy).
   (2) A previous classical cesarean section or extension of a lower-segment incision into the upper segment.
   (3) The type of previous uterine incision is unknown.
   (4) A contracted pelvis or a large soft-tissue mass obstructing the pelvis.
   (5) Abnormal fetal presentation: breech, brow, face
   (6) Overdistended uterus: hydramnios, multiple gestation
c) *Patient education.* The risks and benefits of vaginal delivery in postcesarean pregnancies should be thoroughly explained to the patient. The patient should be allowed to make a choice between a repeat cesarean section and an attempt at vaginal delivery.
d) *Management of labor and delivery*
   (1) Preparations for cesarean section should be made in case the procedure proves necessary. Two to four units of whole blood should be available.
   (2) The physician must be present at all times during labor.
   (3) Continuous electronic monitoring of fetal heart rate and uterine contractions must be maintained throughout labor. An intrauterine pressure catheter should be placed as soon as possible.
   (4) A cesarean section should be performed for arrest of progress, fetal distress, or suspicion of uterine rupture.
   (5) Most authorities consider oxytocin induction or stimulation to be contraindicated.
   (6) The second stage of labor should be shortened by low-forceps delivery. Vigorous pushing by the patient in the second stage should be avoided.
   (7) Manual exploration of the uterine scar should be performed after delivery of the placenta.
   (8) The use of conduction anesthesia is controversial

since some authorities feel that it may mask signs of uterine rupture.

3. *Repeat cesarean section.* If an elective repeat cesarean section is to be performed, fetal maturity must be proven before attempting the procedure.
4. *Patient education.* During prenatal visits, the following points should be emphasized to the patient who has previously had a cesarean section:
   1. Report to the hospital immediately if uterine contractions occur (labor) or if severe lower abdominal pain develops (possible rupture).
   2. There is no theoretical limit to the number of cesarean sections that may be performed. With each subsequent cesarean section, however, the risks of intraoperative complications increase.

FORCEPS

The obstetrics forceps are instruments designed to facilitate delivery. They are used for *rotation* and *extraction* of the fetal head.

A. *Description*
   1. *Handles.* Finger grips facilitate applying traction
   2. *Lock.* The point of articulation
   3. *Shank.* Connects the handle to the blade
   4. *Blades.* Enclose the fetal head
      a) The blade may be *solid* or *fenestrated.* Fenestration provides better traction. Solid blades are less traumatic to the fetal head.
      b) All forceps blades have a *cephalic curve* that conforms to the contour of the fetal head. Most forceps blades have a *pelvic curve* that conforms to the curve of the pelvic axis.
   5. *Toe.* The tips of the blades
   6. *Heel.* The inferior portion of the blades at the junction with the shanks

B. *Indications*
  1. Maternal or fetal conditions that necessitate immediate delivery
  2. When forceps procedures are the safest method of delivering the baby.
  3. *Maternal indications*
    a) To affect delivery after cessation of progress in the second stage of labor due to:
      (1) *Inadequate expulsive force.* Inadequate uterine contractions because of maternal exhaustion or regional anesthesia.
      (2) *Fetal factors:* Brow, face, persistent occiput posterior or transverse positions (selected cases)
    b) To shorten the second stage of labor, especially with patients in whom bearing down is contraindicated, such as in the following cases:
      (1) Heart disease
      (2) Hypertension
      (3) Vascular disease, cerebrovascular anomaly, esophageal varices
      (4) Previous uterine surgery
    c) To shorten the second stage of labor in patients with obstetric or medical complications, as in preeclampsia-eclampsia or abruptio placentae.
  4. *Fetal indications*
    a) Fetal distress
    b) To protect the head of the premature infant from compression-decompression injury
    c) To facilitate delivery and to prevent hyperextension of the head in breech deliveries
C. *Classification of forceps procedures.* Forceps procedures are classified according to the station and position of the fetal head at the time of application of the forceps.
  1. *Low forceps.* The fetal head has reached the perineal floor and the saggital suture is in the anteroposterior diameter of the outlet. The fetal scalp is usually visible at the introitus. (*Note:* Because the biparietal diameter of

the head is higher in the pelvis in the occiput posterior position compared to the occiput anterior position, some authors consider the delivery of an occiput posterior on the perineal floor to be a mid-forceps procedure).

2. *Midforceps.* The fetal head is engaged, but the criteria for low forceps have not been met. The biparietal diameter has passed through the inlet and the lowest part of the skull is at or below the level of the ischial spines. The saggital suture may be in any orientation. Any procedure requiring a rotation is classified as midforceps.

3. *High forceps.* The fetal head is unengaged. The biparietal diameter has not entered the pelvic inlet and the lowest part of the fetal skull is above the ischial spines. *There is no indication for a high-forceps procedure.*

D. *Conditions for use.* The following conditions *must be met* for the safe use of forceps:

1. *Fetal head must be engaged.*

2. *Position, attitude, and station of the fetal head must be accurately determined.* Molding, caput succadaneum, and a deflexed attitude may give the impression of engagement though the biparietal diameter remains above the pelvic inlet.

3. The cervix must be completely dilated and retracted over the head.

4. There must be no marked disproportion between the size of the head and the size of the pelvis.

5. There should be no serious soft-tissue obstruction.

6. Membranes must be ruptured.

7. The head must be large enough to be firmly grasped with the forceps.

8. An indication for forceps delivery must exist.

E. *Types of forceps.* The choice of forceps depends on the following factors (Fig. 28–1; Table 28–1):

1. Position of the head

2. The presence and degree of molding

3. Type of pelvis

4. Size of the head

5. Familiarity by the operator

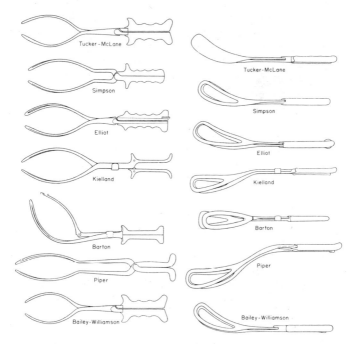

Figure 28–1. Commonly used forceps. (From Quilligan EJ, Zuspan F (eds): Douglas-Stromme Operative Obstetrics, 4th ed. New York, Appleton, 1982, p 439.)

F. *Types of forceps application*
1. *Cephalic application.* The forceps are applied along the occipital diameter of the fetal head. The blades are equidistant from the saggital suture. This application reduces potential compression and laceration injury to the head.
2. *Pelvic application.* The forceps are applied to the sides of the pelvis without regard to the position of the fetal head. This type of application should not be employed, since compression and laceration injuries are common.

G. *Technique.* The basic technique of the low-forceps proce-

TABLE 28–1. FORCEP TYPES, CHARACTERISTICS AND INDICATIONS

Forceps Type	Blade	Lock	Cephalic Curve	Pelvic Curve	Special Indications	Special Characteristics
Simpson	Fenestrated	English	Yes	Yes	Molded head	Small Simpson forceps used for premature infants
Elliott	Fenestrated	English	Yes	Yes	Unmolded head	Shanks cross, less distention of vulva
Kielland	Fenestrated	Sliding	Yes	No	Rotation	Shanks long, no pelvic curve
Tucker-McLane	Solid	English	Yes	Yes	—	Solid blades, shanks cross
Barton	Fenestrated	Sliding	Yes	No	Rotation	Hinged blade, facilitating application
Piper	Fenestrated	English	Yes	No	Delivery of aftercoming head in breech presentation	Shanks long

dure in the occiput anterior position is described below. The reader should see the Bibliography at the end of this chapter for detailed descriptions of other forceps procedures.

1. The patient is placed in the lithotomy position.
2. Anesthesia is administered. Pudendal anesthesia is generally sufficient.
3. The bladder and rectum should be emptied prior to entering the delivery room. Catheterization may be necessary. A distended bladder or rectum may be lacerated during the procedure.
4. *Insertion — left blade*. This blade is inserted first. The handle of the left blade is grasped on the left hand. The fingers of the right hand are inserted along the left lateral wall of the vagina next to the fetal head. The handle of the forcep is held vertical to the patient as the blade is introduced into the vagina at the 5 o'clock position.
5. *Application — left blade*. As the handle of the forcep is gently lowered to a horizontal position, the blade is guided by the vaginal fingers to the optimum position alongside the fetal head.
6. *Insertion/application — right blade*. The handle of the right blade is grasped in the right hand and the fingers of the left hand are inserted into the vagina. The blade is inserted into the vagina at the 7 o'clock position.
7. *Articulation*. The blades are locked in place.
8. *At no time should excessive force be used in application or articulation*. If application or articulation cannot be performed easily, malpositioning of the forceps should be suspected and the appropriate adjustments made. It may be necessary to remove the blades and recheck the position of the head.
9. *The application must be checked for accuracy of blade placement before traction is applied*. Proper application requires that:
   a) The sagittal suture is equidistant from the blades.
   b) The fenestration of the blade (if present) should admit no more than one finger between the fetal head and the angle of the fenestration.

c) The upper borders of the blades should be equidistant from the lambdoidal sutures.

d) The posterior fontanelle should be no more than one finger's breadth above the upper border of the shank.

10. The operator should sit or kneel while applying traction.

11. *Traction* is applied along the axis of the pelvis (Fig. 28–2). The proper sum of vector forces to follow the axis is achieved by horizontal *traction* applied to the handle and downward vertical *pressure* applied over the shanks. Traction should be applied only during uterine contractions and voluntary pushing by the patient to minimize compression of the fetal head. The amount of traction applied is a matter of experience. *Only "gentle force" should be used — and pulling with body weight should be avoided.* The forceps handles should be partially separated between traction attempts to avoid prolonged compression of the skull.

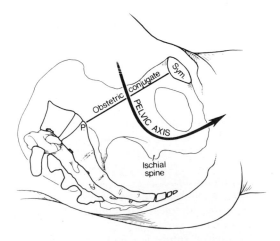

Figure 28–2. Diagram showing the pelvic axis. (From Pritchard J, MacDonald P: Williams Obstetrics, 16th ed. New York, Appleton, 1980, p 277.)

12. If necessary, an episiotomy should be performed as the head distends the vulva. At this time, the forceps may be held by an assistant. If an episiotomy is performed too early, excessive blood loss may occur.

13. As the occiput appears beneath the symphysis, the forceps handles are elevated, recreating the extension mechanism of spontaneous delivery.

14. *Disarticulation.* After the head is delivered, the handles are unlocked.

15. *Removal.* The forceps are removed in the reverse order of insertion.

16. The remainder of the delivery is conducted in the usual fashion.

17. The vagina and cervix should be carefully inspected for lacerations.

H. *Midforceps.* The incidence of midforceps procedures has generally declined in recent years due to the more frequent use of cesarean section as the safest route of delivery. Midforceps procedures, especially those performed at a high station, may result in serious compression and laceration injuries to the fetus and to severe lacerations of the maternal soft tissues. In general, midforceps procedures should be considered only if there is clear indication for immediate delivery.

1. *Evaluation of the patient and fetus*
   a) The pelvis must be thoroughly evaluated by manual examination, and x-ray pelvimetry if feasible. Suspected inlet or midpelvic contraction contraindicates a midforceps procedure.
   b) The size of the infant should be evaluated. Previous ultrasound determinations of the biparietal diameter of the skull should be reviewed.
   c) The adequacy of uterine contractions should be assessed. If uterine contractions are judged ineffective, oxytocin stimulation should be started.

2. *Technique.* The reader is referred to the texts cited at the end of the chapter for specific midforceps techniques and choice of instruments.

I. *Failed forceps.* A forceps procedure is termed "failed" when an atraumatic delivery is not possible. Failed forceps may be due to either:
  1. Failure to obtain proper application
  2. Failure of head extraction after forceps are properly applied
J. *Complications*
  1. *Maternal*
     a) Lacerations of the vulva, vagina, and cervix
     b) Extension of the episiotomy
     c) Rupture of the uterus
     d) Injury to the bladder and rectum
  2. *Fetal*
     a) Skull fracture
     b) Soft-tissue laceration
     c) Peripheral nerve injury
     d) Cephalohematoma
     e) Intracranial injury (especially bleeding)

VACUUM EXTRACTOR

The various types of vacuum extractors employ either a metal or a plastic cup that is applied to the fetal head. The cup is connected to either a manual or an automatic suction pump. Traction is applied by either a chain or a flexible plastic handle.

A. *Indications.* Similar to the indications for use of the forceps.
B. *Classification of procedures.* There is no standard classification for procedures performed with the vacuum extractor. As with forceps procedures, they may be classified as *high, mid-,* or *low pelvic applications* according to the station and position of the fetal head.
C. *Conditions for use.* Similar to those for use of forceps.
D. *Advantages*
  1. The vacuum extractor occupies less space in the pelvis and does not increase the volume of the presenting part as with forceps.

2. There is less potential damage to the mother and fetus in most cases. Head compression does not occur. Maternal lacerations are infrequent. Compared to forceps, more traction can be applied with smaller increases in fetal intracranial pressure.

3. The fetal head is not fixed as with forceps, allowing normal rotations within the pelvis to occur.

E. *Disadvantages*
1. Rotations are often not possible.
2. Axis traction cannot be applied.
3. Not suited in conditions of deflexion of the fetal head.
4. Should not be used with premature infants.

F. *Complications*
1. Cephalohematoma
2. Scalp injury, abrasion, avulsion, necrosis

G. *Technique*
1. The cup is placed over the occiput, avoiding the fonatanelle.
2. Negative pressure is then developed by the pump apparatus to the optimal range of -0.5 to -0.7 kg/cm^2.
3. Traction is applied along the pelvic axis.
4. Traction should be applied only during uterine contractions and voluntary pushing by the patient.

DÜHRSSEN'S INCISIONS (Hysterostomatomy)

Multiple incisions are made into an incompletely dilated cervix to facilitate immediate delivery.

A. *Indications. Dührssen's incisions are rarely indicated in modern obstetrics.* Cesarean section should generally be employed when immediate delivery is necessary in the presence of an incompletely dilated cervix. *Dührssen's incisions may be necessary during breech delivery when the head is trapped by an incompletely dilated cervix.*

B. *Prerequisites*
1. Fully effaced cervix.
2. Cervix dilated at least 7 cm.

C. *Technique*
   1. The cervix is grasped with ring forceps.
   2. Incisions are made at the 2, 6, and 10 o'clock positions about the cervix. The incisions are extended to the cervico-vaginal junction.
   3. Delivery is usually performed using forceps.
   4. The cervical incisions are closed using a running, locking stitch of #0 or #1 chromic catgut.
D. *Complications*
   1. Hemorrhage
   2. Extension of the incisions into the rectum, bladder, or major blood vessels
   3. Poor healing often occurs. Deep cervical defects or adhesions to the vagina may occur.

DESTRUCTIVE OPERATIONS ON THE FETUS (EMBRYOTOMY)

The purpose of destructive operations is to reduce the size of a dead fetus to enable vaginal delivery. This may be necessary in cases of transverse lie, hydrocephalus, entrapped head after breech delivery, conjoined twins, and severe congenital anomalies. Complications are frequent and include maternal soft-tissue laceration, uterine rupture, hemorrhage, and infection. These procedures are rarely performed today. In the past, the morbidity and mortality of cesarean section were greater than with destructive procedures. With modern techniques, the opposite is true. For details regarding technique, the reader is referred to the Bibliography.

BIBLIOGRAPHY

General

Oxorn H: Human Labor and Birth, 4th ed. New York, Appleton-Century-Crofts, 1980

Pritchard JA, MacDonald PC: Williams Obstetrics, 16th ed. New York, Appleton-Century-Crofts, 1980

Quilligan EJ, Zuspan F (eds): Douglas-Stromme Operative Obstetrics, 4th ed. New York, Appleton-Century-Crofts, 1982

Cesarean Section

Barclay DL: Cesarean hysterectomy: thirty years' experience. Obstet Gynecol 35:120, 1970

Bottoms SJ, et al.: The increase in the cesarean birth rate. N Engl J Med 302:559, 1980

Gibbs CE: Planned vaginal delivery following cesarean section. Clin Obstet Gynecol 23:507, 1980

Kerr JM: The technique of cesarean section with special reference to the lower uterine segment incision. Am J Obstet Gynecol 12:729, 1926

Morewood GA, et al.: Vaginal delivery after cesarean section. Obstet Gynecol 42:589, 1973

Waters EG: Supravesical extraperitoneal cesarean section. Am J Obstet Gynecol 39:423, 1940

Forceps

Chez, RA (moderator): Midforceps delivery: Is it an anachronism? (Symposium) Contemp Obstet Gynecol 15:82-100, 1980

Cook W: Evaluation of the midforceps operation. Am J Obstet Gynecol 99:327, 1967

Delee JB: The prophylactic forceps operation. Am J Obstet Gynecol 1:34, 1920

Laufe L: Obstetric Forceps. New York, Harper & Row, 1968

Dührssen's Incisions

Hunt AB, McGee WB: Dührssen's incision. Am J Obstet Gynecol 31:598, 1936

29

Postpartum and Puerperal Infections

Jeffrey C. King, M.D.

PRACTICE PRINCIPLES

The puerperium is usually defined as the six-week period follow-ing delivery. While most infectious complications occur within the first 10 days, mastitis can occur as late as the sixth postpartum week. The Joint Committee on Maternal Welfare has defined *puerperal morbidity as a "temperature of 28.0C (100.4F) or higher, the temperature to occur on any two of the first 10 days postpartum, exclusive of the first 24 hours, and to be taken by mouth by a standard technique at least 4 times daily."* This definition does suggest that all temperature elevations are the result of genital infection without differentiating other possible nongenital causes such as pyelonephritis, upper re-spiratory tract infection, or mastitis.

PREDISPOSING CAUSES

A. *Etiologic associations* for severe postpartum infections
   1. Prolonged rupture of membranes
   2. Increased numbers of vaginal examinations
   3. Prolonged time in labor

    4. Extensive intrauterine manipulation
    5. Greater size and number of incisions and lacerations
       required for delivery of the fetus and placenta
B. Most investigators feel that puerperal infection is more
   common in women of lower socioeconomic classes; however, the reason for this has not been determined.

INVESTIGATION

A. *History. Interrogation of the patient* and complete *review of
   her prenatal record* will show if infection was present before
   labor; whether she was anemic; her nutritional status; or if
   she had a urinary tract infection. *The delivery record* will
   reveal the duration and character of her labor; the time of
   membrane rupture; if the birth was spontaneous, required
   forceps, or was by cesarean section; the amount of blood
   loss; and the extent, if any, of vaginal lacerations.
B. *Examination. A thorough physical examination is mandatory.*
   Particular attention should be paid to the vital signs, throat,
   lungs, heart, breasts, abdomen, abdominal or perineal incisions, and lower extremities.
C. *Studies*
    1. *Complete blood count* with differential
    2. *Catheterized urine for microscopic analysis and culture is
      essential.* While many would argue against routine
      catheterization, the small (3 percent) risk of introducing
      bacteria into the bladder is worth the information gained,
      particularly since there is the possibility of contamination
      with lochia with a voided specimen
    3. *Vaginal speculum examination* is necessary to evaluate
      the lower genital tract and cervix. The cervical canal
      should be probed to eliminate "cervical plug" as a cause
      of retained lochia. A Gram stain and culture (aerobic and
      anaerobic) of a carefully obtained *endometrial swab* may
      be beneficial. There is some question about the cost-

benefit ratio of endometrial cultures, but in general, they are beneficial and should be obtained.

4. Gentle *bimanual examination* is performed to evaluate tenderness or swelling of the uterus, parametria, or adnexea.

5. *Aerobic and anaerobic blood cultures* are also indicated in the evaluation of significant postpartum fever.

BACTERIOLOGY

A. The causative bacteria vary among hospitals, but anaerobic *streptococcus* has been increasing in importance. Other significant organisms are *Escherichia coli, Staphylococcus,* and Group B *streptococcus.*

B. Most cultures result in mixed growth of aerobic and anaerobic organisms; however, pure culture growths from blood, urine, or endometrium usually indicate the offending organism. Antibiotic sensitivity testing is necessary.

C. When a foul, fecal-smelling discharge is present, *Bacillus fragilis* must be suspected. It has been identified in approximately 15 percent of patients with postpartum infections.

ENDOMYOMETRITIS

A. *Diagnosis.* The placental attachment site is an excellent culture medium and provides the most likely portal of entry for bacteria. This is why infection of the endometrium, with occasional spread to myometrium and peritoneum, is the most frequent site of puerperal infection. The infection usually begins between the second and sixth day postpartum. With infection limited to the endometrium (decidua), cases are usually mild and there is only slight temperature elevation. With more severe cases of infection involving deeper structures, such as the parametria or peritoneum, there is often a chill with high fever, ileus, and foul lochia.

B. *Treatment*
1. *Low-grade temperature* elevations (infection limited to the endometrium) can probably be treated with either oral ampicillin or cephalosporin, since these infections often resolve spontaneously.
2. *Serious infections with high-temperature elevations* demand aggressive treatment with IV antibiotics for rapid response and to prevent the development of additional complications such as pelvic abscess.
3. *Because endomyometritis is usually a mixed aerobic and anaerobic infection, a combination of antibiotics is necessary.* In Los Angeles County, DiJerga has shown that treatment with gentamicin plus clindamycin (for *Bacteroides* coverage) resulted in a significantly greater cure rate than penicillin plus gentamicin: 96 vs 71 percent. At Parkand Memorial Hospital, the combination of penicillin G and tetracycline has proven to be effective in approximately 85 percent of patients.
   a) *Dosages*

   - Gentamicin 50 to 80 mg IV q8h
        plus
   - Clindamycin 600 mg IV q6h
        or
   - Penicillin G 5 million units IV q6h
        plus
   - Tetracycline 500 mg IV q6h

   b) Baseline renal function should be evaluated and serum antibiotic levels should be followed if an aminoglycoside is used.
   c) Parenteral antibiotics should be continued until the patient is afebrile for 24 to 48 hours. While many physicians continue treatment with an oral agent (ampicillin or cephalexin, 500 mg, q6h), recent studies have suggested stopping antibiotics completely and observing the clinical course.

4. Careful observation for development of a *pelvic abscess* is necessary. Ultrasound may be helpful in this endeavor. The findings of rebound tenderness and a pelvic mass are almost diagnostic. Drainage, abdominally or transvaginally, is mandatory. Fortunately, this complication occurs rarely.

5. Many physicians administer *methylergonovine maleate,* 0.2 mg p.o.q6h, for two to three days. The theory is that this will increase lochia flow, remove debris within the cavity, and hopefully hasten resolution. Of course, patients who have been preeclamptic or hypertensive should be watched carefully.

URINARY TRACT INFECTION

A. *Diagnosis.* The urinary tract is particularly vulnerable to infection in the postpartum period due to dilatation of the collecting system, slowing of ureteral peristalsis, and increased residual urine. Labor and delivery present significant additional stress. The base of the bladder is traumatized as the fetal head descends. Epidural anesthesia reduces bladder sensation, often making routine and complete emptying unlikely. These factors make the presence of red blood cells and white blood cells in a postpartum urine specimen unreliable for the diagnosis of urinary tract infection. The association of CVA tenderness, pyuria, and fever is very suggestive, but *only a urine culture having greater than 10^5 organisms/ml is diagnostic.*

B. *Treatment*

1. *The most effective treatment is prevention. Attention to bladder care during labor is essential.* The parturient should be encouraged to void frequently and *routine catheterization of the bladder at delivery should be avoided.*

2. The most likely organism is a coliform, and the prenatal history is often helpful in selecting an antibiotic until sensitivities are available.

3. If patients have a history of recurrent urinary tract infection before or during pregnancy, careful consideration should be given to obtaining an intravenous pyelogram and voiding cystourethrogram after the puerperium, since a high number of renal tract abnormalities have been discovered.

ASPIRATION PNEUMONIA

A. *Diagnosis*
   1. Aspiration pneumonia is one of the major causes of death associated with obstetric anesthesia. Gastric emptying during pregnancy is delayed and the gastric contents are not only highly acidic but often mixed with food particles. The enlarging uterus will often exaggerate the effect of a hiatal hernia, making aspiration much more likely to occur.
   2. The patient often complains of chest tightness and difficulty with breathing. Highly acidic fluid can induce bronchospasm, rhonchi, rales, with resulting atelectasis and cyanosis. At this stage, a chest x-ray is often normal but should be obtained for future comparison.

B. *Treatment*
   1. *Suction of gastric contents* is very important, and bronchoscopy may be necessary to remove large particulate matter. However, the damage is done by the contact of acidic material with lung tissue and is almost immediate and nonreversible.
   2. Patients should be carefully *intubated,* and the arterial oxygen should be maintained at no less than 60 mm Hg. Positive end-expiratory pressure is often necessary to help reopen atelactatic lung fields.
   3. The use of *corticosteroids* is controversial, but evidence suggests that 500 mg methylprednisolone every 8 hours for 24 hours may be helpful in maintaining cell integrity.
   4. The use of *antibiotics* is controversial, but if used, adequate anaerobic coverage is necessary.

PELVIC THROMBOPHLEBITIS

A. *Diagnosis*
1. Varying degrees of pelvic thrombophlebitis usually accompany endomyometritis that has extended beyond the confines of the uterus. The veins most commonly involved are the ovarian because of the drainage pattern of the upper uterus, where the placenta is usually attached. The process is most frequently unilateral. The left ovarian vein drains into the left renal vein, while the right ovarian drains directly into the inferior vena cava. Occasionally, large emboli may break loose and reach the pulmonary artery, resulting in sudden death; more commonly, small emboli may reach the pulmonary arterioles and cause abscess, infarct, or pneumonia.
2. Classically, the patient with pelvic thrombophlebitis complains of *diffuse lower abdominal pain* and has a *variable fever curve* that is unresponsive to standard antibiotic therapy. Unfortunately, the diagnosis of pelvic thrombophlebitis is one of *exclusion*.

B. *Treatment*
1. *Heparinization* by the continuous IV route is therapeutic. This should be continued for at least 7 to 10 days while monitoring clinical condition. The patient should not require long-term anticoagulation following resolution of the acute problem.
2. *Recurrent pulmonary emboli* require ligation or occlusion of both the inferior vena cava below the renal veins and of the left ovarian vein, which can be lifesaving.

MASTITIS

A. *Diagnosis*
1. Infection may be introduced into the duct system of the breasts, or into the breast tissue, through *cracked nipples*. The majority of women are probably infected by their own baby during feeding.

   2. The *symptoms* of acute mastitis rarely appear within the first week postpartum. *The development of hard, red, tender breasts with associated chills and temperature elevation is almost diagnostic.* The patient will often complain of intense pain in the affected breast.

B. *Treatment*
   1. If diagnosed early, *breast-feeding should be encouraged* to prevent engorgement and stagnation of milk in the alveoli. Milk should be obtained for culture which frequently reveals *Staphylococcus.* Appropriate antibiotics should be started. Breast-feeding may continue as long as pus is not present.
   2. Warm moist packs and mild analgesics can help relieve breast discomfort.
   3. The use of lanolin or vitamin E has been suggested to help prevent cracking of the nipples while lactating.
   4. If an abscess should develop, drainage is necessary.

WOUND INFECTION

A. *Diagnosis*
   1. Abdominal wound infections may occur following cesarean section and other abdominal surgery. Classically, they develop after the fifth postoperative day, but early (24 to 48 hours) infections can be particularly dangerous due to *Streptococcus* or *Clostridium perfringens.*
   2. The diagnosis is suspected following clinical examination that reveals *erythema, induration, localized pain,* and even *fluctuance of the wound.*

B. *Treatment*
   1. *The mainstay of treatment is drainage.* The wound should be fully explored to ensure that the fascia is intact and that all pockets of infection have been opened. *If the fascia is open, the patient should be returned to the operating room for closure.*
   2. *Antibiotics* are usually not indicated for simple wound infection; however, if spreading inflammation is seen at

the wound edges, antibiotics effective against coagulase-positive *Staphylococcus* should be started.

3. Synergistic *gangrene* and *necrotizing fasciitis* are very rare; but if they develop, wide excision of the infected fascia with replacement by a Marlex graft plus penicillin and clindamycin is often required for cure.

EPISIOTOMY INFECTION

A. *Diagnosis*. Fortunately, episiotomy infections are rare, usually being caused by either the development of a hematoma within the repair or poor technique in closure. The patient with a hematoma will usually complain of severe pain at the episiotomy site or the inability to void within the first 24 hours. A poorly repaired episiotomy will often be noted by the patient, especially if stool or flatus is passed per vagina. This can occur as early as the second day, but may be delayed for many weeks.

B. *Treatment*

1. If a large *hematoma* is discovered, the patient should be returned to the operating room where exploration and drainage may be accomplished. A urinary drainage catheter is usually required for 24 hours.

2. The repair of a *rectovaginal fistula* should be deferred for at least three to six months. During this time, a low-residue diet is prescribed and careful attention to vaginal and perineal hygiene is stressed. When the inflammation surrounding the fistula is minimal, a repair should be attempted by an experienced surgeon.

ANTIBIOTIC PROPHYLAXIS FOR CESAREAN SECTION

A. The clinical situation of a patient undergoing cesarean section seems ideal for the use of prophylactic antibiotics. However, selection of the appropriate group of patients is extremely important. All studies agree that the patient undergoing planned elective primary or repeat cesarean section is at a relatively low risk. Other factors — such as anemia, obesity, duration of membrane rupture, presence of labor — significantly increase the risk of postoperative infection. However, even in the high-risk population there is no easy way to identify those destined to become febrile.

B. Another problem with prophylaxis is the timing of the first dose of antibiotic. Standard prophylaxis requires that the dose be administered prior to the surgical incision so that an effective drug level is present. However, antibiotics easily traverse the placenta, and levels can be achieved that may be misleading in the evaluation of the neonate. This problem can be overcome if the antibiotic is administered after the cord is clamped. This technique avoids drug administration to the fetus, and recent studies suggest that it is as effective as preoperative administration. Three maternal deaths have been reported following post-cord-clamping antibiotic administration. It appears that these mothers had an anaphylactic reaction while under general anesthesia and resuscitation was unsuccessful.

C. The final question concerning prophylactic antibiotics is the effectiveness of this therapeutic modality. Multiple studies have shown a decrease in both degree-hours of fever (febrile index) and clinical morbidity. However, the duration of hospital stay and the development of serious pelvic infections (abscess, etc.) were unaltered. At the present time, it appears that prophylactic antibiotics are effective in reducing *minor* morbidity from cesarean section but do not alter the development of serious infections that require prolonged hospital stay or a repeat surgical procedure.

D. If prophylactic antibiotics are administered, they should be of the broad-spectrum variety, such as ampicillin, cephalothin, cefayolin, cefoxitin, or cefamandole and for no longer than 24 hours following operation. Agents such as clindamycin or the aminoglycosides must be reserved for therapeutic use only.

BIBLIOGRAPHY

Bowes W (ed): The puerperium. Clin Obstet Gynecol 23:971, 1980

Cavanagh D, Rao P, Comas M: Septic Shock in Obstetrics and Gynecology. Philadelphia, Saunders, 1977

Charles D: Infections in Obstetrics and Gynecology. Philadelphia, Saunders, 1977

diZerga G, et al.: A comparison of clindamycin-gentamicin and penicillin-gentamicin in the treatment of post-cesarean endomyometritis. Am J Obstet Gynecol 34:239, 1979

Gibbs R: Clinical risk factors for puerperal infection. Obstet Gynecol (suppl) 55: 178S, 1980

Ledger W: Infection in the Female. Philadelphia, Lea & Febiger, 1977

Monif G, et al.: Postpartum endometritis following cesarean section. Infect Dis Lett Obstet Gynecol 2:19, 1980

Perloe M, Curet LB: The effect of internal fetal monitoring on cesarean section morbidity. Obstet Gynecol 53:354, 1974

Swartz W: Prophylactic antibiotics for cesarean section. Infect Dis Lett Obstet Gynecol 3:67, 1981

Index